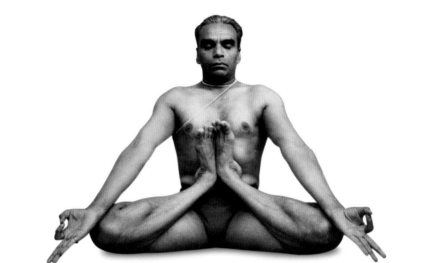

B.K.S. IYENGAR

YOGA

THE PATH TO HOLISTIC HEALTH

London, New York, Melbourne,
Munich, Delhi

ORIGINAL 2001 EDITION: Consultant Dr Geeta S. Iyengar, **Project Editor** Ranjana Sengupta, **Project Designer** Aparna Sharma, **Editors** Dipali Singh, Sheema Mookherjee, **Designers** Ankita Saha, Nikki Duggal, **DTP Designer** Sunil Sharma, **Managing Editor** Prita Maitra, **Managing Art Editor** Shuka Jain

REVISED 2008 EDITION: DK UK **Senior Art Editor** Isabel de Cordova, **Senior Editor** Jennifer Latham
DK INDIA **Design Manager** Arunesh Talapatra, **Designers** Neha Ahuja, Ivy Roy, Mahua Mandal,
DTP Designers Govind Mittal, Pushpak Tyagi, **Editorial Team** Dipali Singh, Alicia Ingty, Aditi Ray, Saloni Talwar, **Head of Publishing** Aparna Sharma

UPDATED 2014 EDITION
DK UK **Project Editors** Elizabeth Yeates, Angela Baynham, **Senior Designer** Tessa Bindloss
Managing Editor Dawn Henderson, **Managing Art Editor** Christine Keilty, **Senior Jacket Creative** Nicola Powling
Jacket Design Assistant Rosie Levine, **Producer, Pre-Production** Sarah Isle, **Senior Producer** Oliver Jeffreys
Art Director Peter Luff, **Publisher** Peggy Vance DK UK **Senior Editor** Shannon Beatty **Editor** Jane Perlmutter DK INDIA **Senior Art Editor** Ivy Roy, **Editor** Janashree Singha, **Art Editors** Sourabh Challariya, Gazal Roongta, Vikas Sachdeva, Neha Wahi **Managing Art Editor** Navidita Thapa, **Deputy Managing Editor** Chitra Subramanyam
Pre-Production Manager Sunil Sharma, **DTP Designers** Satish Chandra Gaur, Anurag Trivedi
Production Manager Pankaj Sharma, **DTP Designers** Nand Kishor Acharya, Arvind Kumar
Yoga Consultant Zarina Mubaraki

Author's Acknowledgments B.K.S. Iyengar would like to thank Dr Geeta S. Iyengar for her expert advice as a consultant, contribution to editing the script, and assisting with the photography; Parth Amin, producer of the CDs *Yoga for You* and *Yoga for Stress*, for his ideas, and perseverance in completing the book; Roshen Amin, Stephanie Quirk, and Uma Dhavale for their contributions; Professor R.N. Kulhali, for drafting and compiling the Yoga text; Harminder Singh for the photography; and models Roshen Amin, Leslie Peters, Ali Dashti, and Jawahar Bangera.

First American edition, 2001
This revised edition, 2014

Published in the United States by
DK Publishing
345 Hudson Street, 4th Floor
New York, New York 10014

16 17 18 10 9 8 7 6
014–196650 – Jan/2014

PUBLISHER'S NOTE Neither the publisher nor the author is engaged in rendering professional advice or services to the individual reader. The ideas, procedures, and suggestions contained in this book are not intended as a substitute for consulting with your physician. All matters regarding your health require medical supervision. Neither the author nor the publisher shall be liable or responsible for any loss or damage allegedly arising from any information or suggestion in this book.

Published in Great Britain by Dorling Kindersley Limited.

A catalog record for this book is available from the Library of Congress.

ISBN 978-1-4654-1583-7

DK books are available at special discounts when purchased in bulk for sales promotions, premiums, fund-raising, or educational use. For details, contact: DK Publishing Special Markets, 345 Hudson Street, 4th Floor, New York, New York 10014 or SpecialSales@dk.com.
Color reproduction by Colourscan, Singapore

Printed and bound in China

Discover more at www.dk.com

B.K.S. IYENGAR
YOGA
THE PATH TO HOLISTIC HEALTH

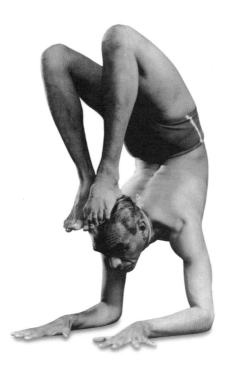

CONTENTS

Foreword 6

CHAPTER 1

B.K.S. IYENGAR'S LIFE AND WORK 8

Iyengar the Guru 10
The Iyengar Approach to Yoga 16
The Iyengar Legacy 24
Message from B.K.S. Iyengar 32

CHAPTER 2

YOGA FOR YOU 34

Aims of Yoga 36
The Way to Health 39
Benefits of Poses 40
Yoga and Stress 41
Yoga and Fitness 42

CHAPTER 3

PHILOSOPHY OF YOGA 44

Meaning of Yoga 46
Philosophy of Asanas 48
State of Mind 50
Eight Limbs 52
Chakras 56
The Guru and the Yogi 58

CHAPTER 4

ASANAS FOR YOU 60

Classic Poses 62
Standing Asanas 66
Tadasana 68
Utthita Trikonasana 70
Virabhadrasana 2 76
Utthita Parsvakonasana 80
Parsvottanasana 84
Adhomukha Svanasana 88
Uttanasana 92
Virabhadrasana 1 96
Sitting Asanas 100
Dandasana 102
Virasana 104
Baddhakonasana 108
Forward Bends 112
Janu Sirsasana 114
Trianga Mukhaikapada
       Paschimottanasana 118
Paschimottanasana 122
Twists 126
Bharadvajasana 128
Marichyasana 132
Inversions 136
Salamba Sirsasana 138
Salamba Sarvangasana 144
Halasana 150
Back Bends 154
Ustrasana 156
Urdhva Dhanurasana 160
Reclining Asanas 164
Supta Virasana 166
Savasana 170

CHAPTER 5

YOGA FOR STRESS 174

Understanding Stress 176
The Modern World 177
Food and Nourishment 178

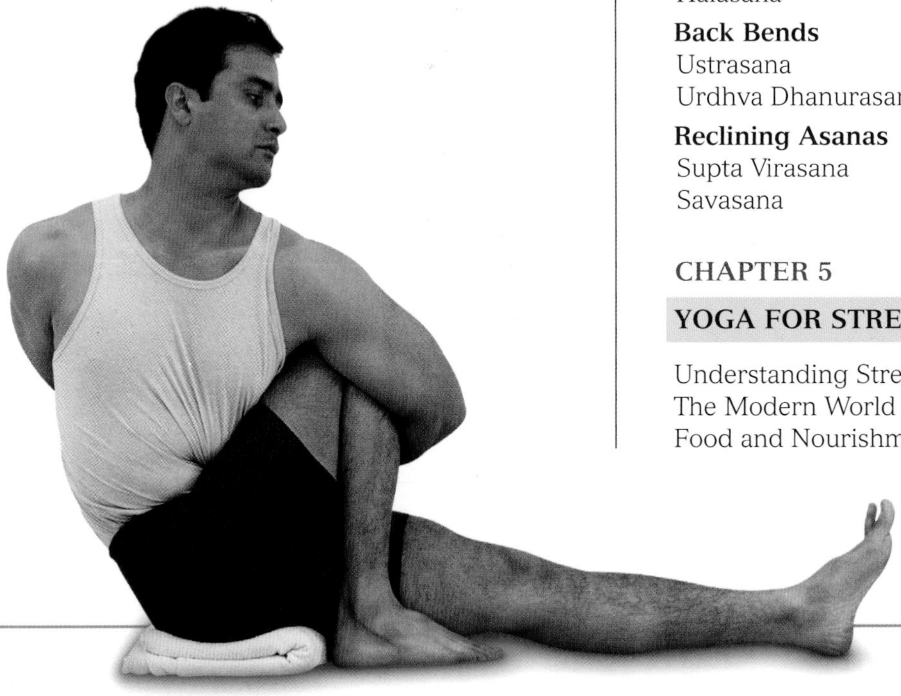

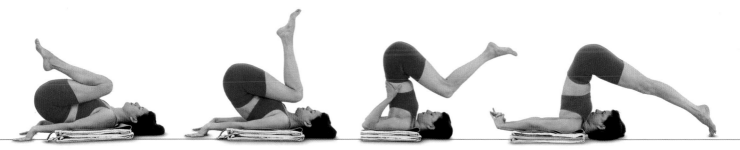

Positive and Negative Stress	179
Asanas and Stress	180
Asanas with Props	182
Props	184

Asanas for Stress

Tadasana Samasthithi	186
Tadasana Urdhva Hastasana	187
Tadasana Urdhva Baddanguliasana	188
Paschima Baddha Hastasana	189
Tadasana Paschima Namaskarasana	190
Tadasana Gomukhasana	191
Utthita Trikonasana	192
Utthita Parsvakonasana	194
Ardha Chandrasana	196
Uttanasana	197
Prasarita Padottanasana	200
Adhomukha Svanasana	202
Dandasana	205
Virasana	206
Urdhvamukha Janu Sirsasana	207
Baddhakonasana	208
Swastikasana	209
Paripurna Navasana	210
Upavista Konasana	213
Paschimottanasana	214
Adhomukha Paschimottanasana	217
Janu Sirsasana	218
Adhomukha Virasana	220
Adhomukha Swastikasana	222
Bharadvajasana	223
Marichyasana	225
Utthita Marichyasana	226
Parsva Virasana	228
Salamba Sarvangasana	230
Halasana	232
Viparita Karani	234
Setubandha Sarvangasana	236
Viparita Dandasana	238
Ustrasana	240
Supta Padangusthasana	242
Supta Baddhakonasana	244
Supta Virasana	246
Savasana	248

CHAPTER 6

PRANAYAMA WITH PROPS 250

The Importance of Pranayama	252
Ujjayi Pranayama	254
Viloma 2 Pranayama	256

CHAPTER 7

YOGA FOR AILMENTS 258

Yoga Therapy	260
Heart and Circulation	264
Respiratory System	276
Digestive System	285
Urinary System	300
Hormonal System	302
Immune System	308
Muscles, Bones, and Joints	312
Skin	344
Brain and Nervous System	351
Mind and Emotions	359
Women's Health	378
Men's Health	397

CHAPTER 8

Iyengar Yoga Course 406

Guide to your Yoga Practice	408
20-Week Yoga Course	410

Anatomy Guide	424
Glossary	426
List of Asanas	427
Index	428
Acknowledgments	432
Useful Addresses	432

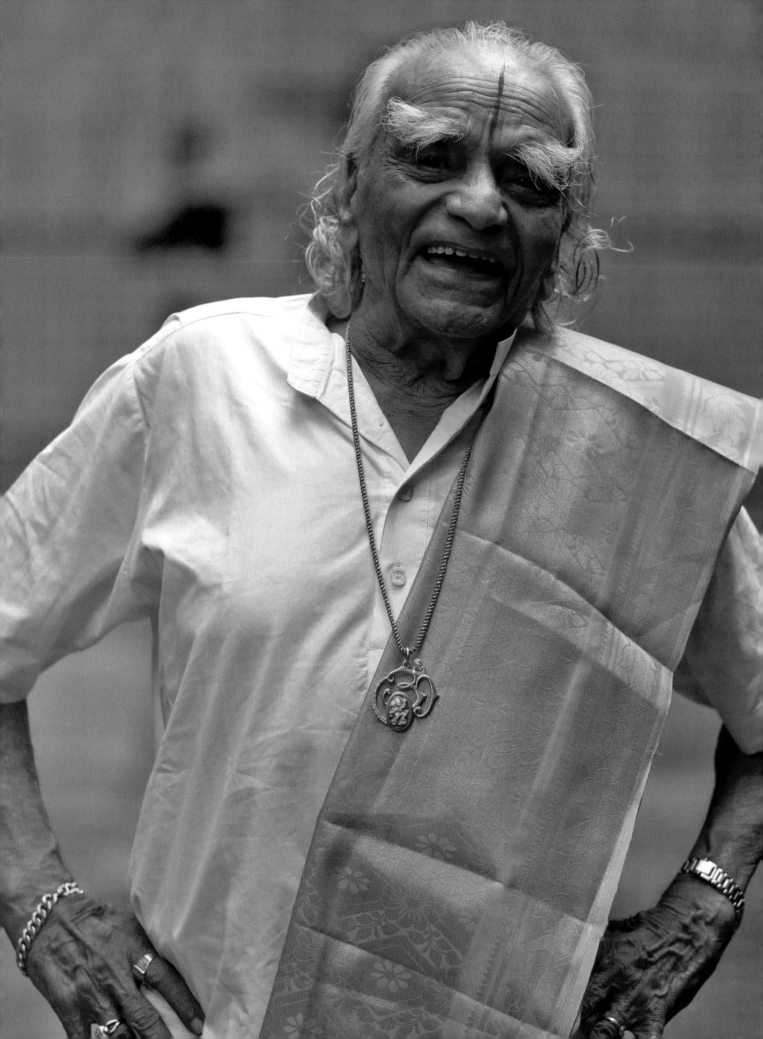

Foreword

by Yogacharya B.K.S. Iyengar

Yoga is for everyone. You need not be an expert or at the peak of physical fitness to practice the asanas described in this book. The strain of modern life can lead to physical pain and illness, as we neglect our bodies in the race for material success. The stress of modern life can also lead to mental suffering: feelings of inadequacy, isolation, or powerlessness. Yoga helps to integrate the mental and the physical plane, bringing about a sense of inner and outer balance, or what I term alignment. True alignment means that the inner mind reaches every cell and fiber of the body.

During seventy-three years of teaching and practicing, I have observed that some students pay attention only to the physical aspect of yoga. Their practice is like a fast-flowing stream, tumbling and falling, which lacks depth and direction. By attending to the mental and spiritual side, a sincere student of yoga becomes like a smoothly flowing river which helps to irrigate and fertilize the land around it. Just as one cannot dip into the same river twice, so each and every asana refreshes your life force with new energy.

My effort in this book has been to focus on techniques, so that even the beginner will have a thorough understanding of how to practice asanas in order to obtain the maximum benefit. By using a few simple props, students with different capabilities can gradually build up strength, confidence, and flexibility without the threat of strain or injury. The yoga techniques described and illustrated in this book can also help those with specific ailments. Regular practice builds up the body's inner strength and natural resistance, helps to alleviate pain, and tackles the root, rather than the symptoms, of the problem. Across the world, there is now a growing awareness that alternative therapies are more conducive to health than conventional ones. It is my hope that this book will help all those who want to change their lives through yoga. May yoga's blessing be on all of you.

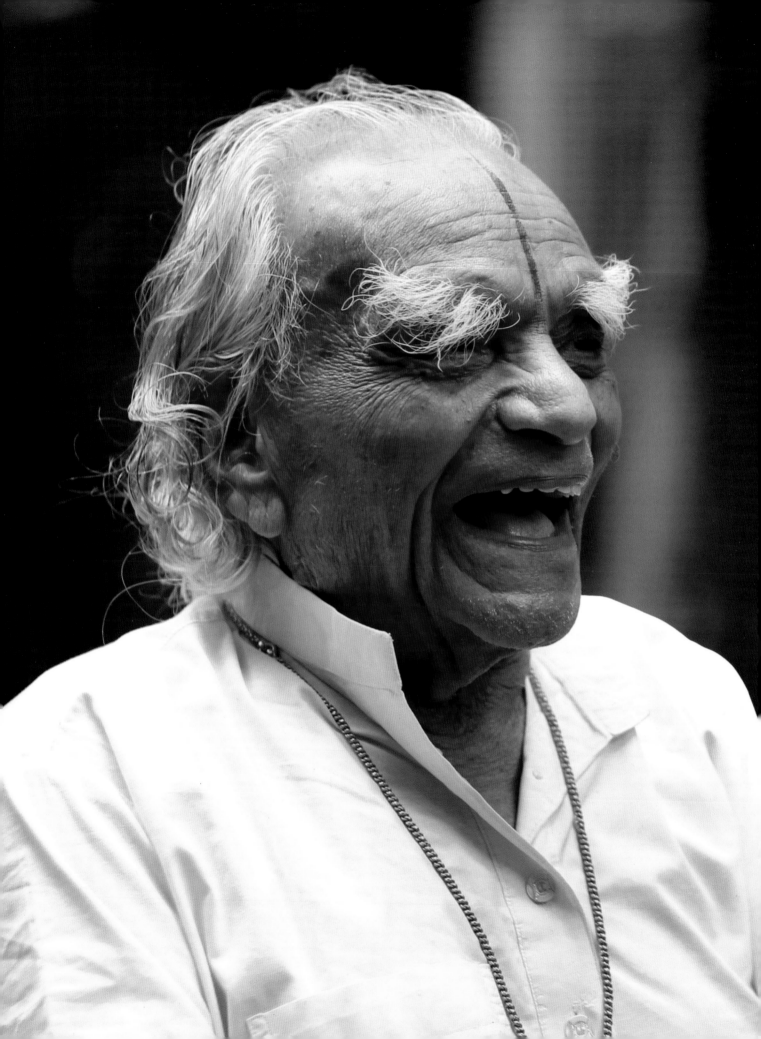

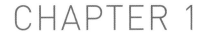

CHAPTER 1

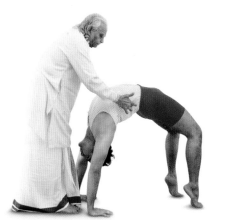

LIFE AND WORK

*"When I **practice**, I am a **philosopher**.*
*When I **teach**, I am a **scientist**.*
*When I **demonstrate**, I am an **artist**."*

It is almost impossible to contemplate the art of yoga without considering the contribution of the revered yoga master, B.K.S. Iyengar. From humble and inauspicious beginnings, Iyengar displayed a truly remarkable fortitude and determination to improve his situation and health through the art of yoga. His genius and insight into mastering and defining the ancient practice has popularized yoga today, making it accessible to millions all over the world and allowing them to discover the enlightenment of spirit enjoyed in the life of a dedicated yogi.

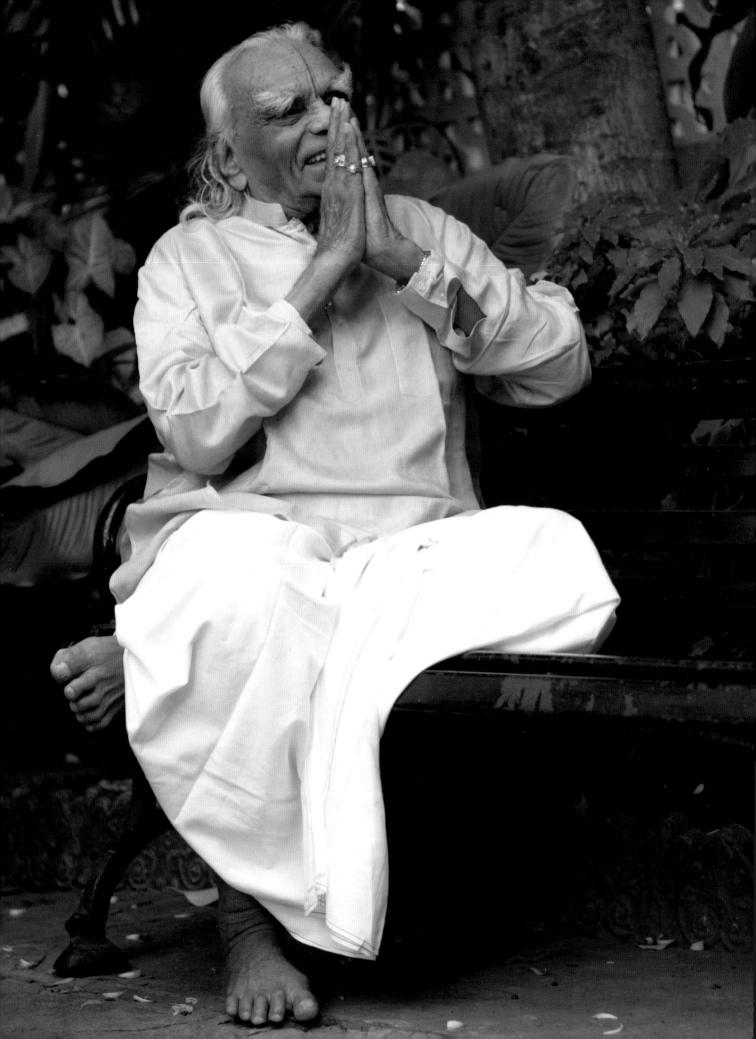

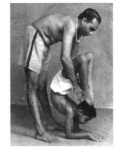

Iyengar the Guru

B.K.S. Iyengar triumphed over poverty and childhood ailments to master and revolutionize the art of yoga. Credited with bringing yoga to the West, he has also made it accessible to millions of people all over the world.

The path to greatness, to becoming a legend, is strewn with disappointments, failures, and anxieties. Enduring and surviving testing times demands unrelenting persistence, dedication, and focus. B.K.S. Iyengar, who has been awarded two of India's greatest civilian awards, the Padma Shri and Padma Bhushan, remembers such times. Today, he is living testament to the triumph that can follow adversity.

"After many strides forward, when one looks back, things seem to fit," says Mr. Iyengar. He is at the Ramaamani Iyengar Memorial Yoga Institute in Pune, India, waiting for a cup of coffee. It is late afternoon and the evening classes are about to begin. The students are trooping in, but stop when they spot their guru sitting near the office. They sit down on the floor, to listen; it isn't often that you get to hear a legend talk about his life, his successes, and his journey toward conquering the body, intellect, and mind.

At 95 years old, B.K.S. Iyengar is a living legend; a simple man who sought to master and immortalize the ancient discipline of yoga, and became a guru. His rise to success can only be described as an act of strong willpower, extreme perseverance, burning determination, and sheer obstinacy.

Humble beginnings
Bellur Krishnamachar Sundararaja Iyengar was born on December 14, 1918, in the tiny village of Bellur, close to Bangalore, a city that is now India's IT hub. He was a sickly child with thin arms and legs, a protruding stomach, and a heavy head. "My appearance was not prepossessing," Mr. Iyengar says. His father died in 1927, when he was eight, leaving the family in absolute poverty. "There was a time when we couldn't pay the school fees and I was not allowed to sit the exams. My brother took me begging for money," he recalls. Despite his present successes, he clearly remembers these challenges from the past. "Poverty acted as a garland for knowledge. If I hadn't been born into such a poor family, I probably wouldn't have gained anything. I am grateful that poverty followed me for years. Knowledge was born from this poverty."

Introduction to yoga
In 1934, Mr. Iyengar received an offer he couldn't refuse from Tirumalai Krishnamarcharya, a respected yoga scholar, who was married to his sister Namagiri. Krishnamarcharya, considered the father of modern yoga, ran a yoga school at the Jaganmohan palace of his patron, the Maharaja of Mysore. He asked Mr. Iyengar to move to Mysore to help Namagiri with household chores, securing his destiny.

Krishnamarcharya was a taskmaster. "I don't think he saw any real potential in me. He told me to practice asanas to improve my health," Mr. Iyengar says. "I jumped at the offer. Health had been a perennial problem for me since I was born." It took three years of practicing yoga before Mr. Iyengar noticed a distinct

(top) **B.K.S. Iyengar** adjusting his son Prashant's posture while he does the Vrschikasana (Scorpion pose), 1960–1961.
(left) **B.K.S. Iyengar** at the Ramaamani Iyengar Memorial Yoga Institute in Pune, 2008.

> *"An **inner voice** urged me to **persist** and
> **carry on**. My **will** alone **held on**."*

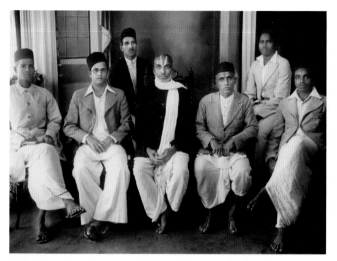

B.K.S. Iyengar (extreme right) with his guru Professor
Tirumalai Krishnamarcharya (center) and the Prince of Mysore
(second from left) in the early days (1937).

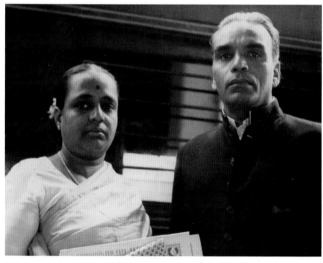

Mr. Iyengar with his wife Ramaamani in 1960. She became
his student and one of his strongest supporters.

change in his health and this encouraged him. "My
guruji (Krishnamarcharya) barely paid me any
attention during this time. Later, he taught me just
the outline for the basic asanas—the classic yoga
postures. I grasped the rudiments of each asana and
practiced on my own. I learned the difficult postures,
such as Vrschikasana (Scorpion pose) and hand
balancing, during the public performances we used
to participate in! I don't know what Guruji really saw
in me, but I think he recognized that I had guts."

In 1935, the Maharaja of Mysore arranged a yoga
demonstration. Mr. Iyengar was getting ready to
present some of the asanas, but Krishnamarcharya
threw him a challenge. He asked Mr. Iyengar to
perform the Hanumanasana (Great Split, where the
legs are split forward and backward). "I had no
knowledge of this asana. My guru described the pose
and I realized it was difficult. I told Guruji that my
shorts were too tight. It would be difficult to stretch my
legs. He asked one of his senior pupils to cut the shorts
on each side with a pair of scissors. Then he told me to
do the asana. I did it, but with a resulting tear in my
hamstring that took years to heal. Guruji was
impressed and asked me how I had managed it. He
told me that he didn't think I would be able to do it,
but I did. The token I received from the Maharaja of
Mysore was nothing compared to those words of
praise from my guruji."

The beginnings of Iyengar yoga
"I learned a valuable lesson that day. I realized that
attempting certain asanas suddenly, without preparation,
could harm the body and the mind. I started evolving
the asana sequences scientifically. I developed a
progressive approach from simple to difficult asanas. I
categorized them by their effects, as being purifying,
pacifying, stimulative, nourishing, or cleansing. Guruji
lit the fire of yoga within me. But I did not learn it in
the form that it is today. I struggled with and traced the
missing links of refinement and precision. I evolved
my guru's method, so that a set of asanas could be
practiced followed by another set, using the alignment
of the intelligence in the asanas," Mr. Iyengar says.

Krishnamarcharya had made an indelible
impression on Mr. Iyengar. "In our wheel of yoga, he
was the hub. We, as spokes, rolled the wheel without

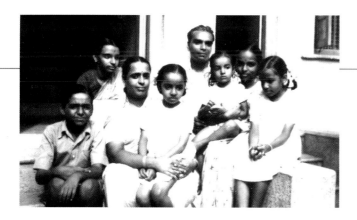

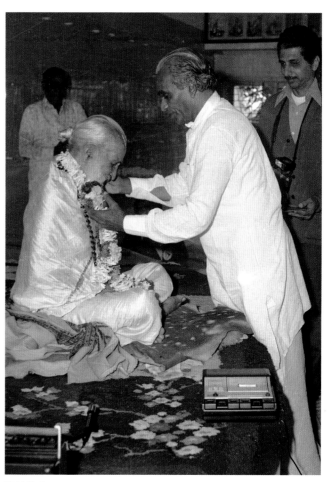

(left) An early family portrait of B.K.S. Iyengar and Ramaamani with their children, 1959.

creating bends or dents in it. Unfortunately for all his intellectual progress, his ways and moods were unpredictable. We were afraid to talk to him, let alone question him. Yet his conduct, firm discipline, perseverance, vast knowledge, and powerful memory left a permanent mark on our lives."

Teaching while learning

In 1936, the Maharaja of Mysore sent Krishnamarcharya and his students on a lecture tour across the state of present-day Karnataka. Soon after this Dr. V.B. Gokhale, a well-known surgeon, asked Krishnamarcharya to send a student to the Deccan Gymkhana Club in Pune, to teach yoga for six months. Mr. Iyengar was 17 and spoke a little English, although he couldn't speak Marathi, the local language. However, he was deemed the obvious choice. "Besides the language barrier, the college students often made fun of me as they were older and better educated," he says. "I suffered from an inferiority complex because of my *shendi* (tuft of hair, typical of orthodox Hindu Brahmins). But I decided I would not be dejected. I worked hard to prove yoga's worth." Mr. Iyengar's term at the Club was extended every six months for a period of three years.

The years that followed would prove to be the darkest period in Mr. Iyengar's life. He lost his job at the Deccan Gymkhana Club and with the exception of two or three students, his teaching had practically come to a full stop. "It was a testing time of tears, failures, and anxieties. In hindsight, it seems that this was the darkest hour before the dawn of prosperity," Mr. Iyengar says." An inner voice urged me to persist and carry on. My will alone held on. I practiced intensely and taught yoga to whoever was interested. I cycled miles to reach students' houses. There were days when I survived on tap water, as everything else was unaffordable. I had no guarantees, no help, and no support from my family. Failures gave me determination and showed me a new light and a fresh way to progress. I used the tool of disappointment as an appointment for a new assignment. Failures, stalemates, and disappointments strengthened my will to pursue this path of yoga with determination, and God graced me in my path."

Amidst this struggle for sustenance and recognition, Mr. Iyengar married Ramaamani in 1943. "My financial

B.K.S. Iyengar felicitates T. Krishnamarcharya on the occasion his 60th birthday.

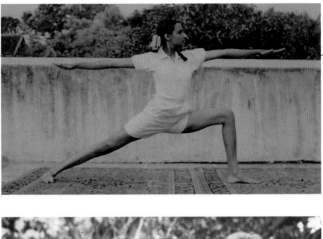

(right) **A young Geeta Iyengar,** Iyengar's daughter, practices the Virabhadrasana 2 (Warrior pose 2).

position was dire, but family pressure prevailed and we were married against my better judgement. We celebrated our marriage on borrowed money," he says. Ramaamani was unfamiliar with yoga in the beginning, but she soon became a dedicated student. "She was quick to help me in my practice. She developed sensitivity and a healing touch. Without Ramaa it is possible that my method of yoga and myself would not be what we are today," he says. "I used to tell Ramaa to observe my posture while I practiced yoga, and to correct me. She was my mirror to achieve accurate form."

There is no doubt, Iyengar says, that Ramaa sacrificed her dreams so that he could pursue his art. "When I left my family to teach in Europe and the US, she faced many problems. For examle, there were massive floods in Pune in 1962, and people rushed to their terraces with their possessions. But Ramaa's sole concern was to keep safe the manuscript for my book *Light on Yoga*."

The rise of Iyengar yoga

Gradually, the number of students who wanted to learn from Mr. Iyengar increased. After he helped a young girl recover from polio of the spinal column, word of B.K.S Iyengar's healing touch spread, too, both locally and within the medical community. The turning point, he says, came in 1946 when both Mr. Iyengar and his wife had similar dreams of divinity. "From that night on, fortune favored us. People suffering from various diseases started coming to me for relief," he says.

It was around this time that Mr. Iyengar was introduced by a student to Jiddu Krishnamurthi, one of India's greatest philosophers. Mr. Iyengar, however, hadn't heard of Krishnamurthi. "I hadn't read his books and I didn't know he was one of the greatest thinkers in the 20th century, but I started to attend his lectures in Pune. He was fond of saying, 'Do not criticize and do not justify.' He taught me not to be disturbed or swayed by people's opinions. Yogis all over the world criticized me for doing what they considered 'physical yoga.' I was very clear about what I practiced. I never felt the need to justify what I was doing. Even now, I do not bother about other people's remarks, but instead focus on evolving my own practice. Nor do I criticize others or their systems.

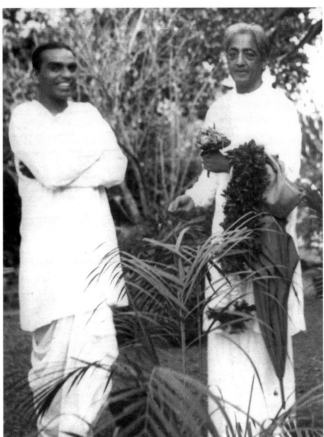

B.K.S. Iyengar with the famous philosopher Jiddu Krishnamurthi (right) who became a loyal student, 1955.

"A **fortuitous meeting** *with Lord Yehudi Menuhin in 1952 introduced the world* **to Iyengar yoga**."

Krishnamurthi paid me a great compliment when he wrote, 'You have taught me yoga for 20 years— whenever someone asks me who is the greatest yoga teacher, I always send him or her to you.'"

Iyengar's dream of making yoga popular, however, was reaching a critical juncture. It was a fortuitous meeting with celebrated violinist Lord Yehudi Menuhin in 1952 that introduced the world to Iyengar yoga. Menuhin was in Bombay and was due to meet Mr. Iyengar but almost canceled the meeting. "I understood the state of his mind and persuaded him to give me five minutes. I made him lie in Savasana (a reclining asana that helps recover the breath and cool the body and mind—see pages 170–172). In that lying position, using my fingers, I guided him in Shanmukhi mudra (the placement of fingers in a particular position on the face to block out the senses). He fell asleep for almost an hour!" says Mr. Iyengar.

"I had never heard of him before. I soon realized that he was a celebrity, but to me he was another human being with a physical ailment that I could cure," he says. Menuhin was exhausted and suffering from hyperextension of the bow arm. Guided by Mr. Iyengar, his condition improved quickly. He was so pleased that he gave Mr. Iyengar a watch with the engraving, "To my best violin teacher."

Tackling misconceptions

That five-minute interview blossomed into a lifelong friendship. Menuhin invited Mr. Iyengar to his home in Gstaad, Switzerland, and later to London, introducing him in Europe and the United States. Iyengar yoga was all set to take off, but this was a difficult time in which to introduce and establish the form. Mr. Iyengar discovered this during his visit to London in 1954. "When I arrived at Victoria Station, the customs officers asked me my profession. When I said yoga, they asked me whether I could walk on fire, chew glass, or swallow blades! Yoga was unknown in the West and the Occidental concept of yoga was next to nothing," he says. Menuhin introduced him to friends interested in learning the form. "It was a tough time. Everyone is interested today, but then it was difficult for any yoga practitioner to teach the local people. Yoga was not respected. A lot of people saw me as a colored man from a former British colony. I faced a

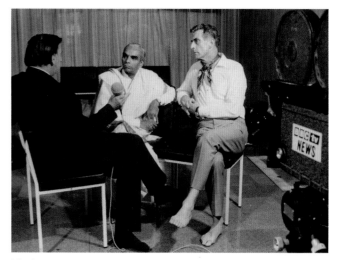

Mr. Iyengar gives a BBC TV interview with Nigel Green (far right), 1962.

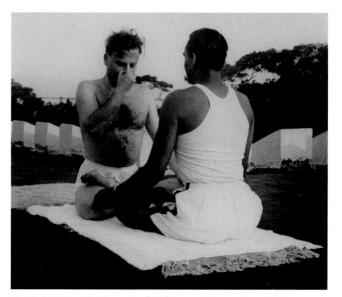

Violinist Yehudi Menuhin (left) learned yoga from Mr. Iyengar, 1956. But the Yogacharya considers Menuhin his guru in the art of Pranayama (the yogic practice of breathing).

*"The **tree** is still spreading. The **winds of yoga** are **blowing everywhere**."*

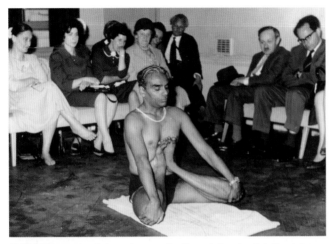

B.K.S. Iyengar gives a demonstration at the Jewish Society during one of his earliest trips to London, 1963.

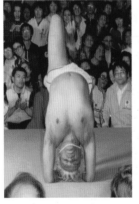

B.K.S. Iyengar
gives a public performance
to an enthralled audience
in Japan, 1984.

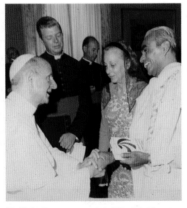

B.K.S. Iyengar with His Holiness
Pope Paul VI at the Vatican in
August, 1966.

certain amount of discrimination in the early days in the UK and the US. Yet, at the same time, there were people who showed me a lot of hospitality and friendship."

Mr. Iyengar started by giving demonstrations in bars or any other place where people gathered and showed interest. "People smoked and drank in my presence. I changed them slowly. I did not demand respect. I earned it. In time, they sought permission to drink wine at the table. Later, they stopped smoking or drinking. It was not a sudden transformation. I was tolerant. My inner voice told me not to criticize. I had gone there to propagate yoga." Mr. Iyengar traveled to the US in 1956 at the invitation of Menuhin's friend Rebekah Harkness, the Standard Oil heiress. His demonstrations were, however, confined to the Harkness family and their friends. It would take more than 18 years for Iyengar yoga to finally make an impact in America.

One of Mr. Iyengar's key encounters took place in 1958 when he met and taught Queen Elisabeth of Belgium. The Queen was 84 when she invited Iyengar to teach her yoga. "I began with simple standing poses and the Halasana (Plough Pose—see pages 150-153). She was not willing to stop. She wanted me to teach her Salamba Sirsasana (Headstand—see pages 138-143). She was frail and I knew by looking at her that she had problems with her heart. When I asked for her medical reports, she said, 'Sir, if you have faith in yoga, why do you want my medical reports? If you are afraid of teaching me the head balance, then you can take the next train to Gstaad, and join your friend Yehudi who recommended you!' I appreciated her courage and persistence. I told her, 'If you have the courage to do the head balance, I have the courage to teach you.' After she did the head balance, I taught her asanas to bring her blood pressure down," he says. Mr. Iyengar continued to teach the Queen until her death in 1965.

Yoga for the people

Mr. Iyengar returned to London in 1960, again on the invitation of Menuhin. This time he wanted to teach everyone and not just celebrities. Menuhin arranged classes for him through the Asian Musical Circle, founded by Mr Ayana Deva Angadi, an Indian settled in London. In the beginning, there were only four students and lack of funds had him turn the backyard of Angadi's house into a classroom. But slowly his practical

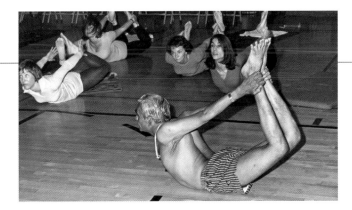

(left) **B.K.S. Iyengar** teaching a class at Ann Arbor in Michigan, 1973.

demonstrations attracted more people.

Iyengar yoga made an important cultural crossover in 1966 when Mr. Iyengar met His Holiness Pope Paul VI. "I was blessed to have an audience with him. Both of us discussed the subject of yoga. It was one of the happiest moments of my life. The Pope caught my hands and blessed my good work. His Holiness praised me with the words, 'You are a professor and director of yoga. I bless you with all my heart and am happy to have met you.'"

This was also the time when Mr. Iyengar's book *Light on Yoga* was first published. It was an instant classic, drawing people to the art of yoga. Menuhin wrote in the foreword, "Whoever has had the privilege of receiving Mr. Iyengar's attention, or of witnessing the precision, refinement, and beauty of his art, is introduced to that vision of perfection and innocence which is man as first created." The book became an international bestseller and has since been translated into 18 languages. It is often called "the bible of yoga."

The Ramaamani Iyengar Memorial Institute

Yoga was finally making an impact across the world. Students started traveling to Pune to learn the form from Mr. Iyengar and his wife Ramaamani recognized the need to create a yoga school. Mr. Iyengar used proceeds from *Light on Yoga* to buy a plot of land in Pune. But three days after the inauguration in January 1973, Ramaamani became ill and died. Work continued and the institute finally opened its doors to students in 1975. "Though she is no more, I am never separated from her— for she is always in my heart. The Ramaamani Iyengar Memorial Yoga Institute is my tribute to her," he says.

Today, thousands of Iyengar students arrive at the Institute to study his unique concept of yoga and to imbibe his rigorous discipline. "I began with two students. Today, millions are practicing yoga," Mr. Iyengar says. "My students teach in schools, colleges, yoga centers, and sports clubs in major US cities. Yoga has breached Apartheid with many South African students attending my classes in London in the early 1960s. I have students in practically every European nation, as well as Russia and China. The tree is still spreading. The number of students influenced by my teaching is impossible to know, but it is certainly in the hundreds of thousands. The winds of yoga are blowing everywhere."

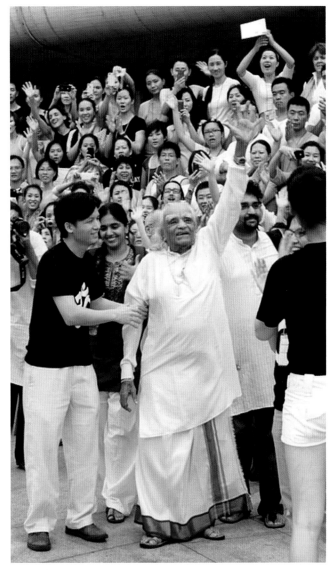

B.K.S. Iyengar being greeted and welcomed by followers in China, in 2011. His books have all been translated into Mandarin.

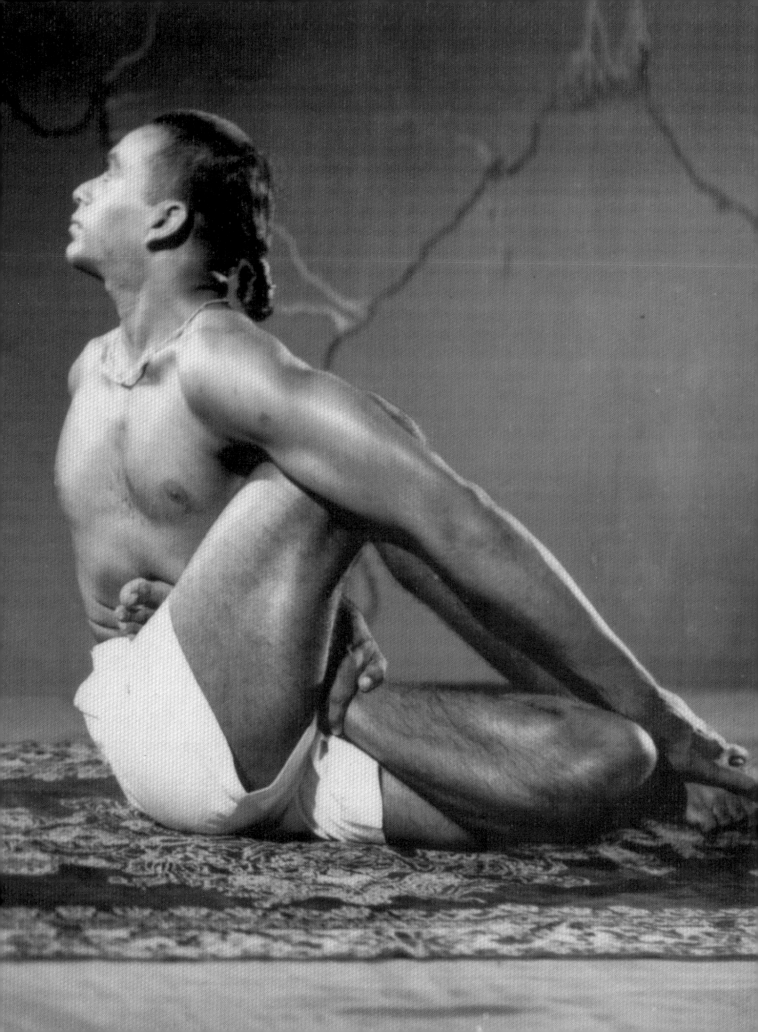

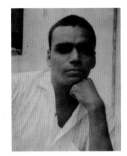

The Iyengar Approach To Yoga

Iyengar yoga is a holistic experience that benefits the body, mind, and emotions. The driving force behind Iyengar yoga is B.K.S. Iyengar's belief that yoga is for everyone, and that it is effective in reducing modern-day stress.

In the early days, while practicing and teaching yoga, B.K.S. Iyengar experienced an inner dryness. He questioned its persistence since he knew his technique was correct, and used his body and intelligence to study himself while practicing. His inner consciousness became his guru. He learned that while practicing any asana, it is important for the body and its organs to work or move in a certain way, without leaving their alignment. He penetrated the organic body by closely examining his outer body, the skin's movement, and the alignment of his physical body. He discovered that perfect symmetry removed undue stress and restored the organic and cellular body to its original state of health. The inner dryness disappeared.

As Mr. Iyengar observed his inner organic body in different asanas, he felt various channels (*nadis*) open from within. These channels allowed the energy (*prana*) to flow, spread, and circulate in every part of the body including the nerves, skin, and brain. He attained a feeling of alignment, sensitivity, and intelligence. This process of performing each asana with microscopic awareness, self inquiry, and mind and body feedback brought a revolution in Mr. Iyengar's practice and, in turn, his teaching.

Aligning the self

Many yoga practitioners are flexible and practice asanas in a habitual manner, without involvement or reflection. Mr. Iyengar teaches his students to understand that asanas are not just about the movement of the physical body; there has to be a microscopic awareness and inner penetration, so that the asana becomes an asana in the real sense. He realized that there is an instrument of awareness in everybody. The average yoga student is aware of his or her body with respect to the asana's technique and outline. However, most do not understand the concept of developing inner awareness.

Mr. Iyengar awakens the intelligence within. This allows practitioners to sharpen their awareness resulting in an inner action. For example, during Tadasana (Mountain posture—see pages 68–69), Mr. Iyengar goes beyond "Stand with your legs and feet joined together." He asks the students to question the need to align the inner and outer foot. Alignment increases the sensitivity in the foot and balances the energy. Now, the practitioner lifts both sides of the knee resulting in a firm grip of the quadriceps, moving it closer to the thigh bone. In Tadasana, the firmness in the thighs leads to a lift in the gastric and lower abdominal region. This, in turn, elates the thoracic and organic region; the breath automatically becomes deeper and more rhythmic with corresponding changes to the senses, mind, and emotions.

Balancing the energy within

Mr. Iyengar's teachings might appear to be physical in nature, but the casual spectator cannot observe the internal workings of the practitioner's mind. He believes awareness brings perfect balance between work output and energy expenditure. Correct utilization of the mind and body ensures that the energy is retained and correctly distributed.

(**top right**) **A young** B.K.S. Iyengar.
(**left**) **Mr. Iyengar,** age 24, practicing the Pari Purna Matsyendrasana (Complete Lord of the Fishes pose).

*"**Energy** can **flow** only when there is **attention** and **purity of breath**."*

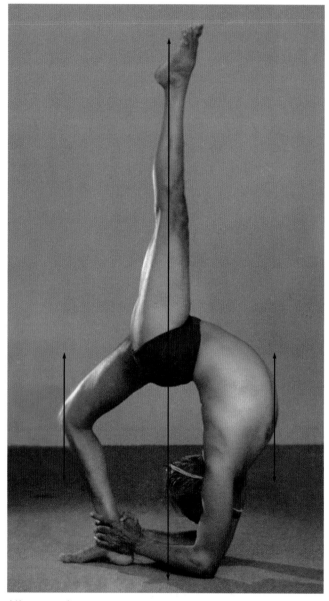

Alignment increases sensitivity and balances the energy within the body. Above, Mr. Iyengar (age 62) demonstrates the importance of alignment as he practices the Eka Pada Viparita Dandasana (One-Legged Inverted Staff Pose).

Every person has two facets of energy: the *pingala* or the *surya nadi* (masculine energy/sun) and the *ida* or the *chandra nadi* (feminine energy/moon). The sun is positive energy representing heat and daytime activity. The moon is negative energy representing coolness and nighttime restfulness. Mr. Iyengar understood the importance of creating the perfect balance between the right (*surya nadi*) and left (*chandra nadi*) sides of the body. Alignment and precision allow the energies to work, interact, intermingle, and unite, bringing about health and balance. Optimum energy is used in the correct practice of yoga and leads the practitioner to a state of equilibrium (*samatvam*). The *Bhagvad Gita* scripture states: *Samatvam yoga uchyate* (Yoga is the state of equilibrium). Sage Patanjali, who wrote the treatise *Yoga Sutras,* explains that the differentiation between the muscles, limbs, joints, organs, mind, intelligence, and self has to disappear to reach this state of equanimity. Mr. Iyengar ensures that students bring more of their consciousness into each asana, through precise instructions and demonstrations. Through this they begin to experience equilibrium.

Mr. Iyengar's inner awareness made him realize that the breath is an instrument to be used at the right time and place, to move inward. Today, asanas are taught with precise breathing instructions. So, to achieve the Padmasana (Lotus pose—see page 54), teachers may say, "Exhale and bend the right knee, and place the right foot on the left upper thigh." But Mr. Iyengar also shows the inner channel of breath. He teaches one to exhale through the nostrils and, as the action takes place, to feel the effect at that point. In Padmasana, the effect of the breath and mind relaxes the knee. When the knee is stiff, the exhalation has to be of a certain quality. It is a surrendering breath that softens the senses of perception, and relaxes the brain, easing the movements in the asana. When the practitioner corrects an adjustment or goes into the asana in the right manner, the attention and breath flow with the action. Energy can flow only when there is attention and purity of breath.

The power of sequences

Sometimes, despite their best efforts, students are unable to perform certain asanas. Mr. Iyengar teaches his students to practice a series of actions before moving on to difficult asanas. Sequencing helps them derive the essence of the asanas, experience their beneficial effects, and elevate the mind's structure. Mr. Iyengar has always taught his students the way the eight limbs (*astanga*), as enumerated by Patanjali, form a whole (see pages 52–53). He says, "*Ahimsa satya asteya brahmacarya aparigrahah yama* (YS II.30)." This means that the five pillars of *yama* are nonviolence, truth, and abstinence from stealing, continence, and greed for possessions beyond one's need. Its principles build the right mannerisms that help us attain the sight of the soul. Mr. Iyengar feels practitioners often apply force (*himsa*) to perform asanas that can lead to sprained muscles, painful joints, shakiness in the breath, and instability in the body. Mr. Iyengar often says, "The brain and body cannot be like dry earth. It is the intelligence or the mind that softens them into clay."

Mr. Iyengar asks each practitioner to use his or her judiciousness while practicing asanas. He teaches the importance of setting goals in order to perfect asanas, but also insists that students be compassionate toward each part of their body. Students should know their capacity. Careful intelligence, like the scales of justice, has to balance violence and nonviolence.

Bringing honesty to the practice

The mind, "I" consciousness, and intellect together form the consciousness (*chitta*). The "I" consciousness contains willpower, ego, and humility. Willpower allows one to stretch the elastic of the "I" consciousness carefully from ego to humility and vice versa. Humility relaxes the brain leading to introspection. Then awareness and sensitivity arise helping the practitioner move toward the self and connect with the soul.

Mr. Iyengar urges his students to practice with sincerity and involvement. This involvement made him a yogi and a master of yoga. Without this element of truthfulness (*satya*), asanas remain mechanical and repetitive. He tells his students to study the awareness and alignment in an asana. If they do not observe the right and the left side as they perform the asana, one side becomes more dominant since it "steals" energy from the other, leaving it weak and dull.

There is enthusiasm and chaos in early practice of yoga, when practitioners often get carried away and aspire to advanced asanas, without practicing the simpler postures that benefit the body and mind. This is a facet of greediness (*steya*) and possessiveness

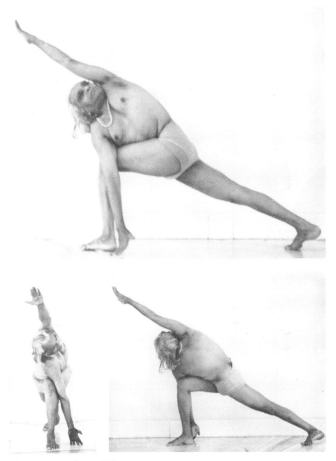

Mr. Iyengar (age 65) demonstrates the correct alignment for the Parivrtta Parshvakonasana (Resolved Side Angle pose). He says, "My way of practice focuses on alignment leading to precision, which is a divine state. This is where the individual soul and the Universal soul intersect."

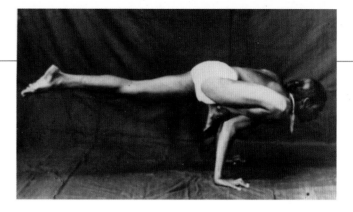

(right) B.K.S. Iyengar, age 17 holds poses with the utmost concentration, stilling and quieting the senses to achieve a state of *dhyana* or meditation.

(*parigraha*). The practitioner unknowingly allows possessiveness to enter the practice. So, the right side of the body may be stronger and better aligned than the left, leading to a dissonance of energy. The right side becomes overnourished, the left undernourished.

Brahmacharya means to know the *Brahma*, to reach the soul. The practitioner should practice yoga with complete involvement, with the purpose of reaching the *Brahma* within. The aim of the practice should always be foremost. The practitioner must follow the principles of restraint (*niyama*): cleanliness (*saucha*), contentment (*santosa*), austerity (*tapas*), self study (*svadhyaya*), and devotion to the Supreme Being (*isvara pranidhana*). Students should observe internal cleanliness and bathe each cell of the inner body through good blood circulation and flow of energy. Good health and healthy living leads to contentment.

This isn't easy, but it helps curb anger, greed, and desire, allowing the practitioner to progress on the yogic path. Mr. Iyengar does not subscribe to the path of easy practice. He demands self-discipline. Ease and comfort are against the principle of yogic discipline and limit the mind. Fear of certain asanas limits the boundaries of the mind. Yoga is meant to purify the body and penetrate the mind. The mind must have that zeal and strength of will to bear physical pain that comes with correct effort. Austere and intense practice of yoga leads the practitioner toward *svadhyaya* and *isvara pranidhana*. The study and practice of yoga with devotional attention on God is meditation. Mr. Iyengar says it is the conscience (*viveka*) and not the brain that tells the practitioner whether the asana has been done with religiosity and judiciousness.

Awakening the inner eye
When Mr. Iyengar guides his students' senses of perception, asking them to allow their organs of action and mind to turn inward, he doesn't expect an automatic cessation of all thoughts and focused inner concentration. Rather, the students need to use their inner eyes—alertness (*prana*) and awareness (*prajna*) —to observe every part of the body. One should exist everywhere in the body. The soul (*atman*) is the owner of the physical, spiritual, and psychological faculties (*indriyas*) but they cannot be used for enjoyment (*bhoga*). They must serve their master in a pure and correct manner.

Pratyahara is a state of bringing control over the *indriyas*. While practicing, one has to focus completely on the inner body, drawing the mind inward and then sharpening the intelligence. The senses of perception are closely allied with the brain. That is why Mr. Iyengar says, "Eyes are the window of the brain and through the ears the brain goes out." While doing asanas, the gaze of the eyes should be inward. In Uthitha Trikonasana (Extended triangle pose—see pages 70–75), the head is turned up, and the student is asked to look up at the ceiling. But the focus should not be a light or a patch on the ceiling. There should be no connection between the eyes and external objects. It is the passive inward gaze that allows the eyes to remain passive. In turn, the skin of the face softens and the brain is freed from tension and anxieties. When the senses of perception are relaxed, the brain becomes void (*shunya*). The thinking process ceases. When the senses of perception turn inward, the energy is balanced evenly in the body and true equilibrium is achieved. Now, the asana is complete.

Achieving a mindless state
Equanimity leads to a state of emptiness in the body and mind, bringing serenity to the body cells and stability to the mind. The practitioner learns to stop invading thoughts from entering the brain. It is a mindless state. Mr. Iyengar often says, "I teach *dharana* in the asana itself. The foundation for *dharana* and *dhyana* (meditation) has to begin from the practice of asana and pranayama. Just as a surge of high voltage can damage electrical equipment, in a similar way luminous energy generated in *dharana* and *dhyana* can damage the nervous system of a person who has not practiced asana and pranayama."

Mr. Iyengar refers to "*Desha bandha cittasya dharana*," which means to fix one's attention on one thing within the body for long periods of time. For example, the mind can be held in the knee in Salamba Sirsasana (Headstand—see pages 138–143). While in this pose students are unable to view the knees with their physical eyes and instead, they have to use their microscopic eyes (*dharmendriya* eyes). This allows the consciousness to spread to the dull areas, correcting different disparities and increasing the span of those microscopic eyes. It creates equanimity in the body. Asanas may look physical

*"In the ultimate stage of yoga, **the seeker** is free from the* **dualities of body and mind,** *and mind and self."*

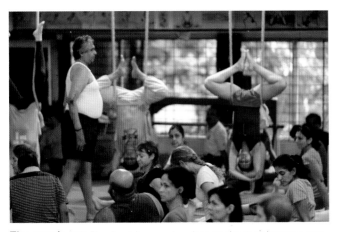

The guru's son Prashant Iyengar teaches students to become one with the asana, during a class at the Institute in Pune.

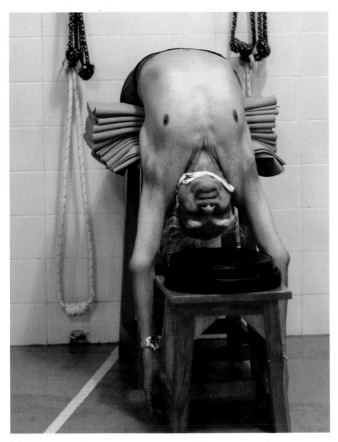

Mr. Iyengar advocates the use of the inner eye to observe every part of the body. "One should exist everywhere in the body," he says.

from the outside, but Mr. Iyengar makes his students aware of the microscopic eyes and builds intelligence in the students. He is strict so his students can achieve this state within the asana. He scolds the student who looks at the clock but allows their leg to remain crooked. He isn't correcting the physical imperfection—he focuses on the dissipation of energy that has to be checked while bringing the wandering mind to a single point of concentration.

Freedom from dualities

In the ultimate stage of yoga, the seeker is free from the dualities of body and mind, and mind and self. Mr. Iyengar explains that dualities have a direct connection with the *tri gunas* (three qualities), *tamas, rajas,* and *sattva.* By nature, the body is *tamasic* (dull and sluggish), the mind is *rajasic* (active and dynamic), and the self, *sattvic* (illuminative). *Tamo guna* (fear and pain) manifests itself in the form of vices and bad habits. Mr. Iyengar uses asanas to challenge his students and the Iyengar approach destroys the sluggishness in the body. It is not just a technically accurate asana appearing to have the right presentation; it is the awakening of the intelligence and the surfacing of a sense of purity (*sattva guna*).

Mr. Iyengar does not pamper his students and urges them to practice daily for an hour, to challenge the body and mind. He advocates the use of props (see pages 182–185) to learn the right alignment and action in the asana. When discernment sets in, he believes, one should practice independently with introspection, comparing the feelings one gets while working with props to those without props and resulting in incorrect movements.

Mr. Iyengar understood that yoga practice must be modified as and when one recognizes one's temperament, to achieve expected results. His method ensures that a *tamo-gunic* asana transforms into a *rajasic* asana by applying the right techniques. In the beginning, there are many movements and adjustments to be made. Once that is done, true steadiness comes. A vibrant asana is one of calm and poise; this is *sattvic* asana.

The process of meditation is dependent on the *sattva guna.* It brings calmness, and the practitioner becomes one with the asana. The dualities between the body and mind fade. This disappearance (*pratiprasava*) happens only for yogis who have reached the highest state of *samadhi* (self-realization). But the seed is sown in the practice of asana and pranayama.

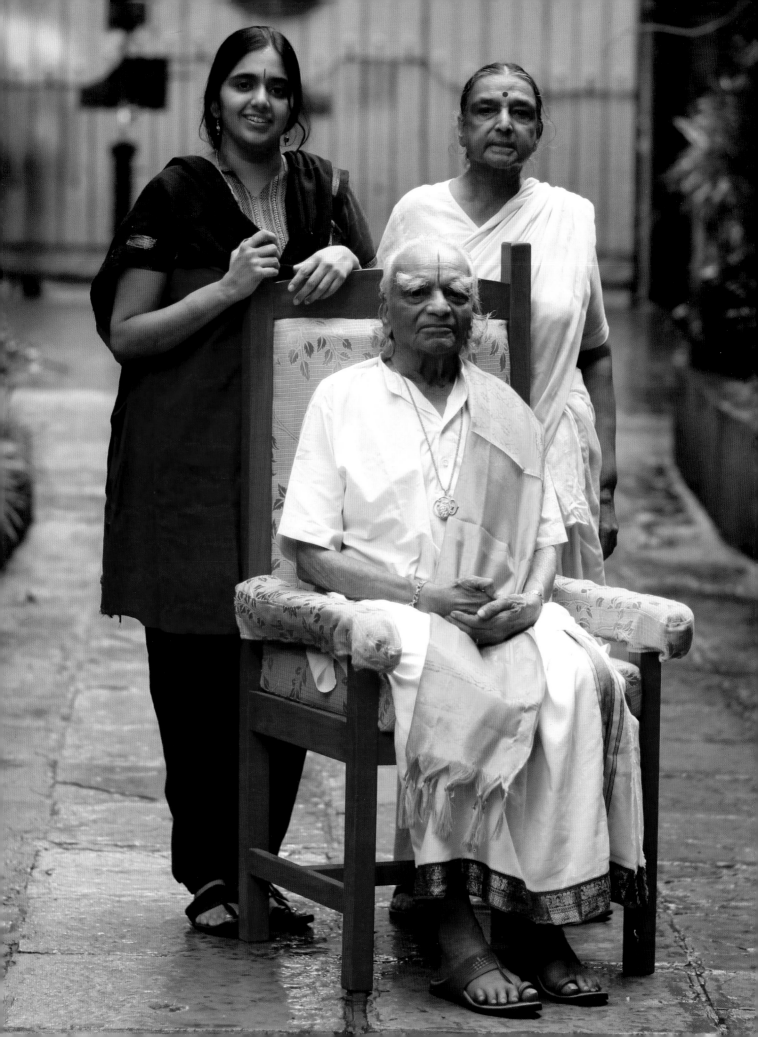

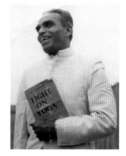

The Iyengar Legacy

B.K.S. Iyengar's unique vision for yoga continues to flourish through his family and his students. His passion for bringing positive changes to the lives of others can be seen in his charitable work at his birth place, Bellur.

It's a Tuesday morning in the city of Pune, India. The incessant rain has taken a short break. The Ramaamani Iyengar Memorial Yoga Institute seems empty, but the large, first-floor hall is busy. A group of students go through their ritual practice, with careful determination and focused intensity. They contort their bodies using ropes, blocks, and towels as aids and props to gain the perfect posture.

B.K.S. Iyengar is practicing yoga in a quiet corner, near the window. His skin ripples as he settles into postures, pushing his body to unimaginable limits, but with beauty and grace—poetry, almost. Mr. Iyengar slips into the final posture. It looks complicated. The Dwi Pada Viparita Dandasana, or the Two-Legged Inverted Staff Pose, is an advanced back bend. But there is no exertion, just a seamless flow. The students, an eclectic mix of people from different parts of the world, have stopped practicing. They sit around their Guru, in a semicircle, watching in complete silence.

Mr. Iyengar comes out of the posture and sits up to catch his breath. The students break into spontaneous applause, cheering and whistling. He smiles as the applause continues. "Hope you are inspired," he says. "God bless you."

The students stand up, stretch, and go about their practice. Many of them are dedicated Iyengar yoga teachers, certified and working at centers and schools across the world. They come to Pune in the thousands, throughout the year, to study under Guruji (as his students lovingly call him), to learn the philosophy behind Iyengar yoga, and imbibe his rigorous discipline.

A family of teachers

Mr. Iyengar is now retired, but his children Geeta and Prashant continue his work, as does his granddaughter Abhijata Sridhar. They teach extensive classes, molding students to become practitioners who truly understand the meaning and purpose of Iyengar yoga.

Abhijata grew up watching her grandfather practice yoga. She would travel to Pune during her summer vacation. "We would play on him during his practice. He would be in an asana and we would go under him or jump over him. But when I realized what he did and the way he did it, I was in awe," she remembers. The fascination for yoga stayed and her understanding of the form developed, as she recognized that yoga was not just for the elderly. "I began to realize that yoga is for me, too," she says. Today, when she isn't teaching, Abhijata works with Mr. Iyengar, honing and understanding the intricacies of each posture.

The family comes together for the medical classes, working with students suffering from medical conditions. Guruji is a tough teacher; a disciplinarian. He chides and scolds the teachers as he gently corrects the patients' postures. "How are you feeling now?" he asks one of them, a woman lying, propped with bolsters under her back. "Much better," she says.

(top) **First published** in 1966, *Light on Yoga* contains invaluable teachings from B.K.S. Iyengar and is called "the Bible of yoga."
(left) **B.K.S. Iyengar** with granddaughter Abhijata Sridhar (left) and daughter Geeta Iyengar (right) at the Ramaamani Iyengar Memorial Yoga Institute, Pune.

"**You** can go **anywhere** in the **world** and practice **Iyengar yoga**."

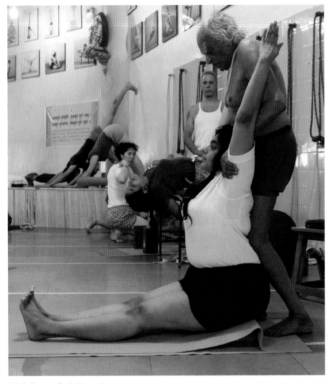

Abhijata Sridhar learns the correct yoga posture from her grandfather and guru B.K.S. Iyengar.

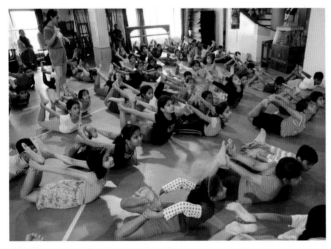

Children practice yoga under Mr. Iyengar's guidance at the Ramaamani Institute in Pune.

Complete surrender

This fierceness is a manifestation of Mr. Iyengar's passion for yoga, according to Penelope Chaplin, founder member of the Iyengar Yoga Institute in Maida Vale, London. She is one of the seven "Most Senior Leading Teachers of the UK," a special designation awarded by Mr. Iyengar in 2009. Penelope first met Mr. Iyengar in 1971 while attending a class he was teaching on Paddington Street. She used to suffer from a bad back and an extreme lack of confidence. "He stood behind me and said, 'As long as you are afraid I cannot help you.'" That's when she realized that the only way she could learn from Mr. Iyengar was through complete surrender, without challenge or resistance. Iyengar yoga has since formed the core of Penelope's life for 45 years.

"For me, his work has been like cement keeping the mind and body together. I was very supple, but he taught me to work from within rather than just from a physical action, although that understanding took quite a few years to develop," she says.

Abhijata almost echoes Penelope when she says, "Guruji teaches us yoga using the metaphor of the body. It's our habit to not look at the bigger picture. We need to develop the sense to understand Guruji's language," she says. "We need to develop receptors to yoga. This is the way our asanas can evolve. This is the way our living can change." The Iyengar form of yoga has changed her life, she says. "It has changed the way I think… the sacred lesson he has taught me, is to do what I do fully, wholly, and completely, with my heart and head. Guruji taught me the binary system in life; he has taught me the meaning of zero and one."

Crossing borders

There is no doubt that Iyengar yoga has transformed how the world views the form. It has transcended cultures, borders, and religions. The Institute has more than 3,800 certified teachers across more than 40 countries, from the US and the UK, to Italy, Spain, Germany, and now China.

"You can go anywhere in the world and practice Iyengar yoga," Mr. Iyengar says. "Today, I am the happiest man on earth, because with all the damnations and frustrations, I have not only earned name and fame for myself, but I have brought back respect and majesty to this art and science called yoga.

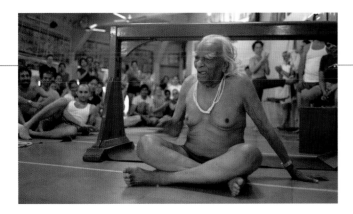

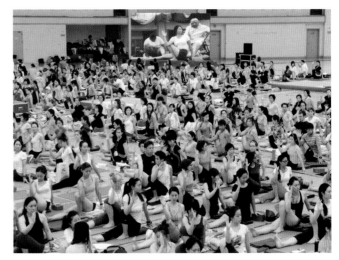

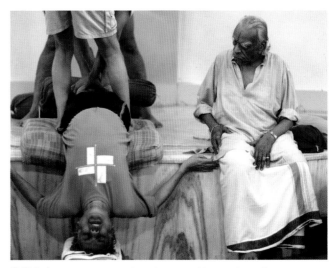

(left) It's rare for the students to watch B.K.S Iyengar practice yoga, but when they do, they get a rare glimpse of the man who is a legend.

If I had not given more than 15,000 lectures and demonstrations single-handedly, I think yoga would not have become popular."

The influence Iyengar yoga has in the world today is evident, whether in Mr. Iyengar's famous meeting with Pope Paul VI, his first visit to South Africa as a guest of the government, the yoga demonstration he gave for Nikita Krushchev during the Premier's visit to India, or more recently, his visit to China in 2011. "When I arrived in China, I did not know what to expect. The response was unbelievable. It was only during the China-India Yoga Summit that I discovered that most of my books have been translated into Mandarin and are widely read," Mr. Iyengar says. There are a large number of yoga schools across 57 cities in 17 provinces across China, all inspired by his books *Light on Yoga* and *Light on Pranayama*.

He believes that yoga's popularity stems from his methodology—its practical approach and in-depth understanding of the relationship between the body and the mind. "The growth of the body is the culture of the mind," Mr. Iyengar says. "It is the culture of intelligence itself. Therefore there are no barriers." He believes that now, as his students move from the "world of materialism to the shores of emancipation," it is time to look inward. "I want my countrymen to carry the light of yoga to our own people in the villages and lift them to general health and happiness. They represent the roots of our Indian culture, untouched by external influences", he says.

The Bellur Initiative

It was this desire to give back to his society and his home that propelled Mr. Iyengar toward Bellur—a tiny village, 40 kilometers from Bangalore and his birthplace. After all, this village is the B in B.K.S. Iyengar's name. Bellur used to be a poor village—there were no schools, hospitals, or even clean drinking water. Having missed out on a formal education himself, Mr. Iyengar valued it the most. Determined to bring change, he and his pupils organized yoga demonstrations in England and Switzerland, raising a total of $1,500. Bellur's first elementary school, Sri Krishnamachar-Seshamma Vidyamandir was built in 1967–68. Venkataswamy and Krishnappa, the chairpersons of the village panchayat, the local governing body, have since watched their

China has embraced the Iyengar method of yoga. B.K.S. Iyengar's 2011 master classes met with great response.

B.K.S. Iyengar is a tough taskmaster. He monitors the yoga instructors in the medical class, helping them work with the students to ensure accurate postures for maximum benefit.

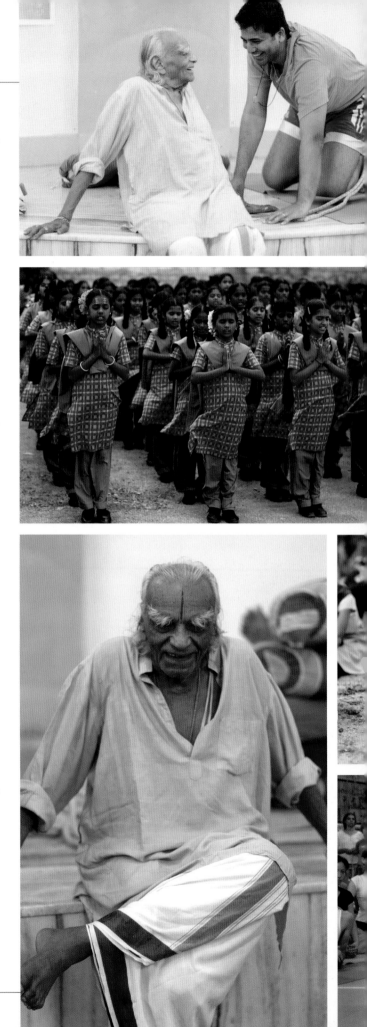

"Guruji *loves the children* and is really *attached* to them."

home transform. They remember the launch of the school and watched the building come up. "It was the first of its kind in the entire region—a school with a roof. We had never seen anything like this. The villagers were excited at this new opportunity, and soon flocked to the school. There were 200 children initially. Guruji (Mr. Iyengar) got the building extended to accommodate more students," Krishnappa says.

In January 2005, the foundation stone of the Smt Ramaamani Sundararaja Iyengar High School was laid, and classes started in June the same year. Iyengar sat through the interviews of the children and teachers on the first day of admissions. Then, two years ago, the Smt Ramaamani Sundararaja Iyengar College opened its doors to the people.

Delivering education

Change has come to Bellur. Today, the village that has a population of 4,000 people includes Ramaamani Nagar, as the adjoining area is now called, which is home to the high school, college, and the hospital. Every morning, the musical chant of Sanskrit *shlokas* (prayers) rings out across the village. The 320 school and 160 college students then troop into a sports field nearby where they work on their yoga postures. Some of the students work on intricate asanas—they are the best of the group who also participate in competitions.

Venkataswamy remembers how Mr. Iyengar showered the schoolchildren with candy every time he visited the village." Guruji loves the children and is really attached to them. Our village is on the way to Tirupati, the holy shrine of Lord Venkateswara. Guruji would visit our village and always bring candy from Tirupati for the children," he says.

Mr. Iyengar has taken care of every aspect of a child's education. He is sensitive to the fact that most of the students come from financially poor backgrounds and travel by their own means from 13 surrounding villages. The school even provides them with a free midday meal that comes all the way from Bangalore. It is obvious that the school and college have increased the opportunities for the children. Krishnappa says,

It is easy to see the vast impact B.K.S. Iyengar and his approach to yoga has had in the world, whether it is in the tiny village of Bellur or at the Institute in Pune.

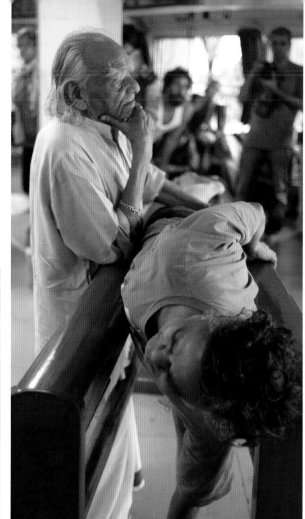
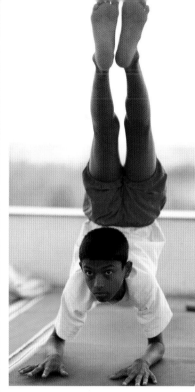
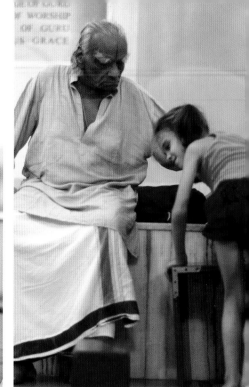
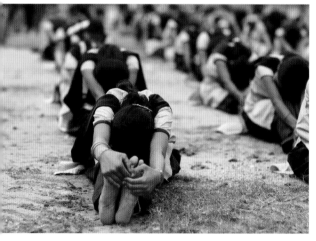
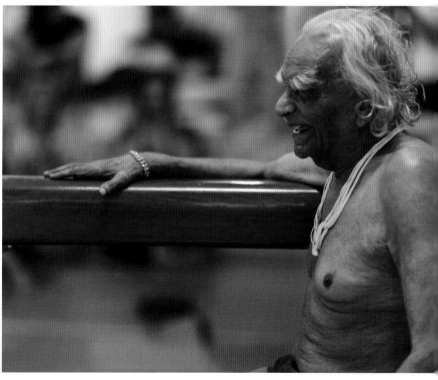
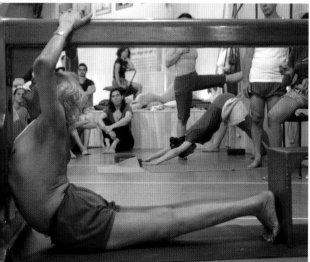
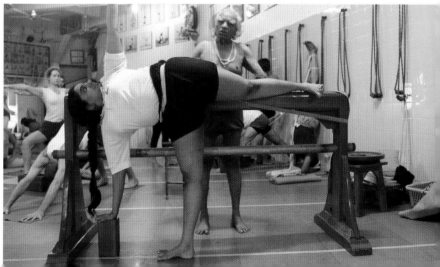

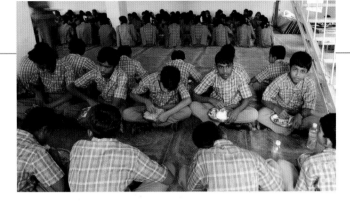

(right) **B.K.S. Iyengar** initiated a midday meal project for students at the schools in Bellur.

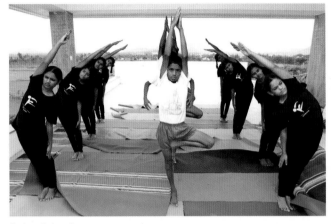

School students in Bellur working on their yoga postures during their daily practice.

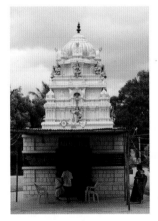

Mr. Iyengar was behind the world's first Sage Patanjali temple, built in Bellur.

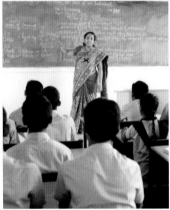

Education has increased opportunities for the people of Mr. Iyengar's birthplace, Bellur.

"The foundation of education has changed our village dramatically. The younger generation has taken up yoga. The students who have graduated from our school have done really well. They work in banks, are lawyers, and there are some who even hold doctorates."

Trust in the future

But education is just one step. The primary concern was to create an infrastructure in the village that would improve quality of life. The Bellur Krishnamachar & Seshamma Smaraka Niddhi Trust (BKSSNT) was formed with this very vision in 2003. The intention was to bring about a silent revolution, since Mr. Iyengar believes that good health and education form a firm foundation for social and economic reform.

One of the Trust's first tasks was to locate pure ground water. Today, a water storage tank with the capacity of 50,000 gallons supplies the village with clean drinking water. A rainwater harvesting initiative was also set up. A malaria epidemic in 1920 and the lack of timely and easily available medical facilities made Mr. Iyengar determined to set up primary health care in the village. The Smt. Ramaamani Sundararaja Iyengar Primary Health Center started in 2007 and treats over 30 villages across the region. So far, more than 18,500 patients from Bellur and the surrounding villages have benefited from the free medical services that the hospital offers. It has 20 beds and the management is now hoping to gain support from more established hospitals. So far, the hospital has two doctors, six nurses, and a lab assistant. The hospital runs a fully equipped daycare service. Medical services, surgical procedures, and medication are free for the village.

Bellur has also become a mecca for Iyengar yoga students. They visit the village for workshops, or on a pilgrimage to see the birthplace of the man who has changed their lives. On the way, they pay their respects at the village temple complex. It is here that Mr. Iyengar has built the world's first Sage Patanjali temple to honor the man who wrote the Yoga Sutras. The trust was also responsible for the renovation of an 800-year-old Hanuman temple and the restoration of a temple dedicated to Lord Ramaa and Rishi Valmiki. Valmiki was the author of the epic Ramaayana transformed from a fierce bandit to a learned Sage. It is significant that the local villagers worship Valmiki; they too have

*"It gives me **great contentment** to **give** to others what **God** has **given me**."*

transformed from a people without hope to a community with a future." Guruji is responsible for putting Bellur on the map of the world," says Krishnappa.

Mr. Iyengar considers Bellur's success as a culmination of his life's work. "It gives me great contentment to give to others what God has given me," he says. "I have taken up the task of uplifting my native village, Bellur and other poor villages in India through educational, cultural, social, and health-related projects. It has not been an easy task. But the transformation that the BKSSNT has achieved in a relatively short period of time is a remarkable. It is obvious that the benefits are not restricted to the people of Bellur, but are shared by a wider geographical region. The quality of life, the overall cleanliness, and the positive attitude among the community, especially the youth, is already showing a change for the better. I am sure that after me, my family, my pupils, their children, and the next generation will carry the message of yoga to every nook and corner of the globe, so that all may live as one human race without geographical division or division of race, religion, color, or gender."

Building the legacy

Abhijata knows that the way forward could be difficult. "What he (Mr. Iyengar) gives is so pure and so vast. As it gets transmitted, more people will benefit. But we know so little compared to what he knows. I am afraid it will get diluted." It is a fear she shares with many yoga teachers. Penelope Chaplin adds, "Part of Guruji's legacy is that he has given precise knowledge and discipline selflessly and patiently to his senior teachers, which means they have been able to reflect something of his essence through their own teaching. 'Iyengar yoga' is therefore available and accessible to everyone in a pure form. We must be careful we don't allow it to be diluted."

But Iyengar yoga's impact on our lives today has never been in question. Abhijata quotes Mr. Iyengar when she says, "Humans innately resist change because we feel safe with what is familiar and fear the insecurity that comes with something new. We seek freedom, but cling to bondage. Guruji's *parampara* (legacy) is about how we change the way we live, using our body and mind for this transformation. Yoga is a *darshana*. *Darshana* also means 'mirror,' a mirror to see oneself. It will always be relevant. It is always contemporary."

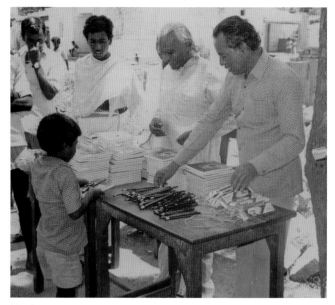

Mr. Iyengar would often visit Bellur to distribute books and encourage the students who attended the school.

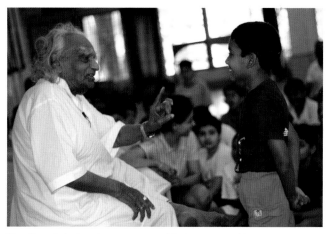

Pupils relish the chance to meet Mr. Iyengar and learn from his message.

Message from B.K.S. Iyengar

" Yoga is eternal. It is evergreen and timeless. It is the answer to the infinite stresses modern-day life brings us. Yoga brings balance to our lives, calms the restless mind, and brings us to a point of complete quiet. It is then that we discover our true selves.

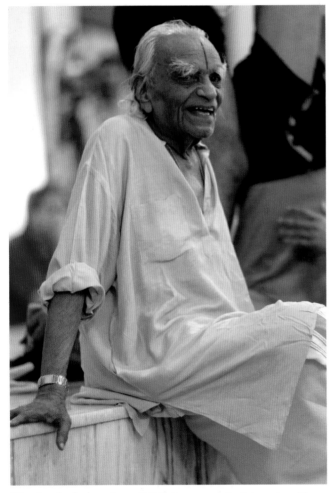

Words of wisdom from B.K.S. Iyengar as he interacts with students at the Ramaamani Iyengar Memorial Yoga Institute.

We are instinctively caught in a web of violence, anger, and greed. It is natural then that these instinctive weaknesses lead us to act violently, directly, indirectly, or because of the pressures of society. The practice of yoga transforms or changes these instinctive weaknesses. They are not eradicated immediately, but they are certainly minimized. It is then that a person's life changes for the better in the art of living. He looks in a different direction, from the direct perception of growth, both mentally and intellectually. Yoga allows us to reach the goal of life that is to live worthily.

I was not an educated person. I was educationally, financially, and emotionally poor. When I was born, I was nowhere in this world. I came from an impoverished family. In my early days, I was attacked by bouts of diseases. I suffered from tuberculosis, influenza, malaria, and typhoid. Somehow I survived. However, my physical body was in a zero state of development. This state did not allow me to develop my physical or mental power. As a result, there were a lot of disturbances in my life, a lot of emotional restlessness. It did not allow me to think of a future. It did not allow me to live a present life.

Yoga brought me to this level of inner bliss through practice, though I was not taught anything theoretically. Whatever I speak and teach today is from my experienced knowledge. It is more stable, because I speak from the intelligence of my heart.

Today, children are highly educated and qualified. Unfortunately, however, there is carelessness in the younger generation because they live intellectually, neglecting their foundation—the body that supports the intelligence within. Their brawn is neglected while their brain is developed to a great extent. So, naturally, there is a tremendous disparity within each individual,

*"**Yoga** allows us to **reach** the **goal of life** that is to **live worthily**."*

which creates psychological and emotional problems. The practice of yoga builds the inner strength needed to endure problems experienced in today's age.

Stress, a common factor today, doesn't come into the field of yoga at all. Negative stress is an enemy, but positive stress is growth. The word stress can be used to describe a person who is negative and sees everything negatively. That person is bound to suffer a great deal. Then, there is another form of stress, where the brain proudly functions while neglecting emotional intelligence and the power of the body's strength. That stress is an enemy, too. Yoga nullifies these two types of negative and hyper-tensed stresses. It balances the person and harmoniously blends the intellect of the head and the intelligence of the heart. This brings poise and peace to each individual.

Those who practice yoga must understand that we may know the external world, but we don't know the internal world. Yoga teaches us about the internal world, about the contents of our body—the liver, spleen, pancreas, respiratory system, neurological system, and so forth. It helps us understand how they function and at what time they cause disturbances within us. Yoga makes us realize the upheavals of day-to-day living and creates balance in our body and mind through its practice.

There are many ways in yoga and each can be adapted to suit the need of the day. There are yoga positions that work purely on the physical level. There are positions that stabilize a person emotionally. If a person feels that there is restlessness in the brain, then yoga has poses that can help him gain restfulness immediately. However, people have to know what they need to do according to their individual environment. This is what the practitioner gains from yoga, but only if it is practiced honestly, with integrity and sincerity.

People believe that the body is finite, so they begin the search for the infinite. However, there is no need to hunt for it—it's not outside but inside us. Yogic practice helps one see the infinite in the finite. When one recognizes all the contents of the body, from the cells of the skin to the self, the finite dissolves and what remains is the infinite self.

I never stop learning, never stop thinking of the practice of yoga. I don't think of my body when I am practicing. I only think if I can expand myself to each and every corner of my body. I ask myself, do I exist there or not? I observe myself during my practice. I see where there is dormancy in my body and where there is fullness. I ask myself, why is there fullness or dormancy in that particular area. I question every second and see that the mind is spread evenly everywhere. For, when the mind is spread evenly through my body without any deviation or refraction, then the mind dissolves. It is like a silence in the ocean. I am completely silent in the ocean of my body. Only the self exists. And that is what yoga teaches. We can learn objective knowledge through books or from contact in society. But subjective knowledge can only be learned through the contact of your self. That is why it is called *samyoga*, which means the oneness of the body, mind, and intelligence with the self.

In one way, yoga is the golden key for golden health. But health is not just physical fitness. There are seven stages of health: physical, physiological, mental, intellectual, conscious, conscientious, and divine. When all the seven stages of health are in harmony in a person, then, I say he is a worthy human being.

This is my message.

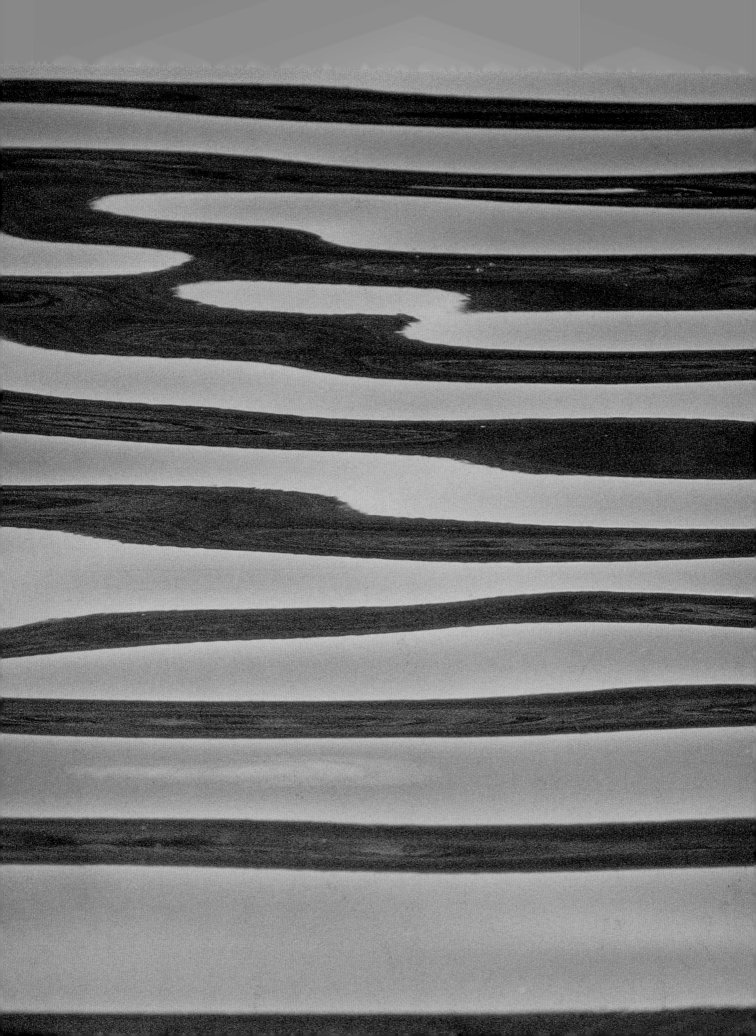

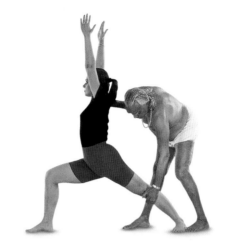

CHAPTER 2

YOGA FOR YOU

"Yoga is a light, which once lit, will never dim. The better your practice, the brighter the flame."

The primary aim of yoga is to restore the mind to simplicity and peace, to free it from confusion and distress. This sense of calm comes from the practice of yogic asanas and pranayama. Unlike other forms of exercise which strain muscles and bones, yoga gently rejuvenates the body. By restoring the body, yoga frees the mind from the negative feelings caused by the fast pace of modern life. The practice of yoga fills up the reservoirs of hope and optimism within you. It helps you to overcome all obstacles on the path to perfect health and spiritual contentment. It is a rebirth.

Aims of Yoga

The practice of yoga aims at overcoming the limitations of the body. Yoga teaches us that the goal of every individual's life is to take the inner journey to the soul. Yoga offers both the goal and the means to reach it.

When there is perfect harmony between body and mind, we achieve self-realization. Yoga teaches us that obstacles in the path of our self-realization indicate themselves in physical or mental indisposition. When our physical state is not perfect, this causes an imbalance in our mental state, which is known in Sanskrit as *chittavritti*. The practice of yoga helps us to overcome that imbalance. Yogic asanas, or poses, can cure *vyadhi* or physical ailments, and redress *angamejayatva* or unsteadiness in the body. *Shvasa-prashvasa*, which translates as "uneven respiration"—an indication of stress—is alleviated by the practice of yoga. Asanas tone the whole body. They strengthen bones and muscles, correct posture, improve breathing, and increase energy. This physical well-being has a strengthening and calming impact on the mind.

Asanas and pranayama

Practicing asanas cleanses the body. Just as a goldsmith heats gold in fire to burn out its impurities, similarly, asanas, by increasing the circulation of fresh blood through the body, purge it of the diseases and toxins which are the consequences of an irregular lifestyle, unhealthy habits, and poor posture. Regular practice of the stretches, twists, bends, and inversions—the basic movements of asanas—restores strength and stamina to the body. Asanas, together with pranayama, or the control of breath, rectify physical, physiological, and psychological disorders. They have a positive impact on the effects of stress and disease. Among the many ailments that benefit from the practice of asanas are osteoarthritis, high and low blood pressure, diabetes, asthma, and anorexia.

Harmony between body and soul
This 10th-century figure, the Yoga Narayan, from Khajuraho, India, depicts the god Vishnu in a state of yogic calm

Mind and body

The body and the mind are in a state of constant interaction. Yogic science does not demarcate where the body ends and the mind begins, but approaches both as a single, integrated entity. The turmoil of daily life brings stress to the body and the mind. This creates anxiety, depression, restlessness, and rage. Yoga asanas, while appearing to deal with the physical body alone, actually influence the chemical balance of the brain, which in turn improves one's mental state of being.

The obstacles to this perfect balance were outlined by the sage, Patanjali, some 2,000 years ago in the *Yoga Sutras*. Historians disagree on the exact dates, but it is known that the *sutras,* or aphorisms on the philosophy and practice of yoga, were compiled sometime between 300 BC and AD 300, and the entire corpus was called the *Patanjala Yoga Darshana*. In the final chapter of the *Yoga Sutras*, the *Samadhi Pada*, Patanjali discusses the disorders that are the root cause of suffering. According to the sage, *vyadhi* or physical ailments, create emotional upheaval. The task of yoga is to tackle both.

The alleviation of pain is, even today, one of the main reasons for the journey into yoga for most people. Yoga asanas work specific parts of the body to soothe and relax the mind as well. Inverted asanas, for instance, simultaneously calm and stimulate the brain. These asanas activate glands and vital organs by supplying fresh blood to the brain, making it alert but relaxed. Yoga possesses the unique ability to calm the nerves. The nerves function as the medium between the physiological body and

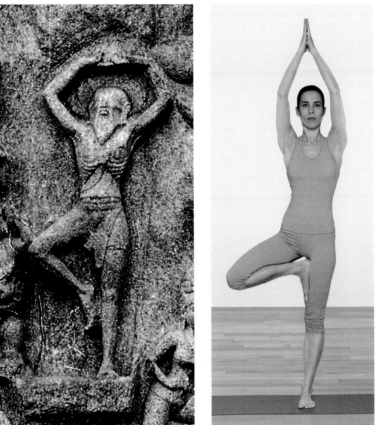

Timeless tradition
The 4th-century figure from Mahabalipuram, India (left), and this modern woman show that certain classic movements are eternal

the psychological body (*see page* 62). Practicing yoga has the holistic impact of relaxing the body and calming the mind.

Stages of yoga

The primary aim of yoga is to restore the mind to simplicity, peace, and poise, to free it from confusion and distress. This simplicity, this sense of order and calm, comes from the practice of asanas and pranayama. Yoga asanas integrate the body, the mind, the intelligence, and, finally, the self, in four stages. The first stage, *arambhavastha*, is one in which we practice at the level of the physical body.

"After a **session** *of* **yoga***, the* **mind** *becomes tranquil and* **passive***."*

The second stage is *ghatavastha*, when the mind learns to move in unison with the body. The third level of *parichayavastha* occurs when the intelligence and the body become one. The final stage is *nishpattyavastha*, the state of perfection (*see page* 62). Spiritual awareness flows into the student of yoga through these stages. *Duhkha*, which is misery or pain, vanishes, and the art of living in simplicity and peace is realized.

Yoga fills the spiritual void

The world today is overwhelmingly materialistic, and this has created a great spiritual void in our lives. Our lifestyles are unduly complex and we become stressed primarily as a result of our own actions. Our existence feels barren and devoid of meaning. There is a lack of spiritual dimension to our lives and in our relationships. This has led many reflective people to realize that solace and inspiration, peace and happiness, cannot come from the external environment but must come from within.

The freedom of yoga

The impact of yoga is never purely physical. Asanas, if correctly practiced, bridge the divide between the physical and the mental spheres. Yoga stems the feelings of pain, fatigue, doubt, confusion, indifference, laziness, self-delusion, and despair that assail us from time to time. The yogic mind simply refuses to accept such negative emotions and seeks to overcome these turbulent currents on the voyage to the total liberation of the self. Once we become sincere practitioners of yoga, we cease to be tormented by these unhappy and discouraging states of mind.

Yoga illuminates your life. If you practice sincerely, with seriousness and honesty, its light will spread to all aspects of your life. Regular practice will bring you to look at yourself and your goals in a new light. It will help remove the obstacles to good health and stable emotions. In this way, yoga will help you to achieve emancipation and self-realization, which is the ultimate goal of every person's life.

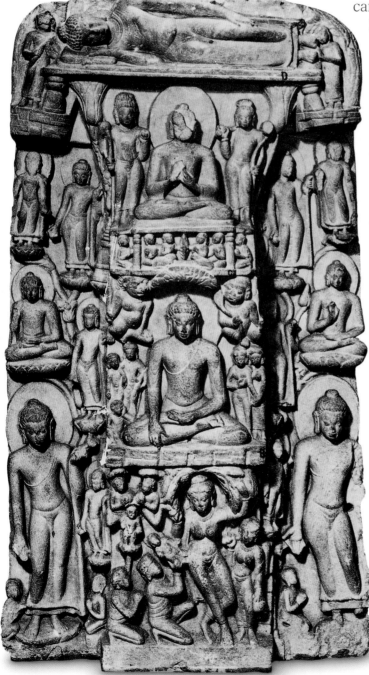

The four stages of the Buddha's journey to self-realization
This 5th-century frieze from Sarnath, India, shows the four defining events of the Buddha's life: (from the bottom) Buddha's birth from his mother's hip; attaining enlightenment in Bodhgaya; preaching to his disciples; the ascent to the celestial realms

The Way to Health

Good health results from perfect communication between each part of the body and mind; when each cell communes with every other. Although yoga is essentially a spiritual science, it leads to a sense of physical and emotional well-being.

Health is not just freedom from disease. For good health, the joints, tissues, muscles, cells, nerves, glands, and each system of the body must be in a state of perfect balance and harmony. Health is the perfect equilibrium of the body and mind, intellect and soul.

Health is like the flowing water of a river, always fresh and pure, in a constant state of flux. Humans are a combination of the senses of perception, the organs of action, the mind, the intelligence, the inner consciousness, and the conscience. Each of these is worked on by the practice of yoga.

Yoga asanas help to ensure an even distribution of bio-energy, or life-force, which brings the mind to a state of calm. A practitioner of yoga faces life not as a victim, but as a master, in control of his or her life situations, circumstances, and environment.

Asanas balance the respiratory, circulatory, nervous, hormonal, digestive, excretory, and reproductive systems perfectly. The equilibrium in the body then brings mental peace and enhances intellectual clarity.

Harmony of body and mind

Asanas cater to the needs of each individual according to his or her specific constitution and physical condition. They involve vertical, horizontal, and cyclical movements, which provide energy to the system by directing the blood supply to the areas of the body which need it most. In yoga, each cell is observed, attended to, and provided with a fresh supply of blood, allowing it to function smoothly.

The mind is naturally active and dynamic, while the soul is luminous. However, unhealthy bodies tend to house inert, dull, and sluggish minds. It is the practice of yoga which removes this sluggishness from the body and brings it to the level of the active mind. Ultimately, both the body and mind rise to the level of the illuminated self.

The practice of yoga stimulates and changes emotional attitudes, converting apprehensiveness into courage, indecision and poor judgement into positive decision-making skills, and emotional instability into confidence and mental equilibrium.

Yoga is for everyone
There are asanas to suit every constitution, irrespective of age or physical condition

Good health
A healthy body is like the flowing water of a river —always fresh and pure

Benefits of Poses

Asanas are based on the three basic human postures of standing, sitting, or lying down. But they are not a series of movements to be followed mechanically. They have a logic which must be internalized if the pose is to be practiced correctly.

The Sanskrit term, *asana*, is sometimes translated as "pose" and sometimes as "posture." Neither translation is wholly accurate, since they do not convey the element of thought or consciousness that must inform each movement of the asana. The final pose of an asana is achieved when all the parts of the body are positioned correctly, with full awareness and intelligence.

To achieve this, you must think through the structure of the asana. Realize the fundamental points by imagining how you will adjust and arrange each part of your anatomical body, especially the limbs, in the given movements.

Then, mold the body to fit the structure of the asana, making sure that the balance between both sides of the body is perfect, until there is no undue stress on any one organ, muscle, bone, or joint.

Importance of practicing asanas

The practice of asanas has a beneficial impact on the whole body. Asanas not only tone the muscles, tissues, ligaments, joints, and nerves, but also maintain the smooth functioning and health of all the body's systems. They relax the body and mind, allowing both to recover from fatigue or weakness, and the stress of daily life. Asanas also boost metabolism, lymphatic circulation, and hormonal secretions, and bring about a chemical balance in the body.

It is important to keep practicing until you are absolutely comfortable in the final pose. It is only then that you experience the full benefits of the asana. The sage Patanjali observes in *Yoga Sutra* 11.47, "Perfection in an asana is achieved when the effort to perform it becomes effortless, and the infinite being within is reached."

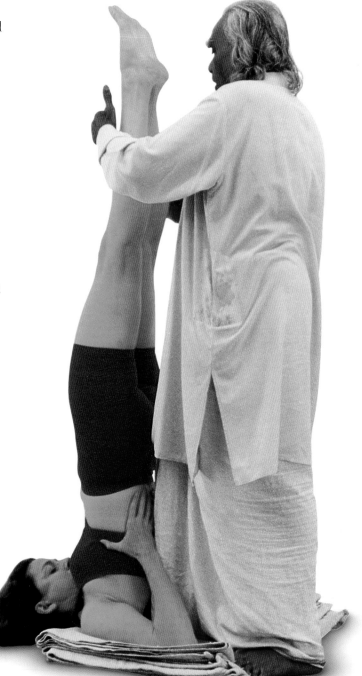

Perfect balance
Yogacharya Iyengar supports a student in Salamba Sarvangasana

Yoga and Stress

Yoga minimizes the impact of stress on the individual. Yogic science believes that the regular practice of asanas and pranayama strengthens the nervous system and helps people face stressful situations positively.

We have all experienced the way unrelieved tension results in both mental disorders and physical ill-health. This is not a modern phenomenon. In the centuries-old *Yoga Sutras*, the sage Patanjali attributed the causes of mental affliction to the ego, spiritual ignorance, desire, hatred of others, and attachment to life. He called these *kleshas* or "sorrows."

Origins of stress

Through advances in science and technology, modern civilization has been able to conquer ignorance in many fields, but its pride in technological achievement is excessive and misplaced. It has triggered widespread feelings of competitiveness and envy. Financial tensions, emotional upheavals, environmental pollution, and, above all, a sense of being overtaken by the speed of events, have all increased the stress of daily life.

All these factors strain the body, causing nervous tension, and adversely affecting the mind. This is when feelings of isolation and loneliness take over.

To deal with this, people turn to artificial solutions to cope with the pressures of daily life. Substance abuse, eating disorders, and destructive relationships are some of the substitutes people grasp at in their desperate search for consolation. But while these measures may provide temporary distraction or oblivion, the root cause of unhappiness—stress—remains unresolved.

Yoga is not a miracle cure that can free a person from all stress, but it can help to minimize it. The worries of modern life deplete our reserves of bio-energy, because we draw on our vital energy from the storehouse—the nerve cells. This can, ultimately, exhaust our energy reserves and lead to the collapse of mental and physical equilibrium. Yogic science believes that the nerves control the unconscious mind, and that when the nervous system is strong, a person faces stressful situations more positively. Asanas improve blood flow to all the cells of the body, revitalizing the nerve cells. This flow strengthens the nervous system and its capacity for enduring stress.

Relieving stress

The diaphragm, according to yogic science, is the seat of the intelligence of the heart and the window to the soul. During stressful situations, however, when you inhale and exhale, the diaphragm becomes too taut to alter its shape. Yogic exercises address this problem by developing elasticity in the diaphragm, so that, when stretched, it can handle any amount of stress, whether intellectual, emotional, or physical.

The practice of asanas and pranayama helps to integrate the body, breath, mind, and intellect. Slow, effortless exhalation during practice of an asana brings serenity to the body cells, relaxes the facial muscles, and releases all tension from the organs of perception: the eyes, ears, nose, tongue, and skin.

When this happens, the brain, which is in constant communication with the organs of action, becomes *shunya*, or void, and all thoughts are stilled. Then, invading fears and anxieties cannot penetrate the brain. When you develop this ability, you perform your daily activities with efficiency and economy. You do not dissipate your valuable bio-energy. You enter the state of true clarity of intellect. Your mind is free of stress and is filled with calm and tranquillity.

Yoga and Fitness

Most types of exercise are competitive. Yoga, although noncompetitive, is nevertheless challenging. The challenge is to one's own will power. It is a competition between one's self and one's body.

Exercise usually involves quick and forceful body movements. It has repeated actions which often lead to exertion, tension, and fatigue. Yoga asanas, on the other hand, involve movements which bring stability to the body, the senses, the mind, the intellect, the consciousness, and finally, to the conscience. The very essence of an asana is steady movement, a process that does not simply end, but finds fulfilment in tranquillity.

Most diseases are caused by the fluctuations in the brain and in the behavioral pattern of the body. In yogic practice, the brain is quieted, the senses are stilled, and perceptions are altered, all generating a calm feeling of detachment. With practice, the student of yoga learns to treat the brain as an object and the body as a subject. Energy is diffused from the brain to the other parts of the body. The brain and body then work together and energy is evenly balanced between the two. Yoga is thus termed *sarvanga sadhana* or "holistic practice."

No other form of exercise so completely involves the mind and self with the body, resulting in all-around development and harmony. Other forms of exercise address only particular parts of the body. Such forms are termed *angabhaga sadhana* or "physical exercise."

Stimulative exercise

Yoga asanas are stimulative exercises, while other endurance exercises are irritative. For instance, medical experts claim that jogging stimulates the heart. In fact, though the heartbeat of the jogger increases, the heart is not stimulated in the yogic sense of being energized and invigorated. In yoga, back bends, for example, are more physically demanding than jogging, but the heart beats at a steady, rhythmic pace.

Asanas do not lead to breathlessness. When practicing yoga, strength and power play separate roles to achieve a perfect balance in every part of the body, as well as the mind. After such stimulating exercise, a sense of rejuvenation and a fresh surge of energy follow.

Exercise can also be exhausting. Many forms of exercise require physical strength and endurance and can lead to a feeling of fatigue after 10–15 minutes of practice. Many such exercises improve energy levels by boosting nerve function, but ultimately, this exhausts the cellular reserves and the endocrine glands. Cellular toxins increase, and though circulation is enhanced, it is at the cost of irritating the other body systems and increasing the pulse rate and blood pressure. Ultimately, the heart is taxed and overworked.

Jogging
This form of exercise raises the heartbeat, but can tire you out

An athlete's strong lung capacity is achieved by hard and forceful usage, which is not conducive to preserving the health of the lungs. Furthermore, ordinary physical exercise, such as jogging, tennis, or soccer, lends itself to repetitive injuries of the bones, joints, and ligaments.

Such forms of exercise work with—and for—the skeletal and muscular systems. They cannot penetrate beyond these limits. But asanas penetrate each layer of the body and, ultimately, the consciousness itself. Only in yoga can you keep both the body and the mind relaxed, even as you stretch, extend, rotate, and flex your body.

Yoga, unlike other forms of exercise, keeps the nervous system elastic and capable of bearing stress. Although all forms of exercise bring about a feeling of well-being, they also stress the body. Yoga refreshes the body, while other systems exhaust it. Yoga involves the equal exertion of all parts of the body and does not overstrain any one part.

In other forms of exercise, the movements are restricted to a part or parts. They are reflex actions, which do not involve the intelligence in their execution. There is little space for precision and perfection, without extra expenditure of energy.

Yoga can be practiced at any age

With advancing age, physically vigorous exercises cannot be performed easily because of stiffening joints and muscles that have lost tone. Isometric exercises, for example, cannot be practiced with increasing age, since they lead to sprained muscles, painful joints, strained body systems, and the degeneration of organs. The great advantage of yoga is that it can be practiced by anyone, irrespective of age, sex, and physical condition.

In fact, yoga is particularly beneficial in middle age and after. Yoga is a gift to older people when the recuperative power of the body is declining and resistance to illness is weakened. Yoga generates energy and does not dissipate it. With yoga one can look forward to a satisfying, healthier future, rather than reflecting on one's youthful past.

Unlike other exercises, yoga results in the concentration of immunity cells in areas affected by disease, and thus improves immunity. That is why the ancient sages called yoga a therapeutic as well as a preventive science.

Yogacharya Iyengar in Eka Pada Viparita Dandasana
Yoga enables older people to have better energy and health

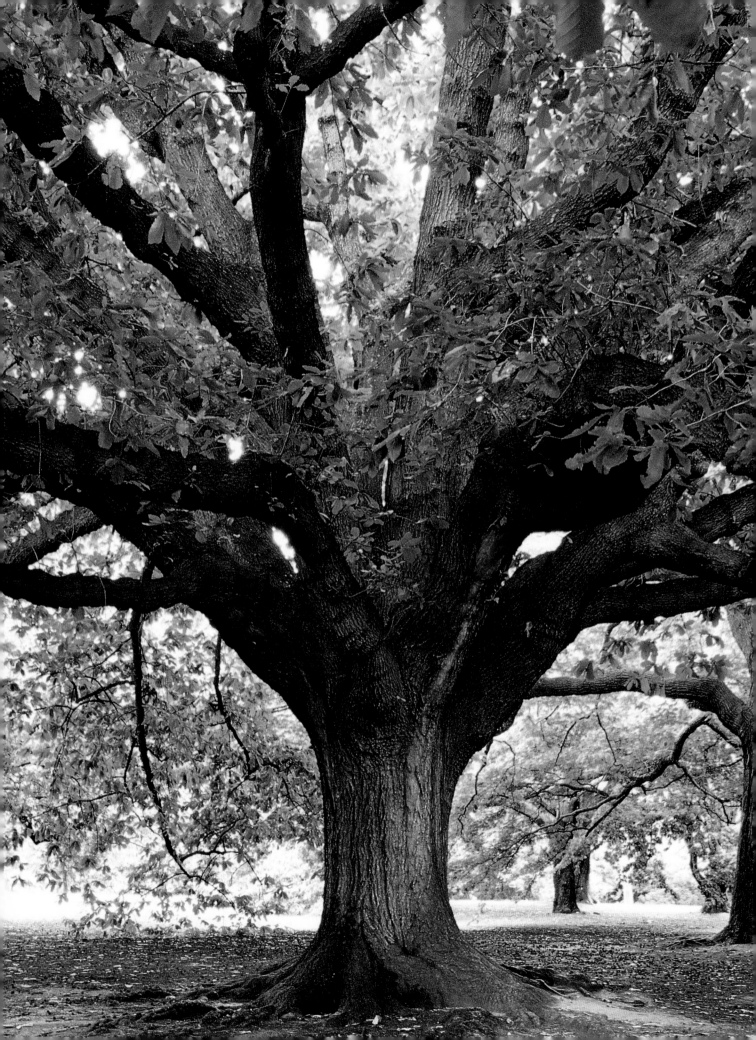

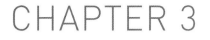

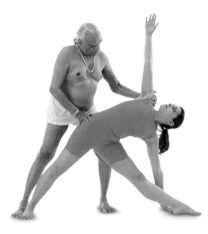

CHAPTER 3

PHILOSOPHY OF YOGA

*"Yoga is the **union** of the **individual self** with the **universal self**."*

Yoga is a fine art and seeks to express the artist's abilities to the fullest possible extent. While most artists need an instrument, such as a paintbrush or a violin, to express their art, the only instruments a yogi needs are his body and his mind. The ancient sages compared yoga to a fruit tree. From a single seed grow the roots, trunk, branches, and leaves. The leaves bring life-giving energy to the entire tree, which then blossoms into flowers and sweet, luscious fruit. Just as the fruit is the natural culmination of the tree, yoga, too, transforms darkness into light, ignorance into knowledge, knowledge into wisdom, and wisdom into unalloyed peace and spiritual bliss.

Meaning of Yoga

Yoga is an ancient art based on an extremely subtle science, that of the body, mind, and soul. The prolonged practice of yoga will, in time, lead the student to a sense of peace and a feeling of being at one with his or her environment.

Most people know that the practice of yoga makes the body strong and flexible. It is also well known that yoga improves the functioning of the respiratory, circulatory, digestive, and hormonal systems. Yoga also brings emotional stability and clarity of mind, but that is only the beginning of the journey to *samadhi*, or self-realization, which is the ultimate aim of yoga.

The ancient sages, who meditated on the human condition 2,000 years ago, outlined four ways to self-realization: *jnana marg*, or the path to knowledge, when the seeker learns to discriminate between the real and the unreal; *karma marg*, the path of selfless service without thought of reward; *bhakti marg*, the path of love and devotion; and finally, *yoga marg*, the path by which the mind and its actions are brought under control. All these paths lead to the same goal: *samadhi*.

The word "yoga" is derived from the Sanskrit root *yuj* which means "to join" or "to yoke"; the related meaning is "to focus attention on" or "to use." In philosophical terms, the union of the individual self, *jivatma*, with the universal self, *paramatma*, is yoga. The union results in a pure and perfect state of consciousness in which the feeling of "I" simply does not exist. Prior to this union is the union of the body with the mind,

and the mind with the self. Yoga is thus a dynamic, internal experience which integrates the body, the senses, the mind, and the intelligence, with the self.

The sage Patanjali was a master of yoga and a fully evolved soul. But this great thinker had the ability to empathize with the joys and sorrows of ordinary people. His reflections and those of other ancient sages on the ways through which every person could realize his full potential were outlined in the 196 *Yoga Sutras*.

Yogacharya Iyengar in Urdhva Dhanurasana
Asanas improve the working of all the systems of the body

Where yoga can take you

According to Patanjali, the aim of yoga is to calm the chaos of conflicting impulses and thoughts. The mind, which is responsible for our thoughts and impulses, is naturally inclined to *asmita* or egoism. From this spring the prejudice and biases which lead to pain and distress in our daily lives. Yogic science centers the intelligence in two areas: the heart and the head. The intelligence of the heart, sometimes also called the "root mind," is the actual agent of *ahankara* or false pride, which disturbs the intelligence of the head, causing fluctuations in the body and mind.

Patanjali describes these afflictions as *vyadhi* or physical ailments, *styana* or the reluctance to work, *samshaya* or doubt, *pramada* or indifference, *alasya* or laziness, *avirati* or the desire for sensual satisfaction, *bhranti darshana* or false knowledge, *alabdha bhumikatva* or indisposition, *angamejayatva* or unsteadiness in the body, and, lastly, *shvasa-prashvasa* or unsteady respiration. Only yoga eradicates these afflictions, and disciplines the mind, emotions, intellect, and reason.

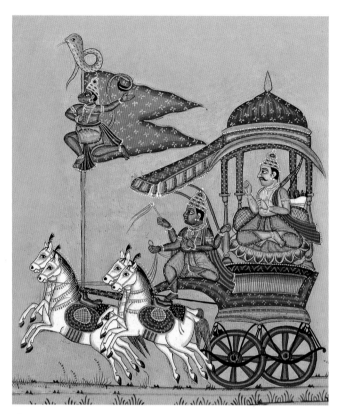

Krishna driving the chariot of the warrior, Arjun
Their discourses are narrated in the *Bhagvad Gita*, the main source of yogic philosophy

Astanga yoga

Yoga is also known as Astanga yoga. *Astanga* means "eight limbs" or "steps" (*see page* 52) and is divided into three disciplines. The *bahiranga-sadhana* discipline comprises ethical practices in the form of *yama*, or general ethical principles, *niyama*, or self-restraint, and physical practices in the form of *asanas* as well as *pranayama*.

The second discipline, *antaranga-sadhana*, is emotional or mental discipline brought to maturity by pranayama and *pratyahara*, or mental detachment. Lastly, *antaratma-sadhana* is the successful quest of the soul through *dharana*, *dhyana*, and *samadhi* (*see page* 52).

In this spiritual quest, it is important to remember the role of the body. The *Kathopanishad*, an ancient text compiled between 300–400 BC, compares the body to a chariot, the senses to the horses, and the mind to the reins. The intellect is the charioteer and the soul is the master of the chariot. If anything were to go wrong with the chariot, the horses, the reins, or the charioteer, the chariot and the charioteer would come to grief, and so would the master of the chariot.

But, writes Patanjali in *Yoga Sutra* 11.28, "The practice of yoga destroys the impurities of the body and mind, after which maturity in intelligence and wisdom radiate from the core of the being to function in unison with the body, senses, mind, intelligence, and the consciousness."

"The **aim of yoga** is to **calm** the **chaos** of **conflicting impulses**."

Philosophy of Asanas

Asanas, one of yoga's most significant "tools," help the sincere student develop physically and spiritually. The ancient sages believed that if you put your whole heart into your practice, you become a master of your circumstances and time.

Asanas are one of the major "tools" of yoga. Their benefits range from the physical level to the spiritual. That is why yoga is called *sarvanga sadhana*, or holistic practice. "Asana" is the positioning of the body in various postures, with the total involvement of the mind and self, in order to establish communication between our external and internal selves.

Yogic philosophy looks at the body as being made up of three layers and five sheaths. The three layers are: the causal body, or *karana sharira*, the subtle body, or *suksma sharira*, and the gross body, or *karya sharira*. Every individual functions in mind, matter, energy, and pure consciousness through five sheaths. These are: the anatomical sheath, or *annamaya kosha*, which is dealt with by asanas; the life-force sheath or *pranamaya kosha*, which is treated by pranayama; the psychological sheath, or *manomaya kosha*, is worked on by meditation; and the intellectual sheath, or *vijnanamaya kosha*, is transformed by studying the scriptures with sincerity and discrimination. Once these goals are addressed, you reach the *anandamaya kosha*, or the sheath of bliss.

Yoga integrates the three layers of the body with the five sheaths, enabling the individual to develop as a total being. The separation between the body and the mind, and the mind and the soul, then vanishes, as all planes fuse into one. In this way, asanas help to transform an individual by bringing him or her away from the awareness of the body toward the consciousness of the soul.

The journey of yoga

The *Hathayoga Pradipika* is a practical treatise on yoga, thought to have been compiled in the 15th century. The author, the sage Svatmarama, gives practical guidelines to beginners on the journey they must make from the culture of the body toward the vision of the soul. Unlike Patanjali, who discusses the sighting of the soul through the restraint of consciousness or *chitta*, Svatmarama begins his treatise with the restraint of energy, or *prana*. Sighting the soul through the restraint of energy is called Hatha yoga, whereas sighting the soul through the restraint of consciousness is known as Raja yoga.

In *Hathayoga Pradipika* 4.29, the author stresses the importance of the breath by saying that if the mind is the king of the senses, the

Samadhi
The Buddha attaining enlightenment at Bodhgaya. The 3rd-century sculpture is from Sarnath, India.

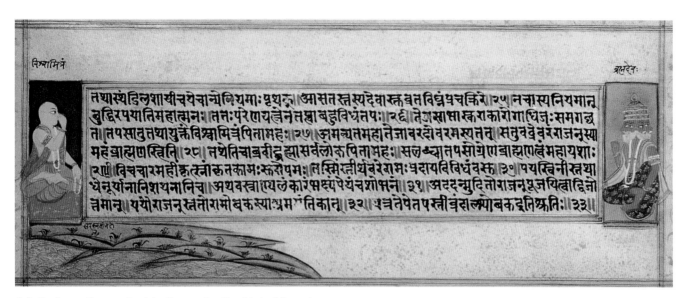

A folio from the ancient indian epic, the Mahabharata
The essentials of yoga philosophy are found in the *Bhagvad Gita*, which forms a part of the epic

master of the mind is breath. If breath is made to move rhythmically, with a controlled, sustained sound, the mind becomes calm. In that calmness, the king of the mind (the soul) becomes the supreme commander of the senses, mind, breath, as well as consciousness. When you learn to focus on the inhaled breath and the exhaled breath, you experience a neutralizing effect on the mind. This reaction led Svatmarama to conclude that the control of *prana* is the key to super-awareness or *samadhi*.

In the chapter *Samadhi Prakarana* of the *Hathayoga Pradipika*, Svatmarama gives glimpses of his experiences of *samadhi*. He says, "If one learns not to think of external things and simultaneously keeps away inner thoughts, one experiences *samadhi*. When the mind is dissolved in the sea of the soul, an absolute state of existence is reached. This is *kaivalya*, the freedom of emancipation."

The goal of yoga is a state of equilibrium and peace. Patanjali warns the student of yoga not to be deceived by this quietness, for it could lead to a state of *yogabhrastha* or "falling from the grace of yoga." He also says, 'The practice of yoga must continue, as it has to culminate in the

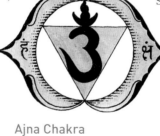

Ajna Chakra
This symbol represents the potential for spirituality in every individual

sight of the soul." This stage, when the individual becomes one with the core of his or her being, is a stage known as *nirbija* (seedless) *samadhi*.

Impact of yoga

In his third chapter of the *Yoga Sutras*, *Vibhuti Pada*, Patanjali speaks of the effects of yoga. Although they seem exotic to our modern conciousness, they indicate the potential of the powers of human nature. These spiritual powers and gifts have to be conquered in their turn. Otherwise, they become a trap, diverting the seeker from the true aim of yoga. When the soul is free from the bondage of body, mind, power, and pride of success, it reaches the state of *kaivalya* or freedom. This aspect is covered in the fourth chapter of the *Yoga Sutras*, *Kaivalya Pada*, the chapter on absolute liberation.

The person who practices yoga regularly will not become a victim but a master of his or her circumstances and time. The yoga practitioner lives to love and serve the world. This is the essence of life. Peace within and peace without, peace in the individual, in the family unit, in society, and in the world at large.

States of Mind

The mind is the vital link between the body and the consciousness. The individual can live with awareness, discrimination, and confidence only once the mind is calm and focused. Yoga is the alchemy that generates this equilibrium.

In yogic terminology, consciousness or *chitta* encompasses the mind or *manas*, intelligence or *buddhi*, and ego or *ahankara*. The Sanskrit word for man, *manusya* or *manava*, means "one who is endowed with this special consciousness." The mind does not have an actual location in the body. It is latent, elusive, and exists everywhere. The mind desires, wills, remembers, perceives, and experiences. Sensations of pain and pleasure, heat and cold, honor and dishonor, are experienced and interpreted by the mind. The mind reflects both the external and the internal worlds, but though it has the capacity to perceive things within and without, its natural tendency is to be preoccupied with the outside world.

Nature of the mind
When the mind is fully absorbed by objects seen, heard, smelled, felt, or tasted, this leads to stress, fatigue, and unhappiness. The mind can be a secret enemy and a treacherous friend. It influences our behavior before we have the time to consider causes and consequences. Yoga trains the mind and inculcates a sense of discrimination, so that objects and events are seen for what they are and are not allowed to gain mastery over us.

Five mental faculties
We have five mental faculties which can be used in a positive or a negative way. These are: correct observation and knowledge, perception, imagination, dreamless sleep, and memory. Sometimes the mind loses its stability and clarity, and is either incapable of using its various faculties properly, or uses them in a negative way. The practice of yoga leads us to use these mental faculties in a positive way, thereby bringing the mind to a discriminative and attentive state. Awareness, together with discrimination and memory, target bad habits, which are essentially repetitive actions based on mistaken perception. These are then replaced by good habits. In this way, an individual becomes stronger, honest, and gains maturity. He or she is able to perceive and understand people, situations, and events with clarity. This seasoned, mature mind gradually transcends its frontiers to reach beyond mundane observation and experience, making the journey from confusion to clarity, one of the greatest benefits of yoga.

Different states of mind
Yogic science distinguishes between five basic states of mind. These are not grouped in stages, nor are they, except the last, unchangeable. According to Patanjali, these states of mind are: dull and lethargic, distracted, scattered, focused, and controlled. Patanjali described the lowest level of the mind as dull or *mudha*. A person in this stateof mind is disinclined to observe, act, or react. This state is rarely inherent or permanent. It is usually caused by a traumatic experience, for

*"The **seasoned, mature mind transcends frontiers** to reach beyond mundane observation."*

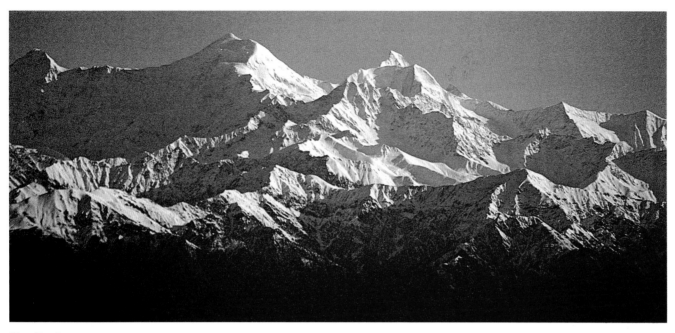

The final stage
The persistent practice of yoga allows you to conquer the lower levels of the mind and reach the peaks of self-realization

instance, bereavement, or when a desired goal presents so many obstacles that the goal seems impossible to attain. After successive failures to take control of their lives, many people withdraw into dullness and lethargy. Often, this is exacerbated by either insomnia or oversleeping, comfort-eating, or the ingestion of tranquilizers and other substances which make the original problem worse. Yoga gradually transforms this feeling of defeat and helplessness into optimism and energy. The distracted state of mind is one where thoughts, feelings, and perceptions churn around in the consciousness, but leave no lasting impressions and hence serve no purpose. Patanjali calls this state, *ksipta*. Someone in a state of *ksipta* is unstable, unable to prioritize or focus on goals, usually because of flawed signals from the senses of perception he or she accepts and follows unthinkingly. This clouds the intellect and disturbs mental equilibrium. Such a state has to be calmed and brought to confront the factual knowledge of reality through the regular practice of yoga asanas and pranayama.

The most common state of mind is the scattered mind. In such a state, though the brain is active, it lacks purpose and direction. This state of mind is known as *viksipta*. Constantly plagued by doubt and fear, it alternates between decisiveness and lack of confidence. The regular practice of yoga gradually encourages the seeds of awareness and discrimination to take root, giving rise to a positive attitude and mental equilibrium.

The ancient sages characterized the focused state of mind, or *ekagra*, as one that indicated a higher state of being. This is a liberated mind which has confronted afflictions and obstacles and conquered them. Such a mind has direction, concentration, and awareness. A person in this category of mental intelligence lives in the present without being caught in the past or future, undisturbed by external circumstances.

The fifth and highest state of mind is *niruddha*, or the controlled, restrained mind. According to Patanjali, *niruddha* is attained through the persistent practice of yoga, which allows an individual to conquer the lower levels of the mind.

At this level, the mind is linked exclusively with the object of its attention. It has the power to become totally absorbed in an activity, allowing nothing to disturb its absorption. When the brain is quiet, the intellect is at peace, the individual is serene and balanced, neither free nor bound, but poised in pure consciousness.

Eight Limbs

The basic tenets of yoga are described in the form of "eight limbs" or "steps" described by the sage, Patanjali. These are aphorisms, explaining the codes of ethical behavior which will ultimately lead to self-realization.

The sage Patanjali reflected on the nature of man and the norms of society during his time. Then, he expressed his observations very systematically in the form of aphorisms, which deal with the entire span of life, beginning with a code of conduct and ending with the ultimate goal, emancipation and freedom. These aphorisms outline the fundamental tenets of yoga, known as the eight limbs or *astanga*.

Astanga yoga

The eight steps are *yama, niyama, asana, pranayama, pratyahara, dharana, dhyana,* and *samadhi.* These are sequential stages in an individual's life journey through yoga. Each step must be understood and followed to attain the ultimate goal of Astanga yoga, that of emancipation of the self. *Yama,* or general ethical principles, and *niyama,* or self-restraint, prescribe a code of conduct that molds individual morality and behavior. Asanas, or yogic poses, and pranayama, or breath control, discipline the body and the mind by basic practices conducive to physical, physiological, psychological, and mental health. Pranayama controls the mind, taming baser instincts, while *pratyahara,* or detachment from the external world, stems the outgoing flow of the senses, withdrawing those of perception and the organs of action from worldly pleasures. *Dharana,* or concentration, guides the consciousness to focus attention rigorously on one point. *Dhyana,* or prolonged concentration, saturates the mind until it permeates to the

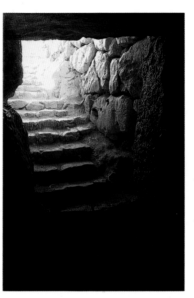

Steps to self-realization
Understand and absorb each stage to reach the ultimate goal

source of existence, and the intellectual and conscious energy dissolves in the seat of the soul. It is then that *samadhi,* when you lose the sense of your separate existence, is attained. Nothing else remains except the core of one's being: the soul.

Yama

Yama and *niyama* require tremendous inner discipline. *Yama* explains the codes of ethical behavior to be observed and followed in everyday life, reminding us of our responsibilities as social beings. *Yama* has five principles. These are: *ahimsa* or nonviolence, *satya* or truthfulness, *asteya* or freedom from avarice, *brahmacharya* or chastity, and *aparigraha* or freedom from desire. *Ahimsa* needs introspection to replace negative, destructive thoughts and actions by positive, constructive ones. Anger, cruelty, or harassment of others are facets of the violence latent in all of us.

These contradict the principles of *ahimsa,* while lying, cheating, dishonesty, and deception break the principles of *satya. Brahmacharya* does not mean total abstinence, but denotes a disciplined sexual life, promoting contentment and moral strength from within. *Parigraha* means "possession" or "covetousness," the instinct within all of us that traps us in the *karmic* cycle of reincarnation after death. However, while you may be able to give up material possessiveness, what about emotional or intellectual possessiveness? This is where Astanga yoga helps to discipline the mind, freeing it from the desire to possess, bringing it into a state of *aparigraha*, freedom from desire, as well as *asteya*, or freedom from greed.

Niyama

Niyama is the positive current that brings discipline, removes inertia, and gives shape to the inner desire to follow the yogic path. The principles of *niyama* are *saucha*, or cleanliness, *santosa*, or contentment, *tapas*, or austerity, *svadhyaya*, or the study of one's own self, which includes the body, mind, intellect, and ego. The final principle of *niyama* is *isvara pranidhana* or devotion to God. Contentment or *santosa* helps to curb desire, anger, ambition, and greed, while *tapas* or austerity involves self-discipline and the desire to purify the body, senses, and mind. The study and practice of yoga with devotional attention to the self and God is *tapas*.

Asanas, pranayama, and pratyahara

According to the *Gheranda Samhita*, a text dating to the 15th century, written by the yogic sage, Gheranda: "The body soon decays like unbaked earthen pots thrown in water. Strengthen and purify the body by baking it in the fire of yoga." Performing an asana helps create and generate energy. Staying in an asana organizes and distributes this energy, while coming out of the pose protects the energy, preventing it from dissipating. In *Yoga Sutra* 111.47, Patanjali explains the effects of an asana as *"Rupa lavanya bala vajra samhananatvani kayasampat."* This means that a perfected body has beauty, grace, and strength which is comparable to the hardness and brilliance of a diamond. While practicing an asana, one must focus attention on the inner body, drawing the mind inward to sharpen the intelligence.

Then, the asana becomes effortless as the blemishes on both the gross and the subtle body are washed off. This is the turning point in the practice of asanas, when the body, mind, and self unite. From this state begins the *isvara pranidhana*, or devotion to God. Asanas and pranayama are interrelated and interwoven. Patanjali clearly specifies that pranayama should be attempted only after the asanas are mastered. *Prana* is "vital energy," which includes will power and ambition, while *ayama* means "stretch, expansion and extension." Pranayama can be described as the "expansion and extension of energy or life-force." Patanjali begins pranayama with the simple movement of breathing, leading us deeper and deeper into ourselves by teaching us to observe the very act of respiration. Pranayama has three movements—prolonged inhalation, deep exhalation, and prolonged, stable retention, all of which have to be performed with precision. Pranayama is the actual process of directing energy inward, making the mind fit for *pratyahara* or the detachment of the senses, which evolves from pranayama. When the senses withdraw from objects of desire, the mind is released from the power of the senses, which in turn become passive. Then the mind turns inward and is set free from the tyranny of the senses. This is *pratyahara*.

Samyama—toward the liberation of the self

Patanjali groups *dharana*, *dhyana*, and *samadhi* under the term *samyama*—the integration of the body, breath, mind, intellect, and self. It is not easy to explain the last three aspects of yoga as separate entities. The controlled mind that is gained in *pratyahara* is made to intensify its attention on a single thought in *dharana*. When this concentration is prolonged, it becomes *dhyana*. In *dhyana*, release, expansion, quietness, and peace are experienced. This prolonged state of quietness frees a person from attachment, resulting in indifference to the joys of pleasure or the sorrows of pain. The experience of *samadhi* is achieved when the knower, the knowable, and the known become one. When the object of meditation engulfs the meditator and becomes the subject, self-awareness is lost. This is *samadhi*—a state of total absorption. *Sama* means "level" or "alike," while *adhi* means "over" and "above." It also denotes the maintenance of the intelligence in a balanced state. Though *samadhi* can be explained at the intellectual level, it can only be experienced at the level of the heart. Ultimately, it is *samadhi* that is the fruit of the discipline of Astanga yoga.

Pranayama

Prana is the life-force which permeates both the individual as well as the universe at all levels. It is at once physical, sexual, mental, intellectual, spiritual, and cosmic. *Prana,* the breath, and the mind are inextricably linked to each other.

The ancient yogis advocated the practice of pranayama to unite the breath with the mind, and thus with the *prana* or life-force. *Prana* is energy, and *ayama* is the storing and distribution of that energy. *Ayama* has three aspects or movements: vertical extension, horizontal extension, and cyclical extension. By practicing pranayama, we learn to move energy vertically, horizontally, and cyclically to the frontiers of the body.

Breath in pranayama

Pranayama is not deep breathing. Deep breathing tenses the facial muscles, makes the skull and scalp rigid, tightens the chest, and applies external force to the intake or release of breath. This creates hardness in the fibers of the lungs and chest, preventing the percolation of breath through the body.

In pranayama, the cells of the brain and the facial muscles remain soft and receptive, and the breath is drawn in or released gently. During inhalation, each molecule, fiber, and cell of the body is independently felt by the mind, and is allowed to receive and absorb the *prana*. There are no sudden movements and one becomes aware of the gradual expansion of the respiratory organs, and feels the breath reaching the most remote parts of the lungs.

In exhalation, the release of breath is gradual, and this gives the air cells sufficient time to re-absorb the residual *prana* to the maximum possible extent. This allows for the full utilization of energy, thus building up emotional stability and calming the mind.

The practice of asanas removes the obstructions which impede the flow of *prana*. During pranayama, one should be totally absorbed in the fineness of inhalation, exhalation, and in the naturalness of retention. One should not disturb or jerk the vital organs and nerves, or stress the brain cells. The brain is the instrument which observes the smooth flow of inhalation and exhalation. One must be aware of the interruptions which occur during a single inhalation and exhalation. Check these, and a smooth flow will set in. Similarly, during retention of breath, learn to retain the first indrawn breath with stability. If this stability is lost, it is better to release the breath, rather than strain to hold it. While inhaling or retaining the breath in a pranayamic cycle, remember to ensure that the abdomen does not swell.

The final goal

Attempt pranayama only when the yoga asanas have been mastered. Patanjali reiterates this several times,

Yogacharya Iyengar in pranayama
Practicing pranayama in Padmasana, the cross-legged Lotus pose, works well for meditation

most emphatically in *Yoga Sutra* 11.49. The next sutra, *Yoga Sutra* 11.50, explains that inhalation, exhalation, and retention must be precise. The sutra begins with control over the movement of exhalation, or *bahya*, and inhalation, or *abhyantara*. Each inhalation activates the central nervous system into stimulating the peripheral nerves, and each exhalation triggers the reverse process. During the retention of breath, both processes take place. The *Hathayoga Pradipika* speaks of *antara-kumbhaka* and *bahya-kumbhaka*, or the suspension of breath with full or empty lungs, as well as inhalation, and exhalation. Pranayama is a complex process composed of all these. It has to be practiced with the greatest sincerity and precision. You cannot achieve pranayama just because you want to—you have to be ready for it.

In pranayamic breathing, the brain is quiet, and this allows the nervous system to function more effectively. Inhalation is the art of receiving primeval energy into the body in the form of breath, and bringing the spiritual cosmic breath into contact with the individual breath. Exhalation is the removal of toxins from the system.

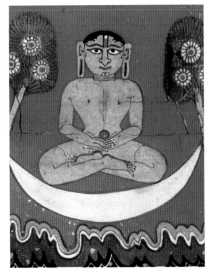

A yogi in pranayama
For more than a thousand years, sages have practiced pranayama, controlling their breath and with it, their mind

Between the material and spiritual world

Pranayama is also the link between the physiological and spiritual organisms of man. At first, pranayama is difficult and requires great effort. Mastery is achieved when pranayama becomes effortless. Just as the diaphragm is the meeting point of the physiological and spiritual body, the retention of energy or *kumbhaka* is realizing the very core of your body. Once the external movements are controlled, there is internal silence. In such a silence there is no thought as the mind has then dissolved in the self.

In the *Hathayoga Pradipika*, the sage Svatmarama gives a detailed description of the ways in which an individual comes to experience the elevated state of oneness with the self through the practice of pranayama. Hence, practicing it is not only very difficult, but also highly absorbing. If you fail after a few cycles, be content with the knowledge that you have practiced three or four cycles with awareness and attention. Do not turn away from failures, but try to accept them and learn from them. Gradually, you will be successful in your attempts and will learn to master pranayama.

Ancient traditions
An illustrated folio from the *Kalpasutra*, 15th-century texts describing the path to health and spirituality

Chakras

Yogic science recognizes that spiritual health is activated by a system of chakras or "nerve" centers, said to be located within the spinal column. Cosmic energy lies coiled within these chakras and has to be awakened for self-realization.

Modern technology has provided us with the means to examine the state of our bodies. But nothing has helped us discern character, personality, or the potential for goodness. The most important aspect of a human being is the part which lies between the outer skin and the innermost soul—the *shakti*, which includes the mind,

intellect, emotions, vital energy, the sense of "I," the powers of will and discrimination, and the conscience. These are different in every human being, and that makes us individually both mysterious and unique. In yogic terminology, the soul is called *purusha shakti*, while *prakriti shakti* or the energy of nature, came to be called *kundalini*

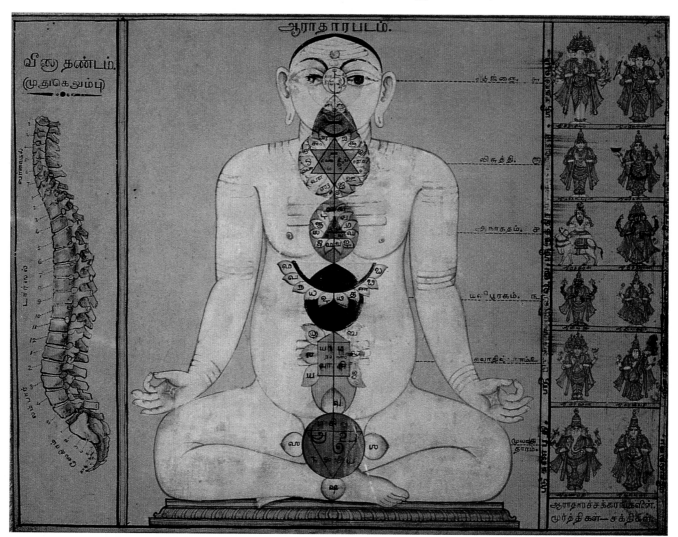

The 7 main chakras of the body Yogic sages believed chakras were located along the spinal column by the ancient yogis. *Kundalini* is the divine, cosmic energy which exists as a latent force in everyone. When the *prakriti shakti* is awakened, it gravitates toward the very core of the soul or *purusha shakti*.

Awakening cosmic energy

This fire of divine, cosmic energy is ignited by *yoga-agni*, the fire of yoga. When a fire is covered with ashes, it goes out. In the same way, if our senses are inert, or if we are motivated by pride, self-indulgence, and envy, the *kundalini* is kept in a dormant state. If we allow such negative qualities to dominate our thinking over long periods, our spiritual evolution is not merely hampered, but actually halted.

We have always known that health is important, but it is time to realize, as proponents of yoga have known for generations, that our physical condition is inextricably linked to our state of mind.

Yogic science recognized this connection from the very beginning. In order to achieve perfect physical health, the ancient sages concluded, you must activate the body's *chakras*. *Chakras* are notionally located along the spine, from the brain to the tailbone. But while the spine is a physical entity, *chakras* are not composed of matter. Although they possess no physicality, they govern all the elements of the body.

The meaning of chakras

Chakra means "wheel" or "ring" in Sanskrit and our personal *chakras* have energy coiled within them. They are the critical junctions which determine the state of the body and mind. Just as the brain controls physical, mental, and intellectual functions through the nerve cells or neurons, *chakras* tap the *prana* or cosmic energy which is within all living beings and transform it into spiritual energy. This is spread through the body by the *nadis*, or channels.

Being invisible, *chakras* are tangible only through their effects. They can be accessed once the student of yoga has achieved all the eight aspects of yoga (*see page* 52), when the human self merges with the divine self.

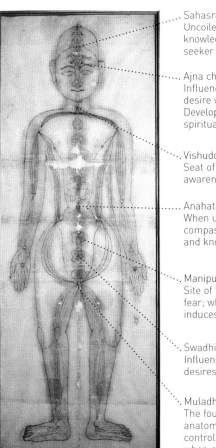

Chakras and nadis of the human body
A 19th-century painting from Rajasthan, India.
Chakras transform cosmic energy into spiritual energy.

Sahasrara chakra
Uncoiled through intuitive knowledge, it allows the seeker to achieve freedom

Ajna chakra
Influences pride and desire when coiled. Develops humanity and spirituality when uncoiled

Vishuddhi chakra
Seat of intellectual awareness

Anahata chakra
When uncoiled, it develops compassion, spirituality, and knowledge

Manipuraka chakra
Site of the sense of fear; when uncoiled, induces calm

Swadhishtana chakra
Influences worldly desires when coiled

Muladhara chakra
The foundation of the anatomical sheath controls sexual energy when coiled

There are 11 *chakras* of which seven are crucial (*see diagram above*), and the others dependent. The most important is the Sahasrara *chakra*, where *prakriti shakti* or energy, unites with *purusha shakti*, or soul.

The practice of yoga is directed at awakening the divine energy within every human being. Asanas and pranayama uncoil and alert the *chakras*. In the process, the *nadis* are activated. This causes the *chakras* to vibrate and to generate energy, which is then circulated all over the body through the *nadis*. The emotions rooted in the *chakras* are transformed as divine energy is awakened and circulated.

To achieve self-realization the sincere student of yoga will, with persistent, rigorous practice, conquer the six main obstacles to happiness— desire, anger, greed, infatuation, pride, and envy.

The Guru and the Yogi

The tradition of the guru, or master, and the yogi, or disciple, is an ancient one. All learning from generation to generation has been handed down this way. The guru must be compassionate, yet exacting. The yogi must be sincere and dedicated.

How do we distinguish between the true guru and the false one? The cult of the guru, or master, is an Asian concept. To other societies, the concept might seem exotic, mysterious, or even abhorrent—a brake on individual freedom or judgment. Some thinkers have declared that a guru is not needed at all, while others believe that you cannot reach your goal without one. Perhaps the importance of the guru can be explained by examining its Sanskrit root. *Gu* means "darkness" and *ru* means "light"— therefore, a guru is one who leads you from darkness to light. Although the *sadhaka* or seeker has to tread the spiritual path to self-realization alone, the guru's guidance is essential to show the right path and to safeguard the yogi, the student of yoga, who decides to follow it.

An ancient tradition

The guru is the voice of consciousness during the process of spiritual awakening. In India, the relationship between a guru and a disciple is an ancient tradition, and has been the foundation of all learning. The *guru-sishya parampara* (*sishya* means "disciple" and *parampara* means "tradition") has been the system through which knowledge has been handed down, generation to generation and age to age. The energy that the guru has imbibed from *his* teacher is passed on to his disciple, keeping the process of communication alive from one epoch to the next. The guru opens the disciple's eyes to awareness. Knowledge exists, but ignorance veils it, and it is the guru who removes this veil from the intellect of the *sishya*.

The guru is the guide who opens the gate of the student's dormant faculties and awakens the latent power and energy within. Being with the guru is like being in the sunlight, and the glow lasts for eternity.

The relationship between the teacher and the disciple is a unique one. It is similar, but not identical, to a mother and child. Just as a mother loves, nourishes, guides, cajoles into obedience, rebukes, educates, and protects her child, the

Yogacharya Iyengar with a student
The guru does not only teach asanas, he teaches you how to live

guru takes the disciple into his care, making it his life's work to mold his student into perfect shape, physically, mentally, and spiritually.

The guru

Yoga is a discipline and the yogic texts aptly begin with the emphasis on discipline or *anusasanam*: "Without discipline, nothing can be achieved." The guru does not enforce discipline with strictness, but builds up an awareness of it in his student, allowing the latter to develop inner discipline. A wise guru does not lay down codes of conduct, but motivates the disciple by precept and example.

The guru does not demand attention, he commands it. In the process of teaching, he creates total confidence in the disciple, and helps him or her develop the will power to face all circumstances with equanimity. The guru constantly improves on his teaching techniques, opening the disciple's eyes, improvising where necessary to create new dimensions in his teaching. The guru is compassionate, but does not expect emotional attachment from his disciple, nor does he become emotionally attached himself.

The guru should be confident, challenging, caring, cautious, constructive, and courageous. The clarity and creativity of his teaching should reflect his devotion and dedication to his subject—in this case, the complexities and subtleties of yoga.

The disciple

An ideal disciple is obedient, earnest, serious, and always ready to follow the teachings of his or her guru. This is not unthinking obedience, but one based on respect and a sincere desire to learn. Disciples can be dull, average, or superior. The dull student has little enthusiasm, is unstable, timorous, and self-indulgent. He or she is unwilling to put in the hard work required which is needed to attain the goal of self-realization.

The average student is indecisive, attracted equally to worldly pleasures as to spiritual matters. While conscious of the highest good, this student

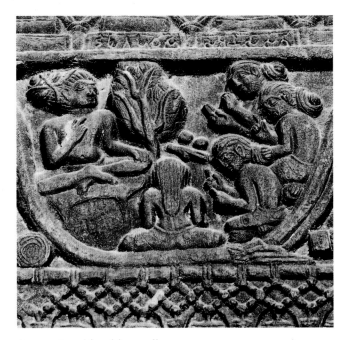

A sage teaching his pupils
This 2nd-century BC frieze from Bharhut, India, points to the antiquity of the guru-yogi tradition

lacks the determination to persevere, and is unable to hold on steadfastly to the yogic path. He or she needs firmness and discipline from his or her guru, a fact the guru recognizes at once.

The superior or intense student, on the other hand, has vision, enthusiasm, and courage. He or she resists temptations and does not hesitate to cast off qualities that distract him or her from the goal. This student becomes steady, stable, and skillful. The guru guides this kind of student to the ultimate goal of self-realization.

While practicing yoga, the disciple must recall and deliberate on each word and action of the guru and consolidate each learning experience. Today's disciple may become the guru of tomorrow. Clarity of mind and firmness of resolve to tread the path to self-realization is essential. The yogi must have *riti* and *niti*—method and morality—to impart to the disciple, the learning, the experience, and wisdom gleaned over the years. Thus, the tradition of the guru and the yogi is carried on for yet another generation.

This book is my attempt to disseminate my knowledge of yoga to all those across the world who wish to become true followers of yoga.

CHAPTER 4

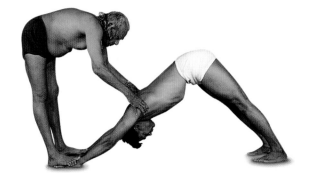

ASANAS FOR YOU

*"The **body** is your **temple**. Keep it **pure** and **clean** for the **soul** to reside in."*

The science of yoga is like the art of music. There is a rhythm within the body, and that can only be maintained by paying attention to each step of the asana, and to the progression between asanas. In your practice of yoga, there has to be a physical, physiological, psychological, and spiritual rhythm. Unless there is harmony and melody, the music will not be worth listening to. The body is a truly sensitive and receptive instrument, and its vibrations, like sound, express the harmony or dissonance within it. Each of these vibrations must synchronize in the movement, which is the asana.

Classic Poses

Yoga asanas cover the basic positions of standing, sitting, forward bends, twists, inversions, back bends, and lying down. The 23 classic poses must be practiced with physical coordination, as well as intelligence and sincerity.

There is more to practicing asanas correctly than merely the physical aligning of the body. The classic poses, when practiced with discrimination and awareness, bring the body, mind, intelligence, nerves, consciousness, and the self together into a single, harmonious whole. Asanas may appear to deal with the physical body alone but, in fact, different asanas can affect the chemical messages sent to and from the brain, improving and stabilizing your mental state. Yoga's unique ability to soothe the nerves—the medium between the physiological body and the psychological body —calms the brain, makes the mind fresh and tranquil, and relaxes the entire body.

I have selected these 23 asanas because they cover all the basic positions of yoga: standing, sitting, forward bends, twists, inversions, back bends, and lying down. The regular practice of these asanas, stimulates and activates all the organs, tissues, and cells of the body. The mind becomes alert and strong, the body healthy and active.

The anatomical body comprises the limbs and the actual parts of the body. The physical body is made up of bones, muscles, skin, and tissue. The physiological body is composed of the heart, lungs, liver, spleen, pancreas, intestines, and the other organs. The nerves, brain, and intellect make up the psychological body. To practice asanas correctly, you have to learn to bring all these levels together.

Stages of learning yoga

Newcomers to yoga approach asanas with "uncultured" minds. They have to learn that at first asanas are practiced at the level of the anatomical body alone—the stage called *arambhavastha*. This beginner's stage is important and should not be hurried through. In order to learn the asanas, beginners should be primarily concerned with getting their movements right. In the step-by-step instructions to the asanas in this chapter, I have highlighted the points you should concentrate on, the important motions and movements in the pose you need to take note of. Beginners have to grasp the whole asana, and not lose themselves in the finer details. It is more important for you to start by striving for stability within a pose. This provides a strong foundation. You will then enter the intermediate stage, or *ghatavastha*, in which the mind is affected by changes in the body. When you reach this stage, you are practicing the movements correctly, your body is under your control, but you must now push your mind to touch every part of your body. In my instructions to the asanas in this chapter, I have pointed out that students of yoga at this stage must

Integrating body and spirit
Yogacharya Iyengar in Adhomukha Svanasana

"*Asanas* keep your **body,** as well as your **mind, healthy and active**."

practice the asanas with reflective and meditative attention. You must become aware of your tissues, organs, skin, and even individual cells. Your mind must flow along with all of these parts.

Parichayavastha, or the advanced stage, comes next. This is the stage of intimate knowledge, when your mind brings your body in touch with your intelligence. Once this happens, the mind ceases to be a separate entity, and the intelligence and the body become one. I have included the concepts that the advanced practitioner of yoga should focus on. Your adjustments are more subtle and discriminating now, and are in the realm of the mental and physiological body, rather than merely in your muscles, bones, and joints. The final stage, *nishpattyavastha*, is the state of perfection. Once the intelligence feels the oneness between the flesh and the skin, it introduces the *atman*—the self or soul. This frees the body and integrates it with the soul in the journey from the finite to the infinite. Then the body, mind, and self become one. At this stage, asanas become meditative and spiritual. This may be termed "dynamic meditation."

What is an asana?

An asana is not a posture that you assume mechanically. It involves a thoughtful process at the end of which a balance is achieved between movement and resistance. Your weight has to be evenly distributed over muscles, bones, and joints, just as your intelligence must be engaged at every level. You have to create space in your muscles and

your skin, fitting the fine network of your entire body into the asana. This helps the organs of perception (the eyes, ears, nose, tongue, and skin) to discern the subtlety of each movement. This conjunction between the organs of action and organs of perception occurs when the student reaches a subjective understanding of an asana, and begins, through instinct as well as knowledge, to adjust his or her movements correctly. Practice with dedication. Be completely absorbed by the asana.

Once both sides of the body become symmetrical, undue stress is removed from the circulatory, respiratory, digestive, reproductive, and excretory systems. In each asana, different organs are placed in different anatomical positions, and are squeezed and spread, dampened and dried, heated and cooled. The organs are supplied with fresh blood, and are gently massaged, relaxed, and toned into a state of optimum health.

Movement and resistance
The final pose of Utthita Parsvakonasana

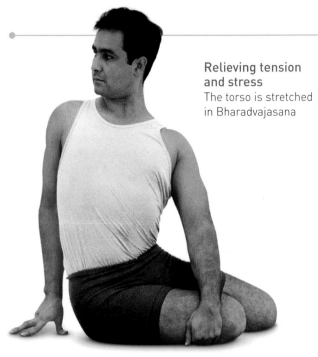

Relieving tension and stress
The torso is stretched in Bharadvajasana

Sitting asanas

All sitting asanas bring elasticity to the hips, knees, ankles, and muscles of the groin. These poses remove tension and hardness in the diaphragm and throat, making breathing smoother and easier. They keep the spine steady, pacifying the mind and stretching the muscles of the heart. Blood circulation increases to all parts of the body.

Standing asanas

Standing asanas strengthen the leg muscles and joints, and increase the suppleness and strength of the spine. Because of their rotational and flexing movements, the spinal muscles and intervertebral joints are kept mobile and well-aligned. The arteries of the legs are stretched, increasing the blood supply to the lower limbs, and preventing thrombosis in the calf muscles. These asanas also tone the cardiovascular system. The lateral wall of the heart is fully stretched, increasing the supply of fresh blood to the heart.

Forward bends

In forward bends, the abdominal organs are compressed. This has a unique effect on the nervous system: as these organs relax, the frontal brain is cooled, and the flow of blood to the entire brain is regulated. The sympathetic nervous system is rested, bringing down the pulse rate and blood pressure. Stress is removed from the organs of perception and the senses relax. The adrenal glands are also soothed and function more efficiently. Because the body is in a horizontal position in forward bends, the heart is relieved of the strain of pumping blood against gravity, and blood circulates through all parts of the body easily. Forward bends also strengthen the paraspinal muscles, intervertebral joints, and ligaments.

Twists

These asanas teach us the importance of a healthy spine and inner body. In twists, the pelvic and abdominal organs are squeezed and flushed with blood. They improve the suppleness of the diaphragm, and relieve spinal, hip, and groin disorders. The spine also becomes more supple, and this improves the flow of blood to the spinal nerves and increases energy levels.

Inversions

Some people fear that if they practice inverted poses, their blood pressure will rise, or their blood vessels will burst. These are complete misconceptions. After all, standing for long periods can lead to thrombosis and varicose veins, but no one is going to stop standing up! Standing upright is a result of evolution. Just as the human body has adjusted to an upright position, it can also learn to perform inversions without any risk or harm. In contrast to the twisting asanas, inverted asanas have a drying effect on the pelvic and abdominal organs, while vital organs like the brain, heart, and lungs are flushed with blood. According to the third chapter of the sage Svatmarama's *Hathayoga Pradipika*, Salamba

Stretching out
Paschimottanasana extends the spine

Sirsasana (headstand, *see page* 138) is the king of asanas, and Salamba Sarvangasana (shoulderstand, *see page* 144) the queen of asanas. The health of your body and mind is greatly enhanced by the practice of these two asanas.

Back bends

All back bends stimulate the central nervous system and increase its ability to bear stress. They help relieve one from stress, tension, and nervous exhaustion. These asanas stimulate and energize the body, and are invaluable to people suffering from depression. In Urdhva Dhanurasana (*see page* 160) and Viparita Dandasana (*see page* 238), the liver and spleen are fully stretched, and can therefore function more effectively.

Reclining asanas

Reclining asanas are restful poses which soothe the body and refresh the mind. While reclining asanas are often sequenced at the end of a yoga session, they are also preparatory asanas, since they help relax the body and strengthen the joints. They give the body the required energy for the more strenuous asanas. Savasana (*see page* 150), for instance, helps recover the breath and cool the body and the mind. Reclining asanas prepare you for pranayama.

Practicing classic poses

Read the instructions for practice (*see page* 408). Practice classic poses when you feel confident of the suppleness of your body and the stability of your mind. In the 20-Week Yoga Course (*see page* 410), I recommend that beginners and those with stiff muscles or joints, or people with specific ailments, might prefer to practice with props for the first six–eight months. If you normally practice classic poses without props, you may, however, wish to use them on days when you are feeling tired, or if a particular part of your body feels stiff. Always sequence your asanas with care. Beginners should follow the order given in the 20-Week Yoga Course. Whenever you practice, take care not to "harden" your brain. This occurs when you hold your breath, and your head becomes tense and heavy, particularly common when practicing standing asanas and forward bends. This can also happen in a standing asana when you use force to descend without fully extending your spine. Since the action is achieved by force, rather than by utilizing the intelligence of the spine, this results in tension in the spine. I call this situation "hardening the brain" because it means you are not allowing your brain to be sufficiently sensitive to your body's actions. Similarly, in back bends, if force, not intelligence is applied while extending the back, the cervical region remains hard. This, too, "hardens the brain."

"Brain" of the pose

In each asana, a specific part of your body is the "brain" of the pose. For instance, the outstretched arm is the "brain" of Utthita Parsvakonasana (*see page* 80), the center of balance in the pose. When you practice, observe this specific part of your body carefully and focus on it. Bring a firmness and steadiness to it. This will then spread to the rest of your body and bring it under your control. Gradually, you will be able to experience the pose at the physiological, and not merely the physical level.

Practice without fear
Inversions, like Salamba Sarvangasana, are good for your body and mind

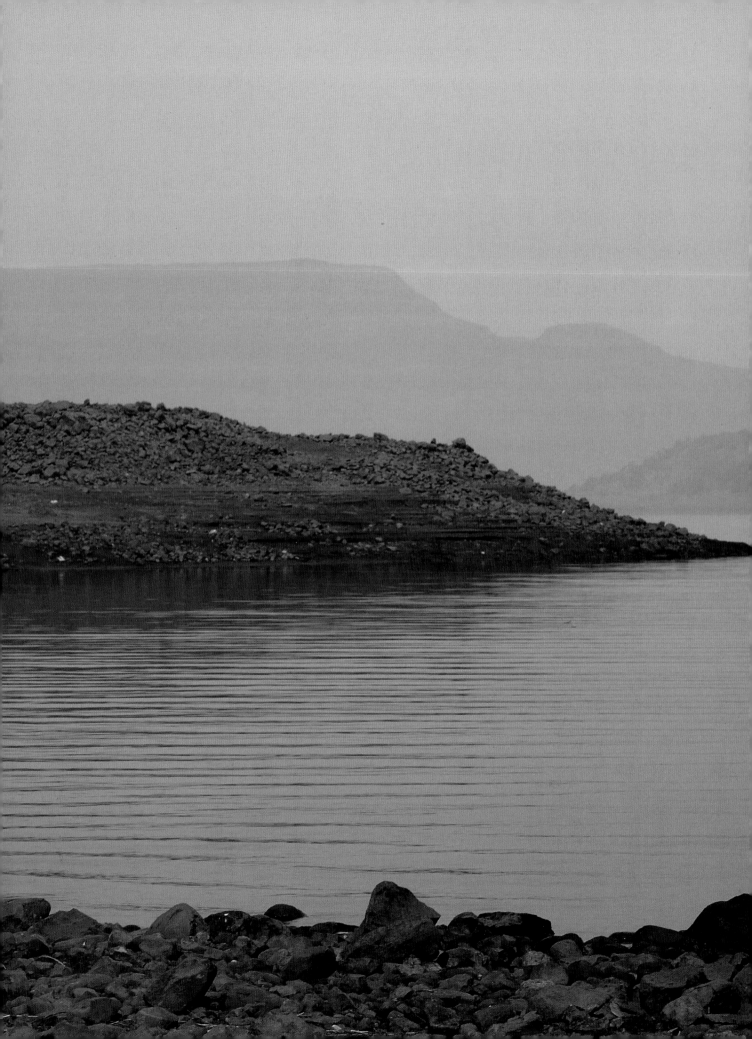

STANDING ASANAS

*"An **asana** is not a posture which you assume **mechanically**. It involves **thought**, at the end of which a **balance** is achieved between **movement** and **resistance**."*

TADASANA
Mountain posture

In this posture you learn to stand as firm and erect as a mountain. The word *tada* in Sanskrit means "mountain." Most people do not balance perfectly on both legs, leading to ailments which can be avoided. Tadasana teaches you the art of standing correctly and increases your awareness of your body.

● BENEFITS

Corrects bad posture by straightening the spine
Improves the alignment of your body
Counters the degenerative effects of aging on the spine, legs, and feet
Tones the buttock muscles

● CAUTIONS

If you have Parkinson's disease or a spinal disk disorder, you may find it helpful to stand facing a wall with your palms placed on it. People with scoliosis should rest the spine against the protruding edge of two adjoining walls.

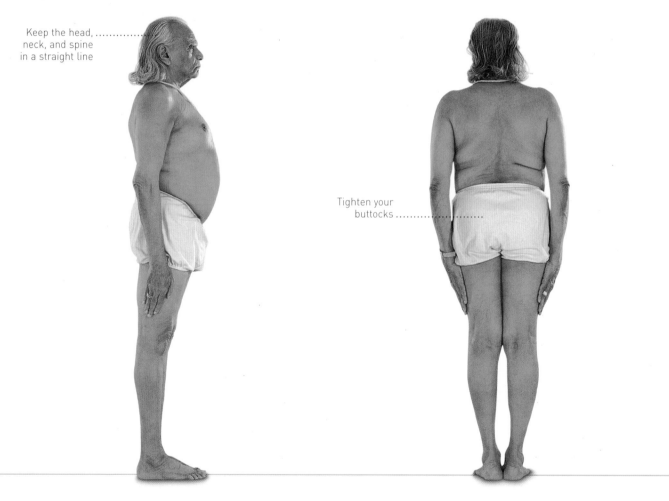

Keep the head, neck, and spine in a straight line

Tighten your buttocks

1 Stand with your feet together on a smooth, uncovered floor. Make sure that your feet are in line with each other, with both the big toes and heels touching. If you find it difficult to keep your feet together, separate them by about 2-3 in (7 cm). Rest your weight on the centers of the arches of the feet. Keep the heels firm and toes extended. Stretch out your toes and keep them relaxed.

2 Press your feet firmly down on the floor and stretch both your legs upward. Keep both ankles in line with each other. Your legs should be perpendicular to the floor and aligned to each other. Tighten your kneecaps and quadriceps and pull them upward. Draw your hips inward by compressing them as well as your buttocks.

"Tadasana is the foundation stone for other asanas. Practicing it gives rise to a sense of firmness, strength, stillness, and steadiness."

Keep your head upright and look straight ahead

Do not lift your shoulders

Raise your sternum

Keep your arms close to your sides

3 Extend your arms along the sides of your body, with your palms facing your thighs and fingers pointing down. Keep the head and spine in a straight line. Stretch your neck without tensing the muscles. Pull your lower abdomen in and up. Lift your sternum and broaden your chest. Breathe normally during all the steps of the asana.

Keep your fingers together

4 Press your heels, as well as the mounds of your toes down on the floor. This will place equal pressure on the outer and inner edges of the feet. Guard against balancing on the front of the feet. Now, consciously rest most of your weight on your heels. Hold the pose for 20-30 seconds.

Stretch your toes from the base to the tips

UTTHITA TRIKONASANA
Extended triangle pose

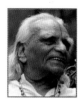

In this asana, your body takes the shape of an extended triangle, giving an intense stretch to your trunk and legs. *Utthita* means "extended" in Sanskrit, *tri* means "three," and *kona* indicates an angle. With practice, you will learn to move from your physical body into your physiological body (*see page* 62).You will learn to activate the organs, glands, and nerves—which form the physiological body—by controlling the movements of your limbs. This pose tones the ligaments and improves flexibility.

● BENEFITS

Relieves gastritis, indigestion, acidity, and flatulence
Improves the flexibility of the spine
Alleviates backache
Corrects alignment of the shoulders
Helps treat neck sprains
Massages and tones the pelvic area
Strengthens the ankles
Reduces discomfort during menstruation

● CAUTIONS

If you are prone to dizzy spells, vertigo, or high blood pressure, look down at the floor in the final pose. Do not turn your head up. If you have a cardiac condition, practice against a wall. Do not raise the arm, but rest it along your hip.

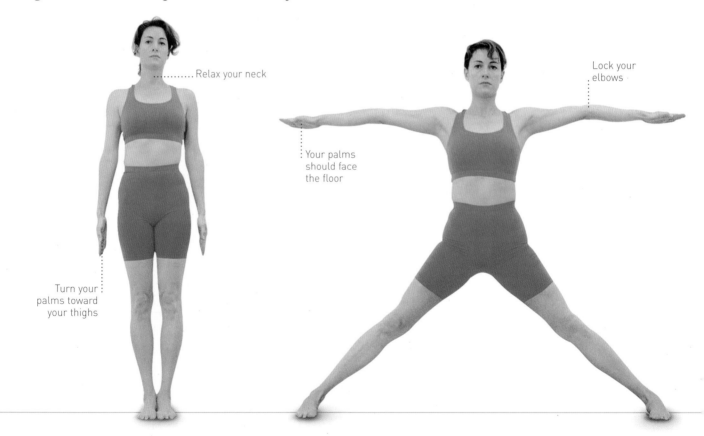

........Relax your neck

Turn your palms toward your thighs

Lock your elbows

Your palms should face the floor

1 Stand in Tadasana (*see page* 68). Distribute your weight equally on both legs. Rest on the center of your arches. Keep the heels firm and the toes extended. Make sure that the inner sides of both feet touch each other. Keep your back straight. Breathe evenly.

2 Inhale deeply and jump, landing with your feet approximately 4ft (1.2m) apart. Your feet should be in line, pointing forward. Raise your arms to shoulder-level (*see inset*), making sure that they are in line with each other. Stretch your arms from the back of your elbows. Lift your chest and look straight ahead.

3 Turn your right foot in slightly to the left, maintaining the stretch of your other leg. Then, turn your left foot 90° to the left, keeping the right leg stretched and tightened at the knee. Make sure that your arms do not waver. Keep them fully stretched.

BEGINNERS To maintain your balance during this step, always keep to the sequence of turning in your right foot first. Once you have done this, turn your left foot out.

INTERMEDIATES For a better stretch in the final pose, press your left heel down on the floor and raise your toes toward the ceiling (*see inset*). Then

tighten the left knee and flatten your foot on the floor again.

CORRECTING YOURSELF

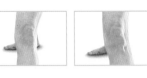

THE RIGHT KNEE

WRONG If your right knee rotates to the right, this will impair your stretch in the final pose.

RIGHT Keep your right kneecap facing front. Make sure that your right thigh does not turn inward.

THE LEFT KNEE

WRONG If the left knee rotates too far to the left, your balance in the final pose will be affected.

RIGHT Keep your left knee tightened, and in line with the center of your left foot, shin, and thigh.

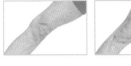

Stretch your shoulders away from your torso

Do not allow your fingers to go up, down, or sideways

Keep your chest lifted

Rotate the muscles of the inner thigh outward

Maintain the stretch of your left leg

UTTHITA TRIKONASANA

THE GURU'S ADVICE

"Look at how I am moving my student's left buttock in with my knee. To help rotate her torso, I grip her right shoulder and slowly revolve her torso upward. Once you are in this position, move your left floating rib forward and extend the length of the right side of your torso toward the right armpit."

CORRECTING YOURSELF

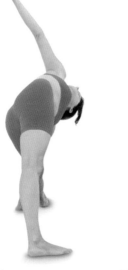

WRONG If your right arm tilts back, you will lose the correct alignment of the hips and buttocks. Your neck and head will jut forward and your weight will fall on your left palm, and not on your left heel.

RIGHT The right arm is stretched straight upward from the armpit and kept steady. Keep the back of your head aligned to your spine, and keep your shoulder blades in line with each other.

Keep your kneecap facing front .

Make sure your right leg is fully stretched ....

4 Exhale, and bend your torso sideways to the left. Place your left palm flat on the floor, and press your left heel down on the floor. Adjust your pose until your weight rests on your left heel and not on your left palm. Raise your right arm up toward the ceiling, in line with your shoulders and left arm. Turn your head, keeping your neck passive, and fix your eyes on your right thumb. Stay in the pose for 20-30 seconds. Do not take deep breaths, but breathe evenly.

BEGINNERS When you bend, first grip your left ankle with your left hand. Bring the left buttock forward slightly. Place your right hand on your right hip. Once you feel steady in this pose, follow the instructions above.

Keep your right palm open and fully stretched

Look at your right thumb

Keep your left shoulder straight

Do not let the left thigh turn inward

Press the inner edge of your left heel down on the floor

UTTHITA TRIKONASANA

ADVANCED WORK IN THE POSE 360° VIEW

Keep your right arm steady, since it is the "brain" of the pose (*see page* 65). Work on your back. Imagine your body is being pulled in opposite directions from the spine. Check that both shoulders are equally stretched out. Make sure that your torso revolves slightly upward and back. Keep the back of your neck in line with your spine—but relax your throat, keeping the muscles of your neck passive. Make sure that your tailbone and the back of your head align with each other, and that your whole body is balanced symmetrically in one plane.

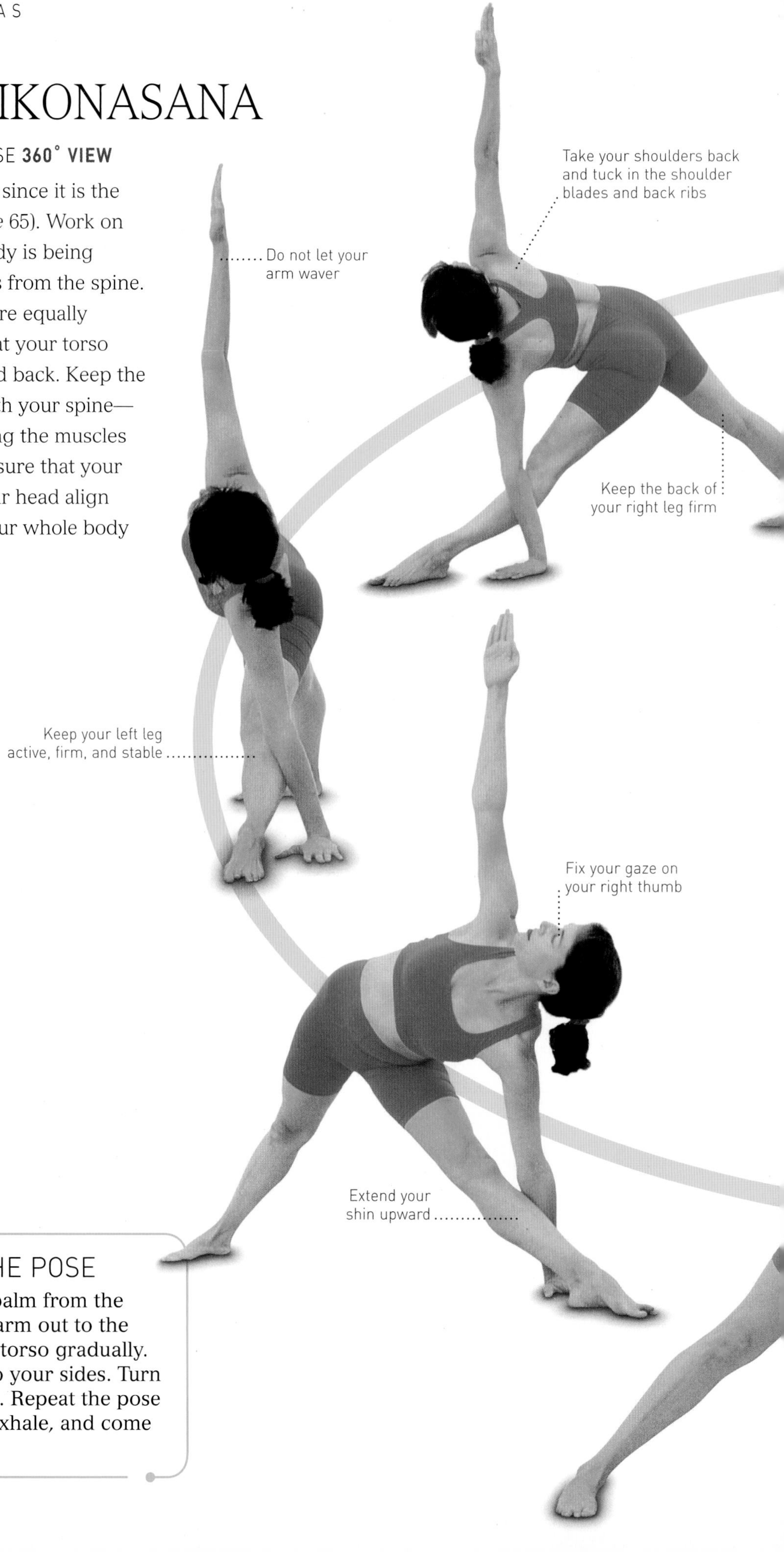

Do not let your arm waver

Take your shoulders back and tuck in the shoulder blades and back ribs

Keep the back of your right leg firm

Keep your left leg active, firm, and stable

Fix your gaze on your right thumb

Extend your shin upward

COMING OUT OF THE POSE

Inhale, and lift your left palm from the floor. Stretch your right arm out to the side and straighten your torso gradually. Bring your arms down to your sides. Turn your feet to face forward. Repeat the pose on the other side. Then exhale, and come back to Tadasana.

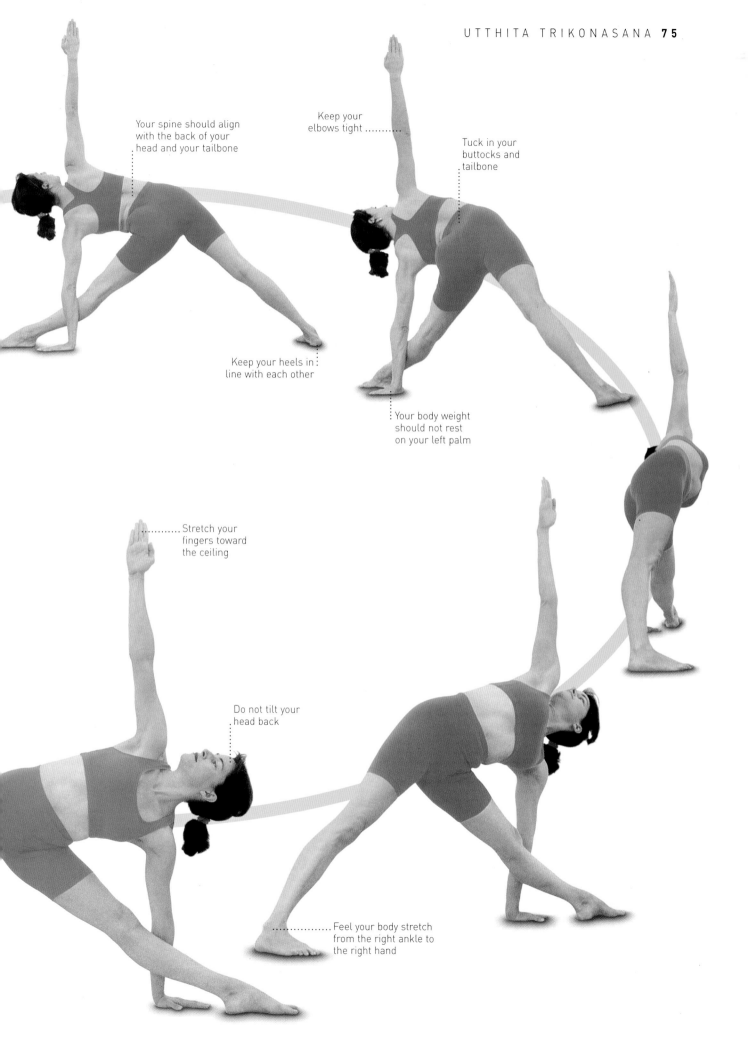

Your spine should align with the back of your head and your tailbone

Keep your elbows tight

Tuck in your buttocks and tailbone

Keep your heels in line with each other

Your body weight should not rest on your left palm

Stretch your fingers toward the ceiling

Do not tilt your head back

Feel your body stretch from the right ankle to the right hand

VIRABHADRASANA 2
Warrior pose 2

This pose is named after Virabhadra, a legendary warrior. His story is told by the famous Sanskrit playwright, Kalidasa, in the epic, *Kumarasambhava*. The steps exercise your limbs and torso vigorously, reducing stiffness in your neck and shoulders. It also makes your knee and hip joints more flexible.

● BENEFITS

Improves breathing capacity by expanding the chest
Helps in the treatment of a prolapsed or slipped disk
Alleviates the condition of a broken, fused, or deviated tailbone
Reduces fat around the hips
Relieves lower backache

● CAUTIONS

Do not practice if you have a cardiac condition, palpitations, heartburn, diarrhea, or dysentery. Women with menorrhagia and metrorrhagia should avoid this asana.

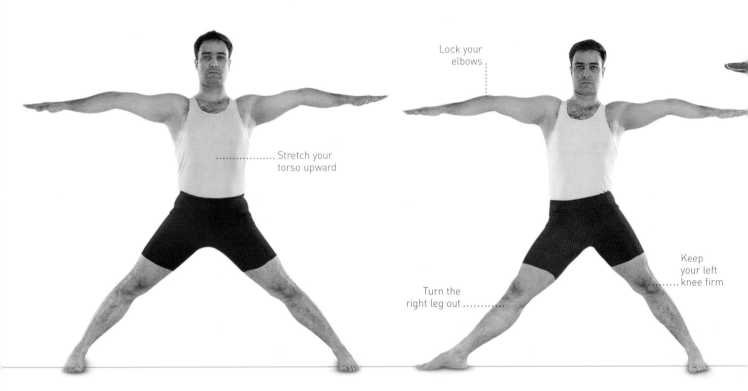

Stretch your torso upward

Lock your elbows

Turn the right leg out

Keep your left knee firm

1 Stand in Tadasana (*see page* 68) and inhale deeply. Jump, landing with your feet approximately 4ft (1.2m) apart. Your toes should point forward. Raise your arms out to the sides, in line with your shoulders (*see inset*). Your palms should face the floor and be in line with each other. Keep your fingers straight and stretched out. Press the little toe of each foot down on the floor. Consciously pull the inner sides of your legs up toward your waist.

2 Exhale slowly, and turn your right leg 90° to the right. Turn in your left foot slightly to the right. Make sure that your body weight is resting on your right heel and not on your toes. Keep your left leg stretched out and taut at the knee. To prevent this leg from slipping, make sure that your weight falls on the last two toes.

BEGINNERS Focus on turning the right thigh out correctly. The thigh should turn at the same time—and to the same extent—as your right foot.

3 Exhale, and bend your right knee. Make sure that your right thigh is parallel to the floor. Keep the shin perpendicular to the floor, in line with your right heel. Pull the muscles of your right calf upward. Turn your head to the right. Stretch the arches and toes of both feet. Hold the pose for 30 seconds. Breathe evenly.

INTERMEDIATES Bend your right knee from the buttock bone and consciously push the flesh and skin of the thigh toward the knee. Stretch your arms out fully. Imagine they are being pulled apart in a tug-of-war.

CORRECTING YOURSELF

Do not allow the torso to either move right or tilt forward. To guard against this, make sure that your left armpit and your left hip are in a straight line. Tuck in the left shoulder blade and keep your eyes on your right arm. Be conscious of the stretched side of your body.

Keep your brain passive

Stretch your arms away from your shoulders

Expand your chest

"*Regular practice of this asana helps to develop your strength and endurance.*"

The right knee should be positioned above the right heel

Tighten the muscles of your thighs

Press down on your right heel

VIRABHADRASANA 2

ADVANCED WORK IN THE POSE **360°** VIEW

Do not bend your knee too rigidly and keep your bent leg relaxed. Consciously keep your brain passive. Your right buttock should be slightly lower than the right inner knee. Tighten your buttocks and broaden the hips. Press the outer edges of both your feet down on the floor. Feel the energy rise from the ankle to the knee. Push your chest out and expand your chest cavity to its full extent. Keep the left knee taut and lifted upward. If it drops, your chest will cave in. Maintain the stretch of your arms and shoulder blades away from your torso.

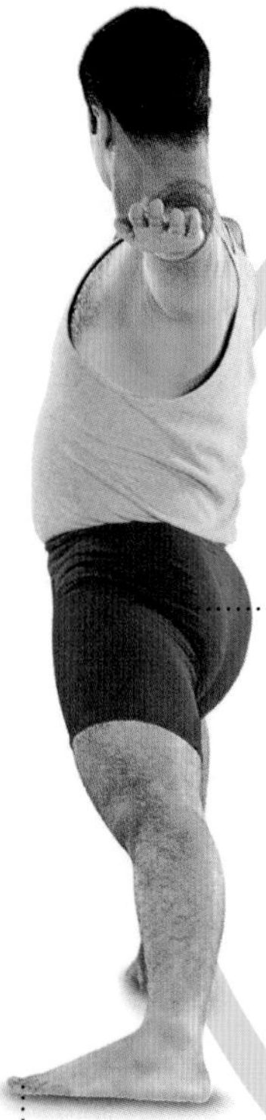

Your right heel should be in line with your right knee

Keep your buttocks taut

Lock your elbows

Keep your toes separated and active

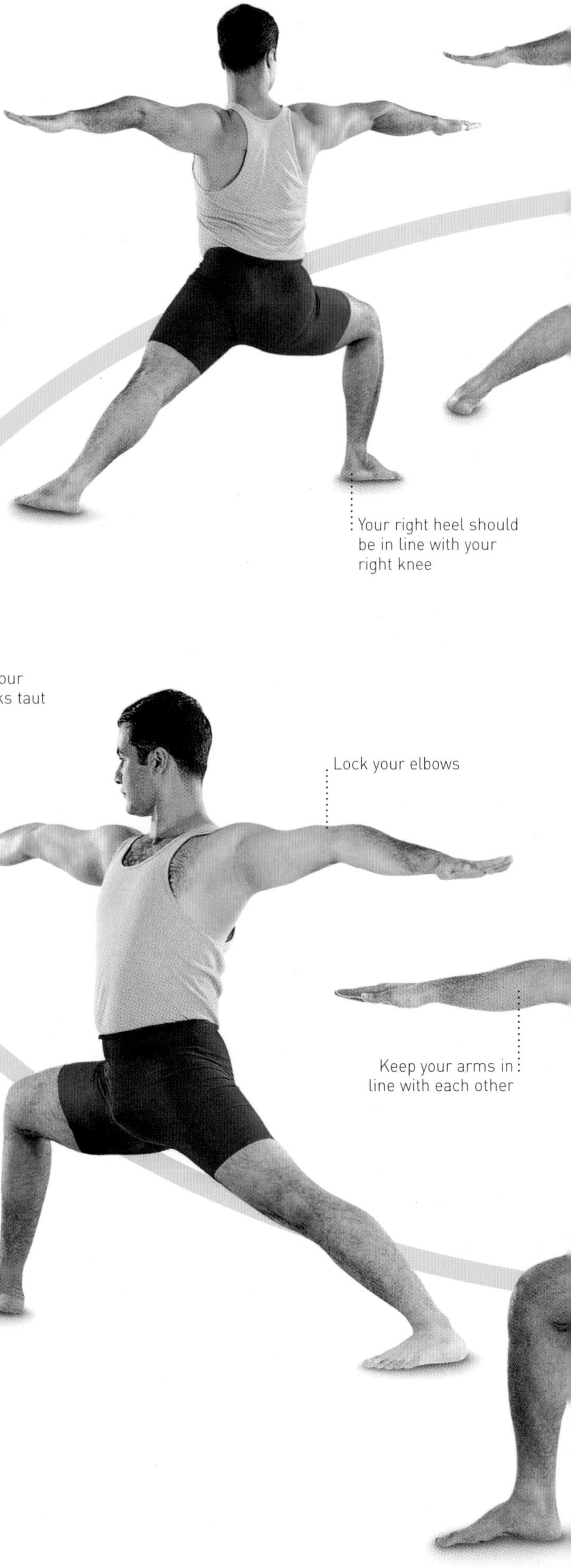

Keep your arms in line with each other

COMING OUT OF THE POSE
Inhale, and straighten your right leg. Turn your feet, so that they face forward. Repeat this pose on the other side. Then exhale, and jump back to Tadasana.

Tuck in your shoulder blades

Pull the flesh of your right buttock into your tailbone

Suck your left kneecap into the back of the knee

Do not allow the torso to move to the right

Stretch both arms from shoulders to fingertips

Stretch both sides of your torso upward

UTTHITA PARSVAKONASANA
Extended side stretch

In Sanskrit, *utthita* means "stretch," parsva indicates "side" or "flank," while *kona* translates as "angle." In this asana, both sides of your body are stretched intensely, from the toes of one foot to the fingertips of the opposite hand.

● BENEFITS

Enhances lung capacity
Tones the muscles of the heart
Relieves sciatic and arthritic pain
Improves digestion and helps the elimination of waste
Reduces fat on the waist and hips

● CAUTIONS

If you have high blood pressure, avoid this asana. If you have cervical spondylosis, do not turn your neck or look up.

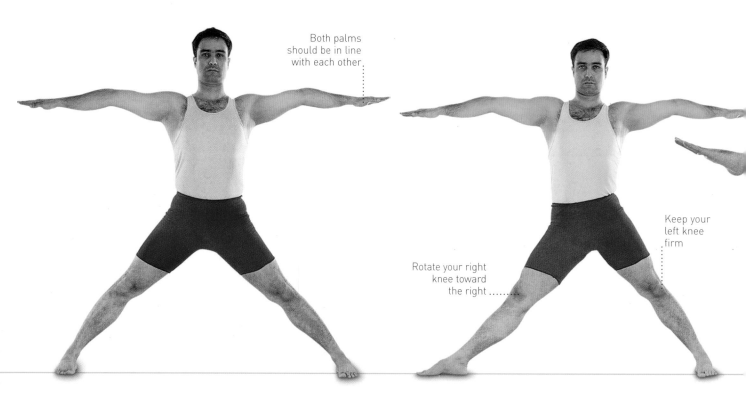

Both palms should be in line with each other

Rotate your right knee toward the right

Keep your left knee firm

1 Stand in Tadasana (*see page* 68). Inhale, and jump your feet about 4ft (1.2 m) apart. At the same time, raise both your arms out to the sides, to shoulder level. Your palms should face the floor. Stretch your arms from the back of the elbows. Make sure that your feet are in line with each other, toes pointing forward. Push down on the outer edges of your feet. Press the little toe of each foot down to the floor.

2 Exhale slowly and simultaneously rotate your right leg and foot 90° to the right. At the same time, turn in the left foot slightly to the right. Stretch your left leg and tighten it at the knee. Make sure that your weight falls on the heel, not the toes, of your right foot. Adjust the distance between your legs, if necessary. Make sure your feet remain in line with each other.

BEGINNERS As you rotate your right leg, focus on turning out your thigh. This reduces pressure on the right knee.

"Remember to keep your body absolutely steady when practicing this asana."

3 Bend your right knee until your thigh and calf form a right angle, and your right thigh is parallel to the floor. Take one or two breaths.

INTERMEDIATES Consciously pull your left knee and ankle upward. Open the back of the left knee from the center to the sides. Pull the muscles of both calves toward your thighs.

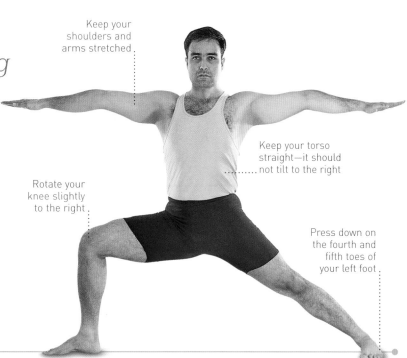

Keep your shoulders and arms stretched

Keep your torso straight—it should not tilt to the right

Rotate your knee slightly to the right

Press down on the fourth and fifth toes of your left foot

4 Exhale, and place your right palm on the floor beside your right foot. Make sure your right armpit touches the outside of your right knee. Stretch your left arm out over your left ear. Turn your head and look up. Hold the pose for 20-30 seconds.

BEGINNERS Exhale, and first stretch your right arm. Then, bring it down to the floor. You can place your fingertips, instead of your palm, on the floor.

Allow your thigh to descend

Keep your left leg stretched out

UTTHITA PARSVAKONASANA

ADVANCED WORK IN THE POSE **360° VIEW**

Your left arm is the "brain" of the pose (*see page* 65), so keep it stable and do not allow it to move. Increase the intensity of the stretch in this arm, pushing it away from the left armpit. Bring your lower shoulder blades into your back. Lift your left thigh slightly—this will help the right hand to descend more easily. Make sure you rest on the back of the right heel and do not allow dead weight to fall on your right thigh or palm. Keep your chest, hips, and left leg in line with each other. Stretch every part of your body, focusing especially on the spine. Feel a single, continuous stretch from your left ankle to your left wrist.

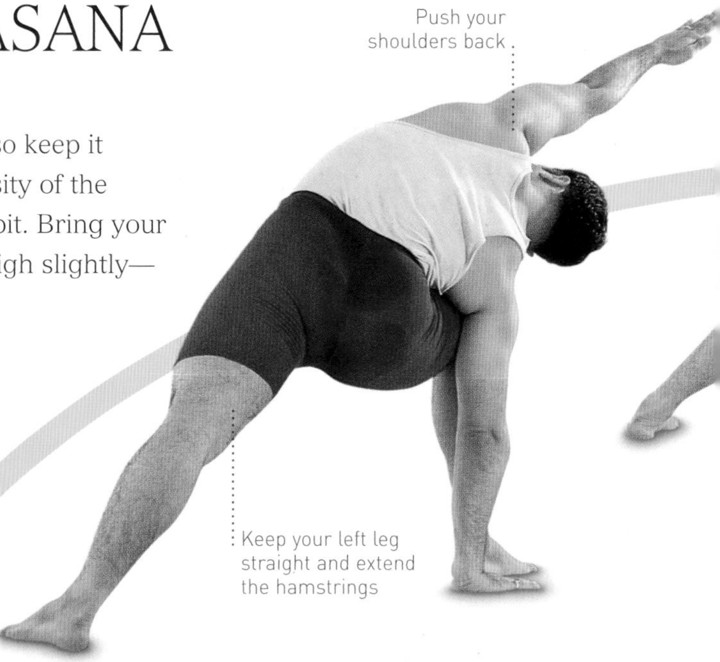

Push your shoulders back

Keep your left leg straight and extend the hamstrings

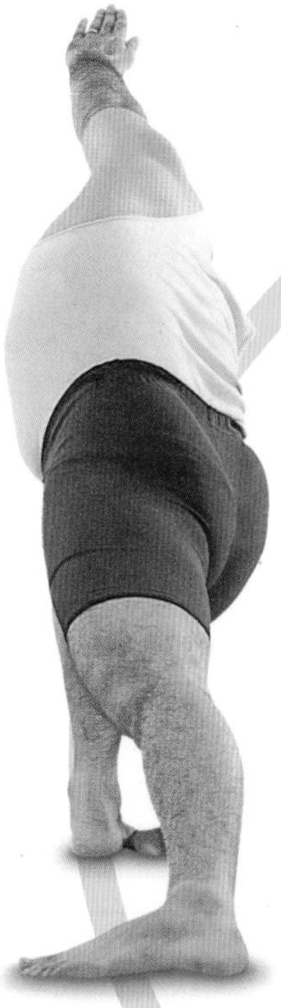

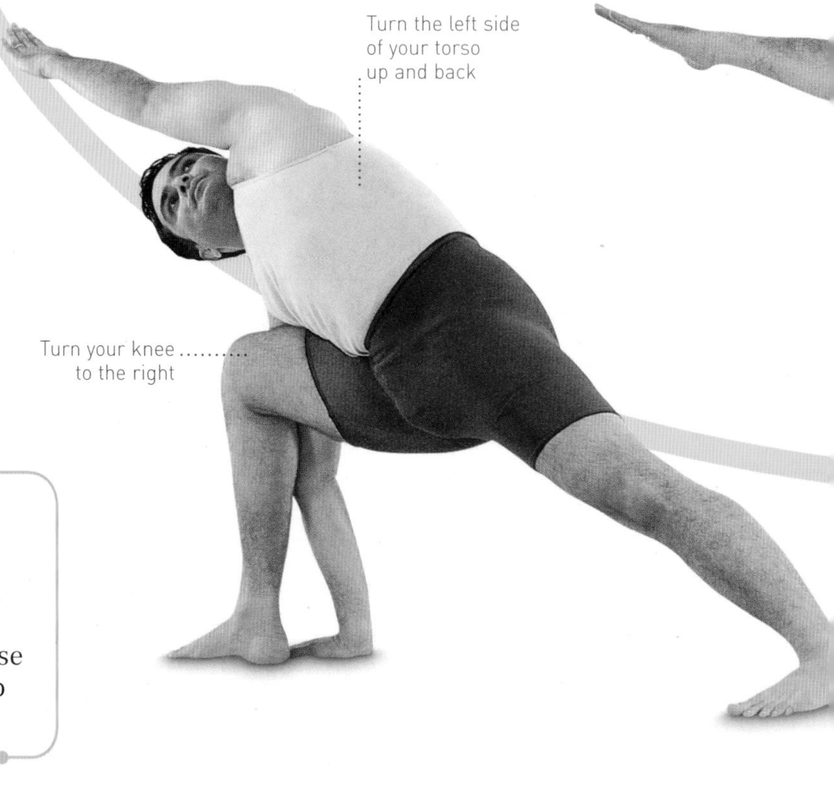

Turn the left side of your torso up and back

Turn your knee to the right

COMING OUT OF THE POSE

Inhale, and lift your right hand from the floor. Bring your arms to your sides and straighten your right leg. Turn both feet so that they face forward. Repeat the pose on the other side. Then exhale, and jump back to Tadasana.

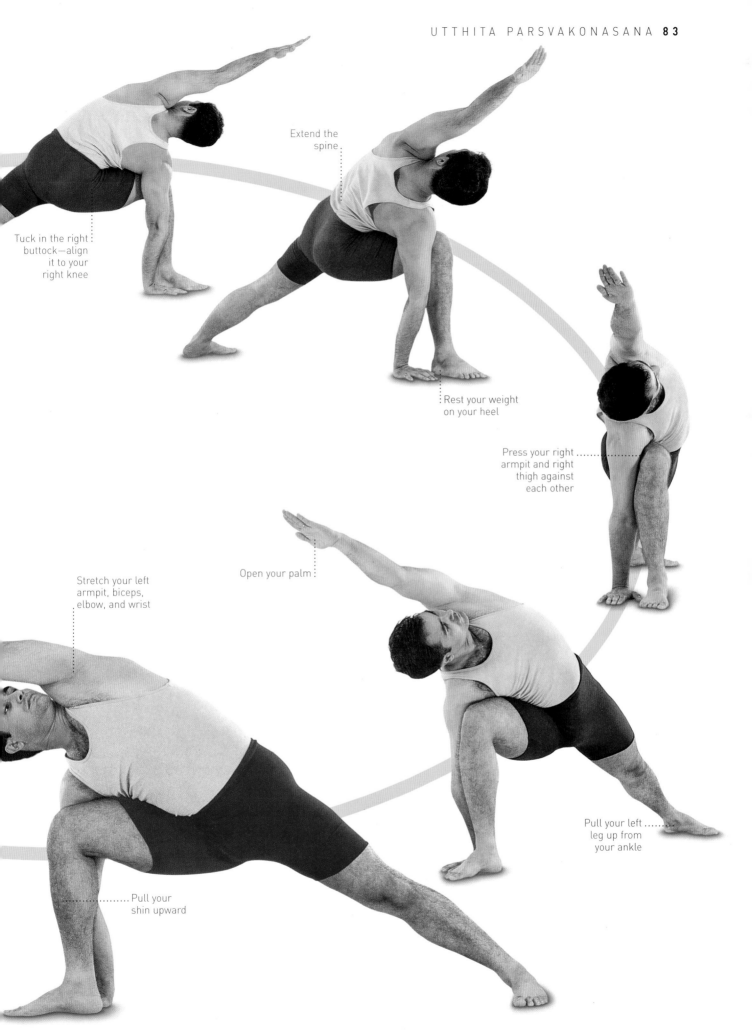

Tuck in the right buttock—align it to your right knee

Extend the spine

Rest your weight on your heel

Press your right armpit and right thigh against each other

Open your palm

Stretch your left armpit, biceps, elbow, and wrist

Pull your shin upward

Pull your left leg up from your ankle

PARSVOTTANASANA
Intense chest stretch

This asana gives an intense stretch to your chest. *Parsva* means "side" or "flank" in Sanskrit, while *uttana* indicates the great intensity of the final stretch. Regular practice of Parsvottanasana stimulates and tones the kidneys, an effect you can feel once you are comfortable in the final pose.

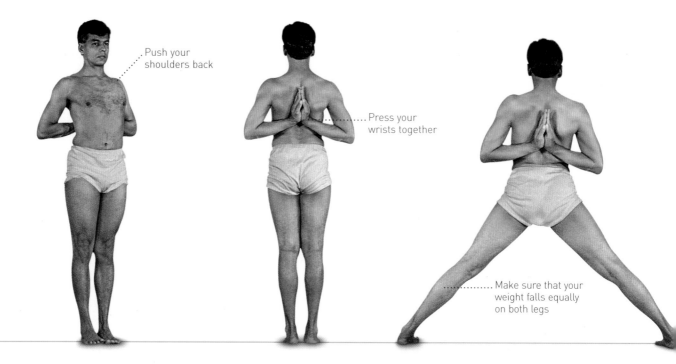

Push your shoulders back

Press your wrists together

Make sure that your weight falls equally on both legs

1 Stand in Tadasana (*see page* 68). Loosen your arms by turning them inside and out several times. Join your fingertips together behind your back, with your fingers pointing down, toward your feet. Then rotate your wrists

(*see inset*), until your fingers point to the ceiling.

BEGINNERS If joining your palms is too difficult, take your arms behind your back, bend your elbows and rest each palm on the opposite elbow.

2 Move your joined palms up to the middle of your back. The little fingers of each hand should touch your back. Then, move your hands up your back (*see inset*) until they rest between your shoulder blades. Press your fingers together. Press your palms together by pushing your elbows inward. This will help to push your

shoulders back and expand your chest even further.

3 Inhale and jump up, landing with your feet about 4 ft (1.2 m) apart. If your legs feel over-stretched or uncomfortably close together, adjust the distance accordingly. When you feel that your body weight is distributed equally—and comfortably—on both legs, you have the distance right. Pause for a few seconds and exhale slowly.

"The asana also helps remove stiffness in the neck, shoulders, and elbows."

4 Inhale, and turn your right foot 90° to the right. Turn the left foot 75-80° to the right. At the same time, rotate to the right from the waist and hips. Make sure that your torso faces front and is in line with your right leg. Rest your weight on the heel of your right foot. Tighten your right knee and extend your chest, waist, and hips. Then, tilt your head and chest back and look up at the ceiling, making sure that you do not strain your throat. Press your palms to your back—do not allow them to slide down.

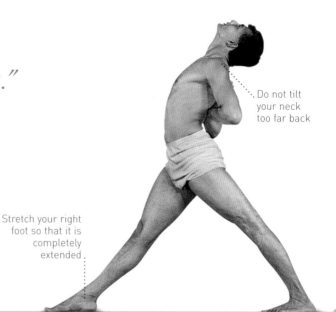

Do not tilt your neck too far back

Stretch your right foot so that it is completely extended

Widen your elbows

5 Exhale, extend the spine, and bend forward from the top of both your thighs. As you bend, lead with your sternum and do not allow your right knee to bend as you come forward. Take care to bend equally from both sides of the waist. Rest your chin on your right knee. Stay in the pose for 20-30 seconds. Breathe evenly.

BEGINNERS If you find the final stretch difficult, then place your palms on the floor on either side of the right foot. Be careful to stretch your back and neck gradually.

Turn in your left kneecap slightly

Keep the right leg fully stretched

PARSVOTTANASANA

ADVANCED WORK IN THE POSE **360° VIEW**

Maintain the stretch of your upper body, from the pelvis
to the collar bones, while holding the pose. Elongate
both sides of your waist evenly, to increase the stretch of
your thighs. Bend down from your groin, keeping
the perineum area passive. To make sure that your torso
rests on the center of your right thigh, move your
abdomen slightly to the right, until your navel rests
on the center of your right thigh. Tighten the leg
muscles and feel the stretch along the back of
both legs. Push your spine down even
further over your right leg.
Move both your shoulders
back, until both sides of your
chest are equally expanded.
Breathe evenly.

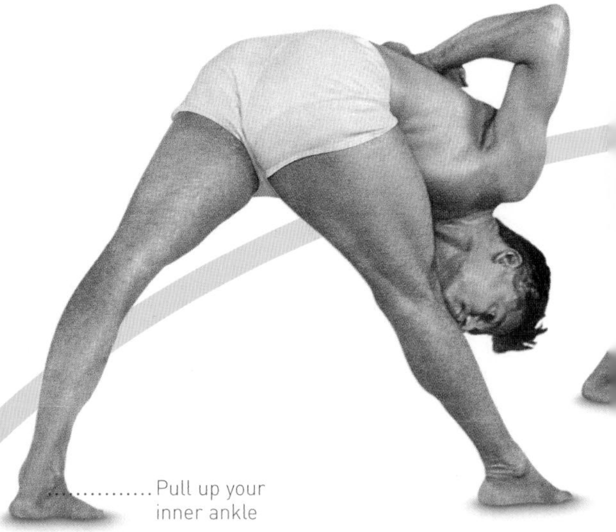

............Pull up your
inner ankle

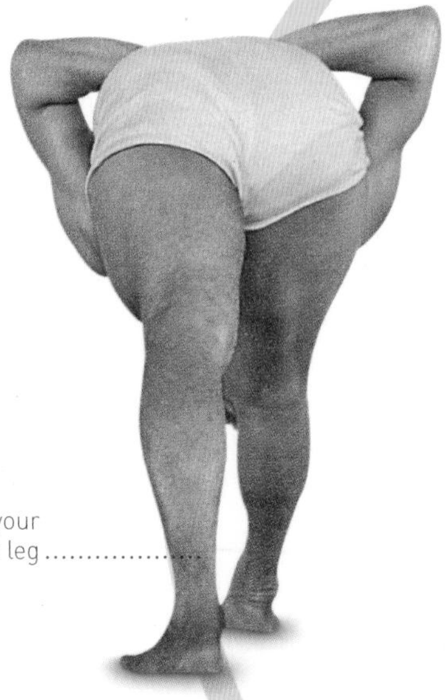

Stretch your
left leg ....

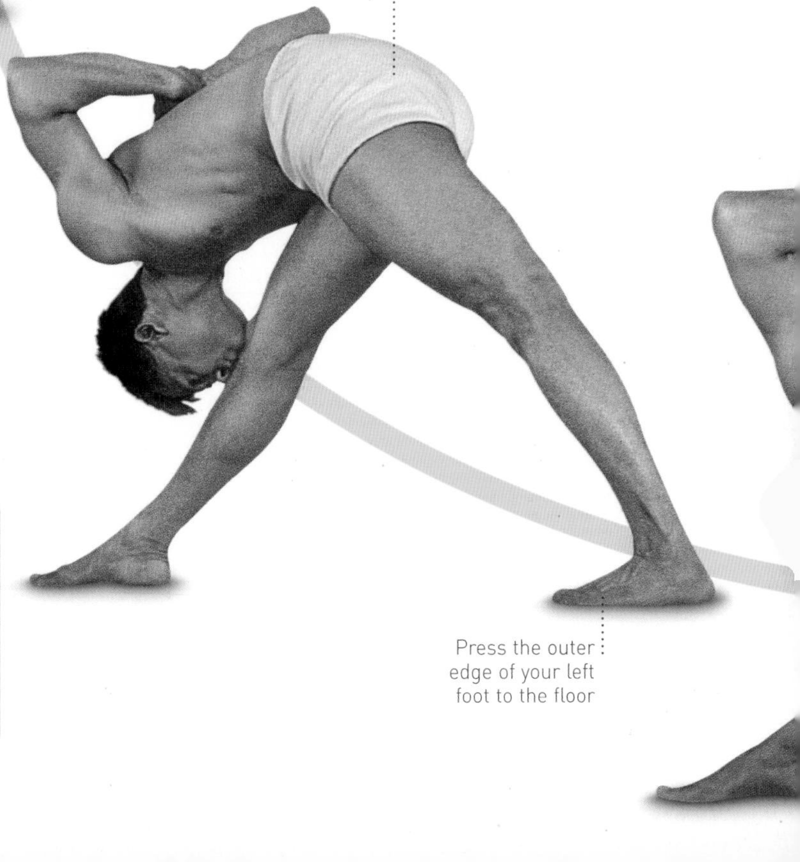

Keep your
buttocks parallel
to each other

COMING OUT OF THE POSE

Inhale, and lift your torso. Come back
to a standing position, but do not raise
your head immediately. Repeat the pose
on the other side. Stretch out your arms
to shoulder level and jump your feet
together. Stand in Tadasana.

Press the outer
edge of your left
foot to the floor

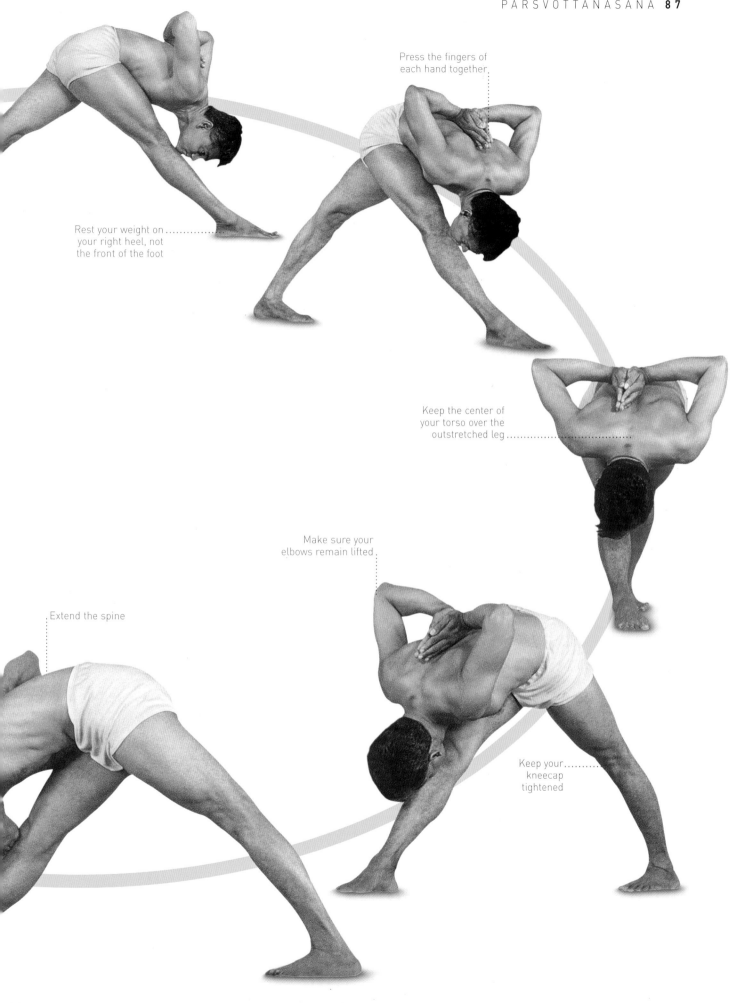

Press the fingers of
each hand together

Rest your weight on
your right heel, not
the front of the foot

Keep the center of
your torso over the
outstretched leg

Make sure your
elbows remain lifted

Extend the spine

Keep your
kneecap
tightened

ADHOMUKHA SVANASANA
Downward-facing dog stretch

In this asana, your body takes the shape of a dog stretching itself. *Adhomukha* means to have your "face downward" in Sanskrit, and *svana* translates as "dog." The asana helps runners, because it reduces stiffness in the heels, and makes the legs strong and agile. Holding the pose for one minute restores energy when you are tired. This asana gently stimulates your nervous system, and regular practice will rejuvenate your whole body.

● BENEFITS
Calms the brain and gently stimulates the nerves
Slows down the heartbeat
Reduces stiffness in the shoulder blades and arthritis in the shoulder joints
Strengthens the ankles and tones the legs
Relieves pain in the heels and softens calcaneal spurs
Checks heavy menstrual flow
Helps prevent hot flashes during menopause

● CAUTIONS
If you have high blood pressure or frequent headaches, support your head with a bolster (*see page* 185). If you are prone to dislocation of the shoulders, make sure that your arms do not rotate outward. Do not practice this asana in an advanced stage of pregnancy.

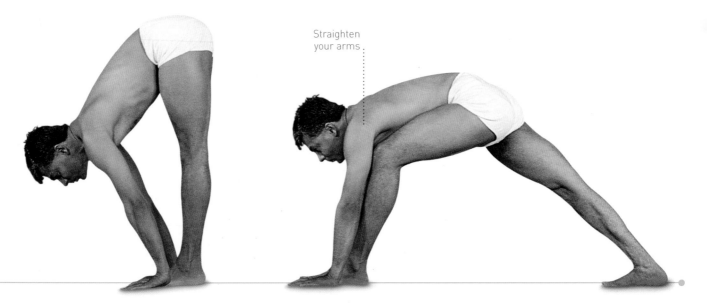

Straighten your arms

1 Stand in Tadasana (*see page* 68). Exhale, and bend from the waist, placing each palm on the floor beside each foot.

BEGINNERS Exhale, and bend from your waist. Bend both knees and place your palms on the floor next to your feet.

2 Bend your knees and step back approximately 4ft (1.2m), one leg at a time. Keep your palms about 3–4ft (1m) apart. Make sure that the distance between your feet is the same as that between your palms.

THE GURU'S ADVICE

"To make sure that my student's arms are straight, I stand on his hands to keep them firmly placed on the floor. Then I press his shoulder blades in, creating a right-angled triangle presentation of the pose. In this position, you should feel an intense stretch from your buttocks, along the dorsal and thoracic spine, right down to your palms."

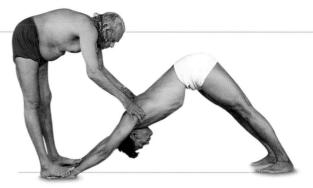

3 Position your right leg in line with your right arm, and your left leg in line with your left arm. Stretch your fingers and toes. Raise your heels, tighten the muscles at the top of your thighs, and pull your kneecaps in. Then stretch the arches of your feet and bring your heels down to the floor again.

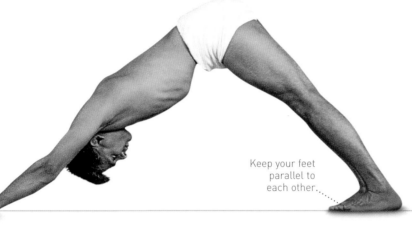

Keep your feet parallel to each other.

4 Pull your inner arms up from the elbows to the shoulders. Move your torso toward your legs. Feel the stretch from your palms to your heels. Now exhale, and stretching the base of your neck, lower the crown of your head to the floor. Hold the pose for 15–20 seconds.

INTERMEDIATES Before you lower your head, move the deltoids deep into the shoulder joints and lift your shoulder blades. Press both your palms down on the floor and pull your sternum up toward your diaphragm.

Push your buttocks upward

Stretch both legs equally

Keep your arms fully stretched

Rest on the front of your crown

Keep your feet flat on the floor with the toes pointing straight ahead.

ADHOMUKHA SVANASANA

ADVANCED WORK IN THE POSE **360° VIEW**

Move your legs as far back as possible. Make sure that both thighs are stretched equally—the inner and outer back edges should be parallel to each other. If your thighs are not parallel, they tend to shorten and lose their stretch. Similarly, keep your spine stretched out and do not compress it. Feel the energy in the spine flowing upward, from the neck to the buttocks, and not the other way around. Tuck in your shoulder blades and broaden your chest. As the chest opens out fully, your breathing becomes deep. Be aware of that depth.

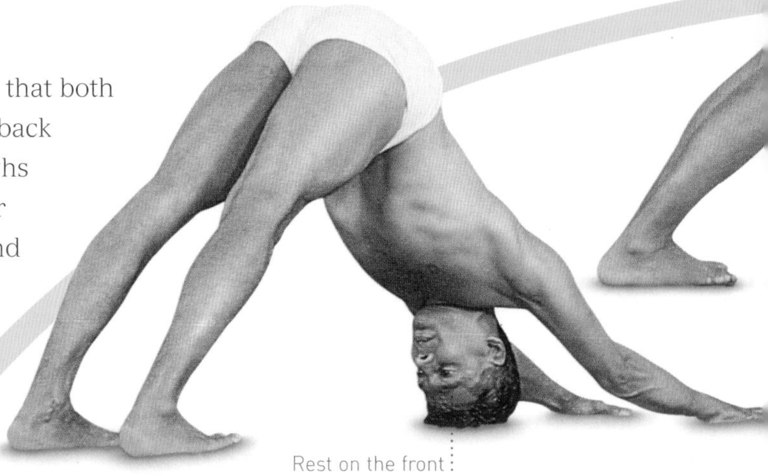

Rest on the front your crown

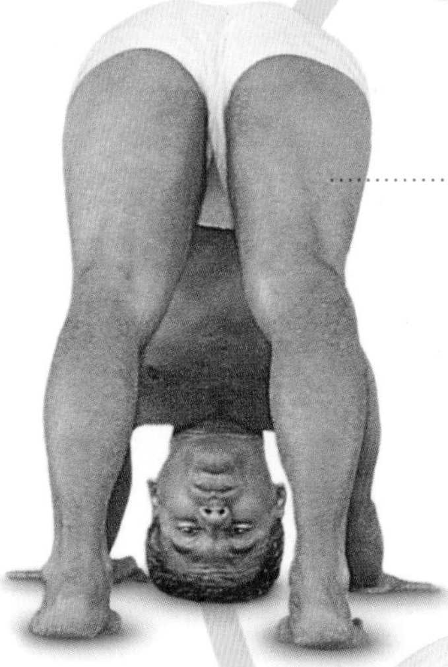

Keep your thighs parallel to each other

*The **long and** of asanas, done with*

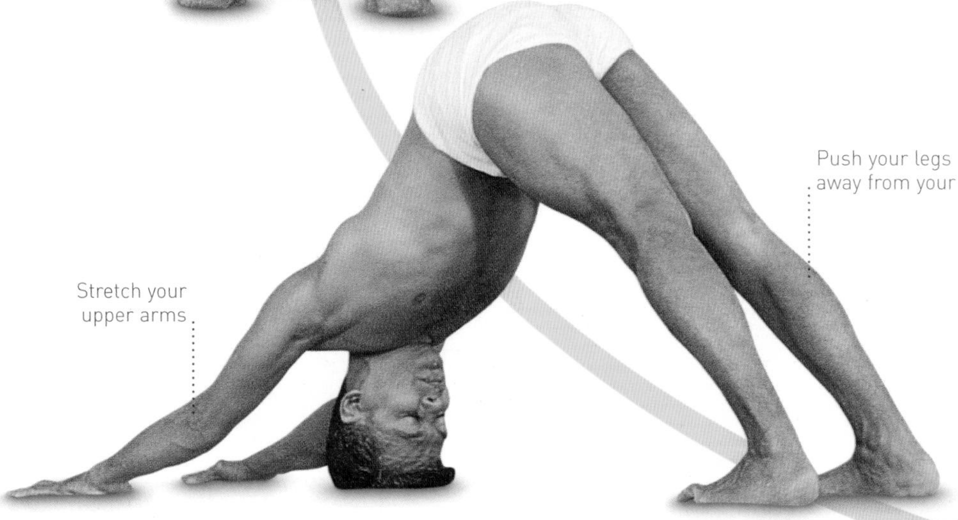

Push your legs away from your body

Stretch your upper arms

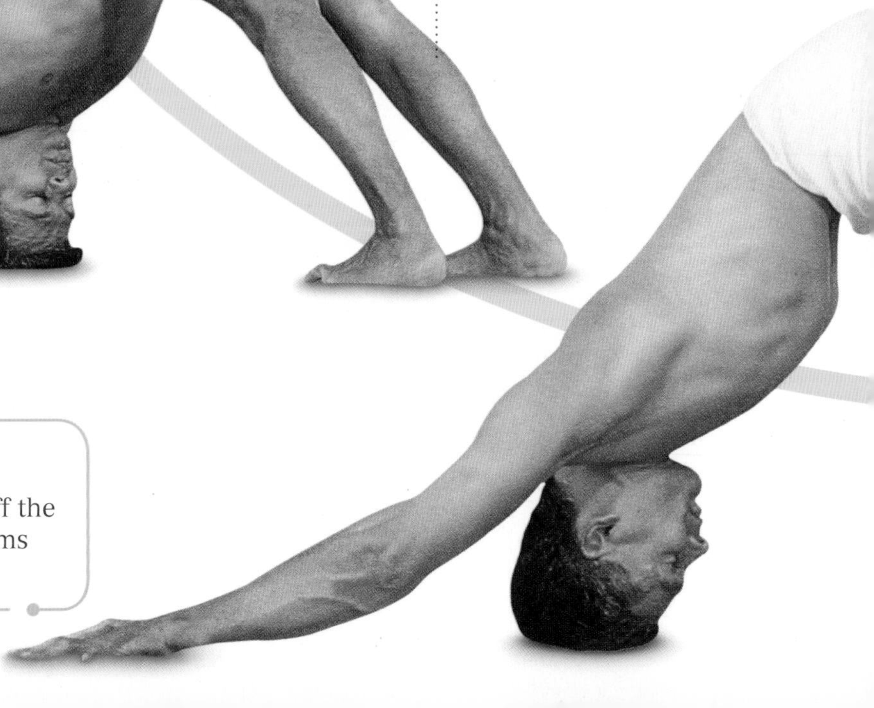

COMING OUT OF THE POSE

Inhale, and gradually lift your head off the floor. Walk your feet toward your palms and come back to Tadasana.

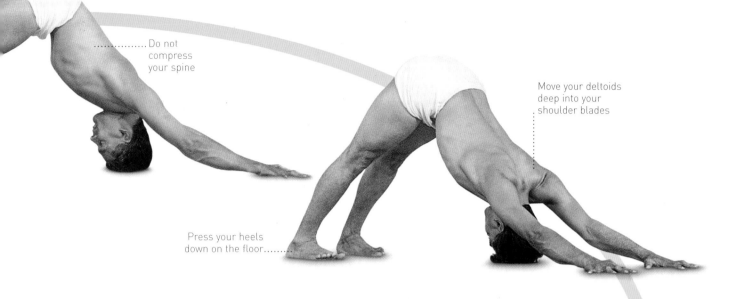

Do not
compress
your spine

Move your deltoids
deep into your
shoulder blades

Press your heels
down on the floor

uninterrupted practice
awareness, brings success.

Keep your
neck soft, but
elongated

Do not bend
your knees

Push your torso
toward your legs

UTTANASANA
Intense forward stretch

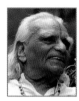

The spine receives a deliberate and intense stretch in this asana. The word *ut* means "deliberate" or "intense" in Sanskrit, while *tana* connotes "stretch." This asana can help those who are prone to anxiety or depression since it rejuvenates the spinal nerves and brain cells. It also slows down the heartbeat.

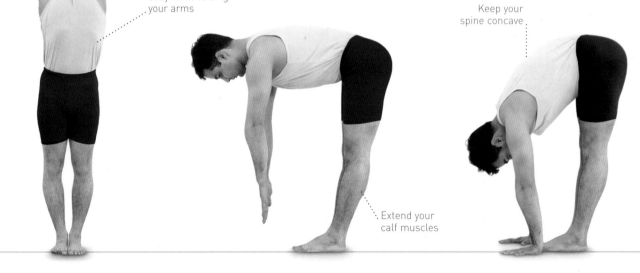

Stretch your entire body while raising your arms

Extend your calf muscles

Keep your spine concave

1 Stand in Tadasana (*see page* 68) with your legs straight and fully stretched. Tighten your kneecaps and then pull them upward. Raise your arms toward the ceiling, the palms facing forward. Stretch your whole body. Take one or two breaths.

2 Exhale, and bend forward from the waist. Keep your legs fully stretched. Make sure that your body weight is placed equally on both feet. Extend your toes.

3 Bend your torso further and place your palms on the floor in front of your feet. Separate your ankles a little, to free your lower back, buttocks, and legs. Consciously stretch the skin at the backs of your knees and thighs.

BEGINNERS Lift your toes and press your heels down on the floor as you bend (*see inset*). Instead of your palms, you can rest your fingertips on the floor, until you are more flexible.

Stretch your
torso forward

4 Move your hands back and place them next to your heels. Rest on your fingers and thumbs, with the palms raised off the floor. Keep your thighs fully stretched—feel the energy flow along the back of your legs, into the waist, and down your spine. Pull your kneecaps into your knees, and keep both knees parallel to each other and fully opened out at the back. The pressure on the inner and outer edges of your feet should be equal.

Press the front of
your soles down
on the floor.

CORRECTING YOURSELF

WRONG If your knees bend, the tailbone juts out, impairing the pose.

RIGHT Stretch your thighs, keeping the kneecaps locked and pushed upward.

Push your
hips forward

5 Exhale, and push your torso closer to your legs until your face rests on the knees. Push your torso and abdomen further down toward the floor until your chin touches both knees. Your chin should not touch your chest, since this will cause your neck and throat to tighten, leading to pressure on the head. Hold the pose for 30-60 seconds, breathing evenly.

Extend your thighs
from the knees
to the hips

Stretch your
arms from
your shoulders

"The practice of Uttanasana helps the body and the brain recover from mental and physical exhaustion."

UTTANASANA

ADVANCED WORK IN THE POSE 360° VIEW

When you place your fingers on the floor, turn your arms out and stretch them downward. Imagine you are pushing the skin of your arms down from your armpits to your fingertips. Focus on your ribs. Consciously stretch each rib, from the bottom of your rib cage right up to your armpits. Then, descend even further from your armpits. This will open the back of your inner thighs. Feel a continuous stretch from your heels to the crown of your head.

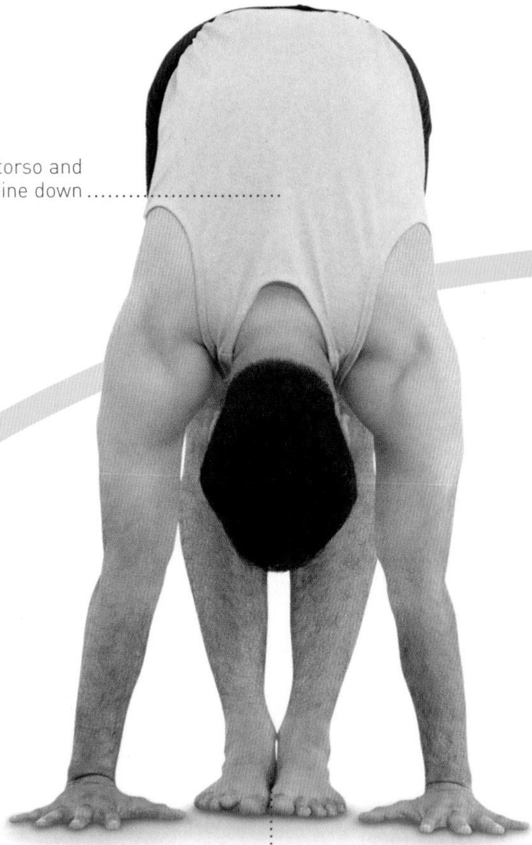

Push your torso and spine down

Keep the inner sides of your ankles, knees, and thighs together

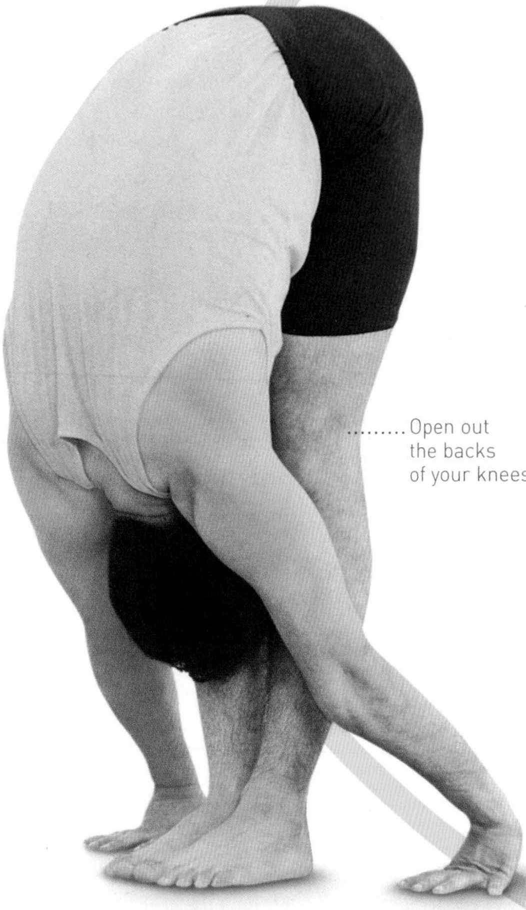

Open out the backs of your knees

*Your **body** exists*
your mind exists in
*they come **together***

COMING OUT OF THE POSE

Inhale, and raise your head without lifting your palms off the floor. Press your fingers into the floor and descend your armpits. Then, raise your torso gradually. Always be sure to come up with your back straight. Stand in Tadasana.

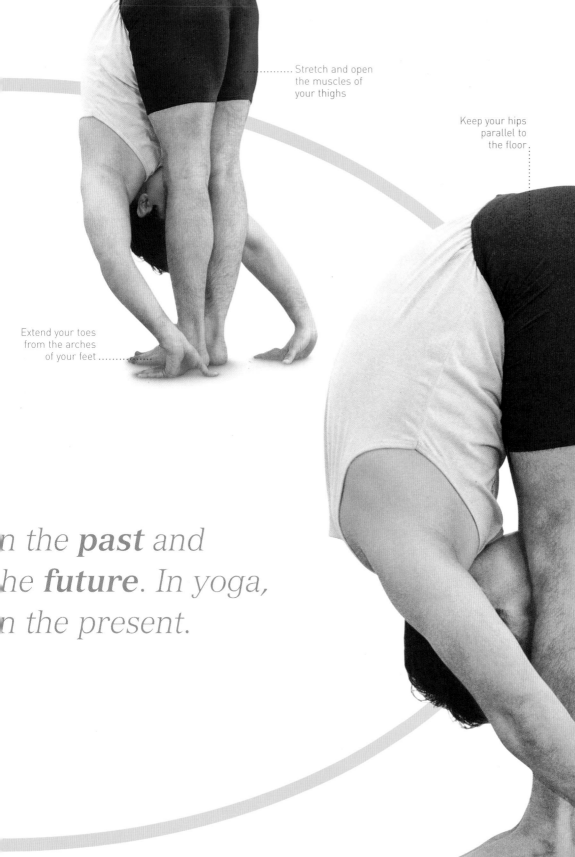

Stretch and open
the muscles of
your thighs

Keep your hips
parallel to
the floor.

Extend your toes
from the arches
of your feet

n the **past** and
he **future**. In yoga,
n the present.

VIRABHADRASANA 1
Warrior pose 1

This asana, based on a warrior pose, is a more intense version of Virabhadrasana 2 (*see page* 76). Both asanas are named after the mythic warrior-sage, Virabhadra. This vigorous asana strengthens your spine and increases the flexibility of your knees and thighs. The arms receive an intense stretch, and this expands the muscles of your chest and enhances the capacity of your lungs.

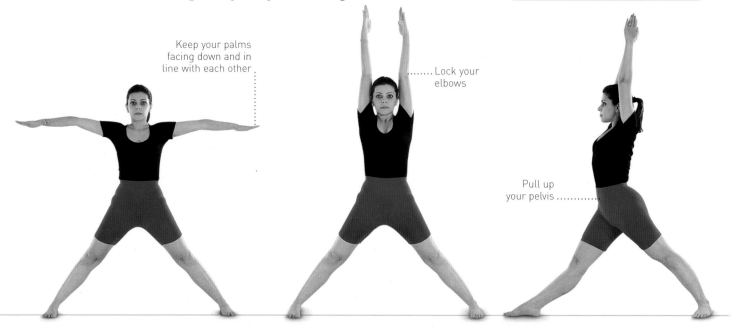

Keep your palms facing down and in line with each other

Lock your elbows

Pull up your pelvis

1 Stand in Tadasana (*see page* 68). Inhale and jump, landing with your feet about 4ft (1.2m) apart. Your feet should be in line, the toes pointing forward. Raise your arms up to shoulder level, parallel to the floor. Lock your elbows. Press the little toes of both feet onto the floor. The outer edges of both feet should rest on the floor.

INTERMEDIATES For a more effective stretch, focus on the inner sides of your legs. Imagine that you are pulling the skin of both legs up from your heels to your waist.

2 Turn your wrists until your palms face the ceiling. Raise both arms until they are perpendicular to the floor and parallel to each other. Lift your shoulder blades and push them into your body (*see inset*).

INTERMEDIATES Your elbows are the "brain" of your arms (*see page* 65). Stretch from your elbows to your fingertips.

3 Exhale, and turn your torso and right leg 90º to the right. Then turn your left leg to the right. Rotate your torso from the chest as well as the waist. The more you rotate to the right and stretch your upper arms, the more effective the pose.

INTERMEDIATES Be conscious of your left leg, and concentrate on the stretch from the back of your heel to the back of your thigh.

THE GURU'S ADVICE

4 Exhale, and bend the right knee from the right buttock bone. The calf and thigh should form a right angle. Go down into the pose with resistance and then stretch the length of your body up to the ceiling. Make sure that the weight of your body does not fall on your right knee. Breathe evenly and stay in the pose for 15-20 seconds.

"You must maintain the lift of the left knee. Simultaneously, adjust your shoulder blades by pushing them in, and then lifting them."

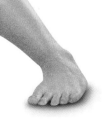

Push out your
upper chest ....

Do not
harden your
shoulders

Your knee should
be in line with
your ankle

VIRABHADRASANA 1

ADVANCED WORK IN THE POSE 360° VIEW

Feel the stretch in your back to experience the pose. Push your shoulder joints into the armpits, stretching your arms up higher. Make sure that the upper part of your body is symmetrical, with both armpits parallel to each other. Your face, chest, and right knee should be in line with your right foot. To avoid straining your right knee, turn your kneecap out toward the little toe of your right foot. Your weight should rest on the inner edge of your left buttock and on the outer heel of the left foot. Focus on your left side because it controls the harmony of the pose. Feel the energy flow up your left leg.

Stretch your arms from the shoulder blades

Turn your left buttock out slightly

Stretch both sides of the waist equally

Extend your spine up from the tailbone

Keep the muscles of the right thigh relaxed

COMING OUT OF THE POSE

Inhale, and stretch your arms out to your sides. Straighten your right knee and bring both your feet together, facing forward. Repeat the pose on the other side. Then exhale, and jump back to Tadasana.

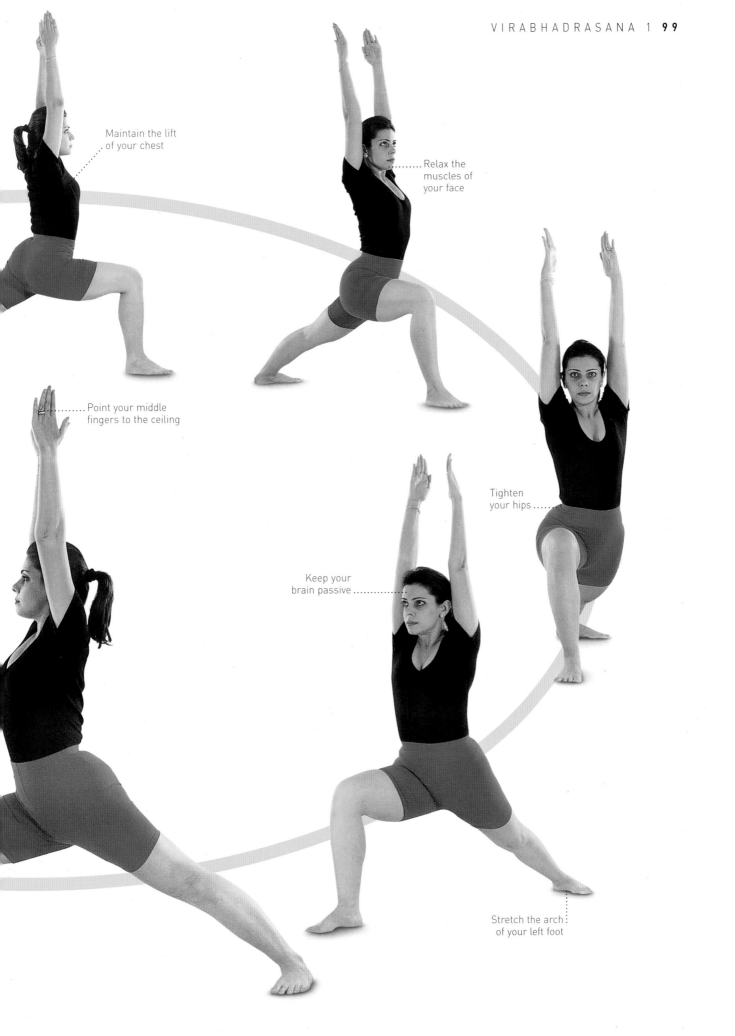

Maintain the lift of your chest

Relax the muscles of your face

Point your middle fingers to the ceiling

Tighten your hips

Keep your brain passive

Stretch the arch of your left foot

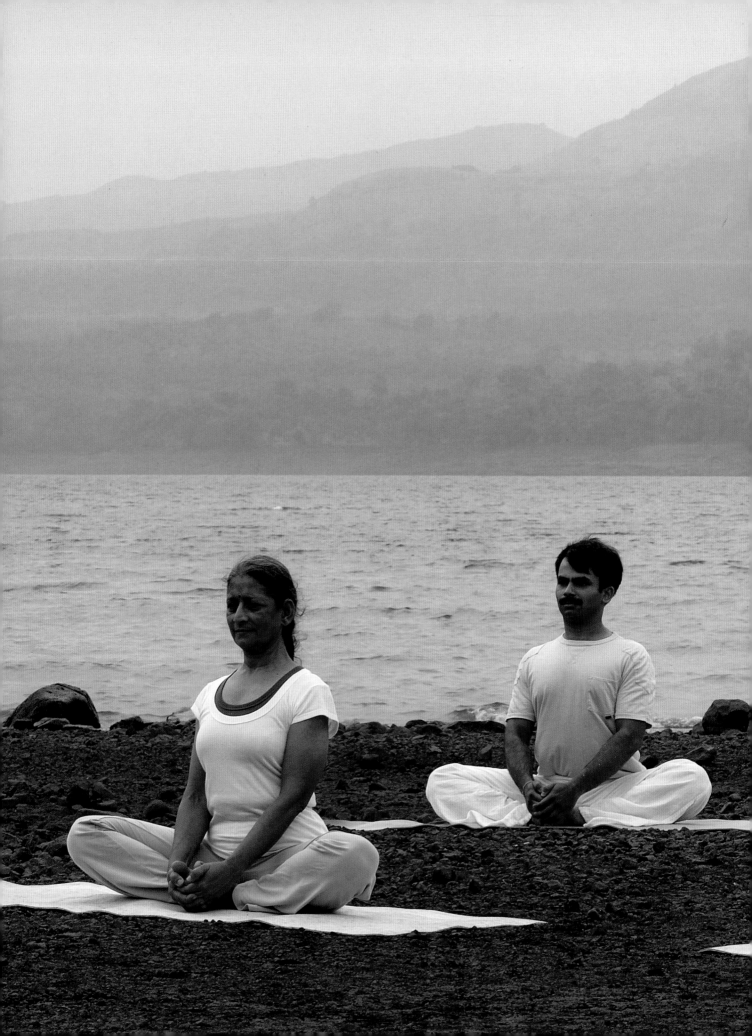

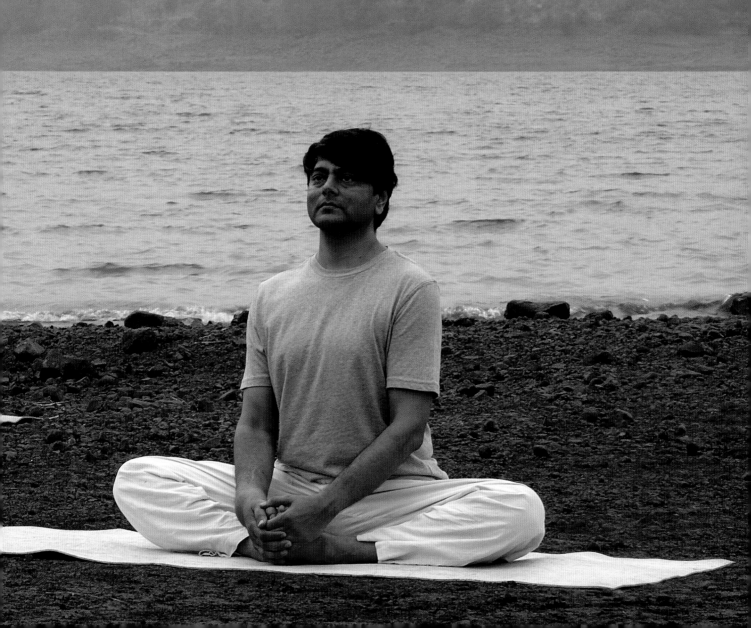

SITTING ASANAS

*"**Classic** poses, when practiced with **discrimination** and **awareness**, bring the **body**, **mind**, and **consciousness** into a single, **harmonious** whole."*

DANDASANA
Staff pose

Dandasana is the basic sitting pose for all forward bends. *Danda* means a "staff" or "walking stick" in Sanskrit, and regular practice of this asana improves your posture when seated. Your legs are rested during this asana, and it is recommended for people with arthritis or rheumatism of the knees and ankles.

● BENEFITS

Relieves breathlessness, choking, and throat congestion in asthmatics
Strengthens the muscles of the chest
Tones the abdominal organs and lifts sagging abdominal walls
Reduces heartburn and flatulence
Tones the spinal and leg muscles
Lengthens the ligaments of the legs

● CAUTIONS

If your spine has a tendency to sag, or if you are experiencing a severe attack of asthma, practice this asana with the length of your spine supported against a wall.

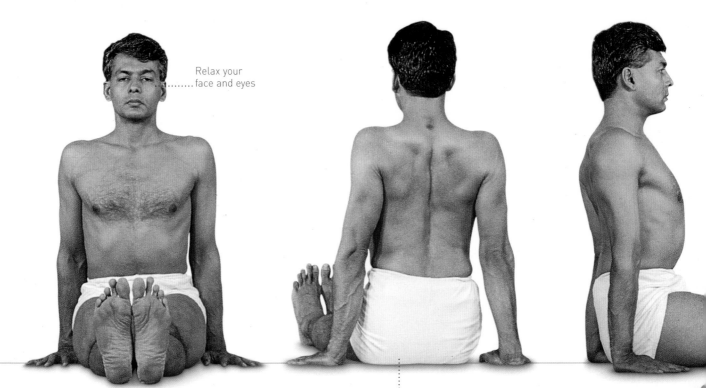

Relax your face and eyes

Rest on your buttock bones

Spread out the soles of your feet

1 Sit on the floor with your legs stretched out. Move the flesh of each buttock out to the side with your hands (*see inset*), so that you are resting on the buttock bones. Keep your thighs, knees, ankles, and feet together. Place your palms on the floor beside your hips, with your fingers pointing forward. Lift your chest. Lock your elbows and straighten your arms.

"If you are prone to anxiety or mood swings, practicing this asana helps to increase your willpower and enhance your emotional stability."

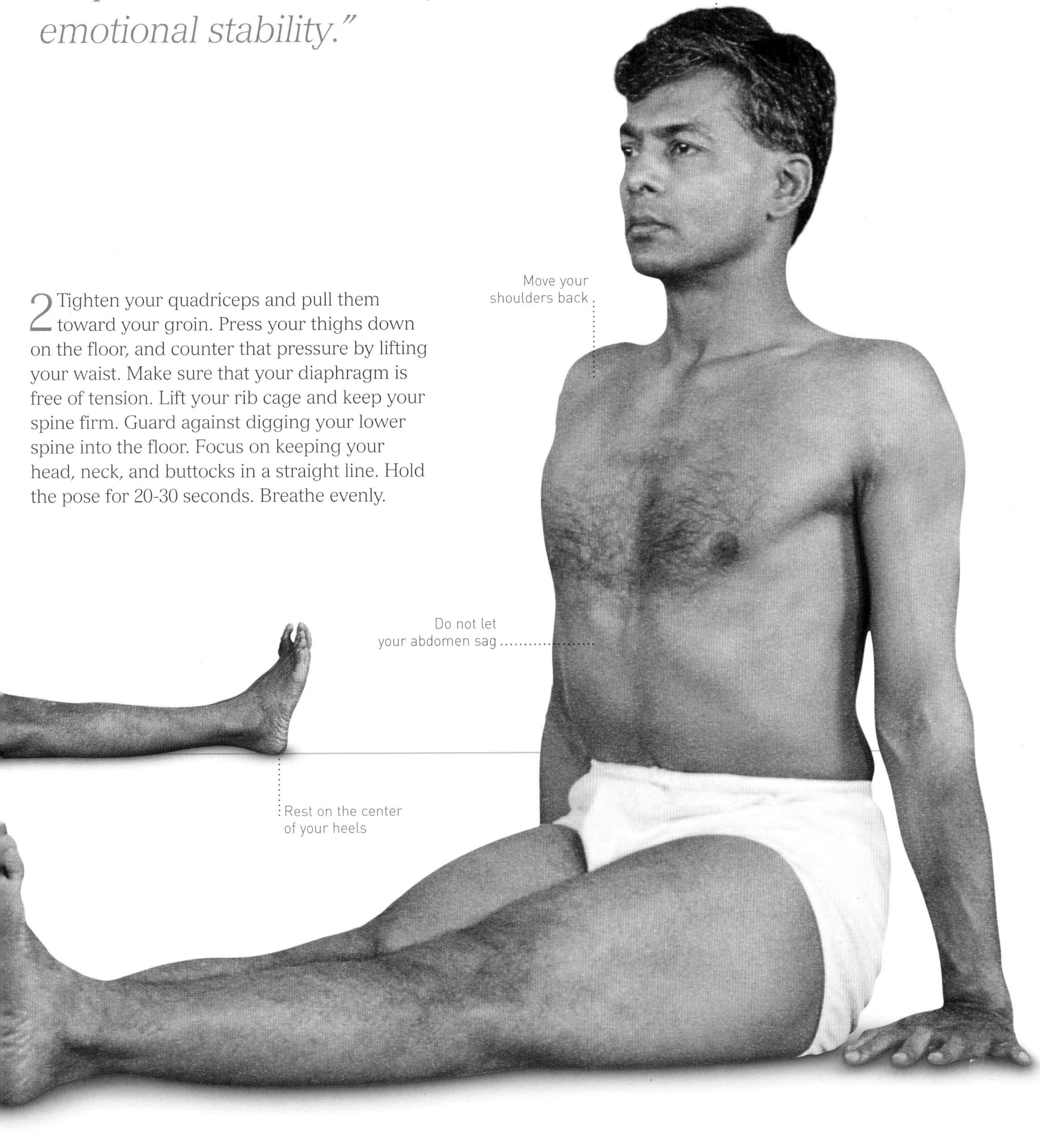

Keep your head
and neck erect

2 Tighten your quadriceps and pull them toward your groin. Press your thighs down on the floor, and counter that pressure by lifting your waist. Make sure that your diaphragm is free of tension. Lift your rib cage and keep your spine firm. Guard against digging your lower spine into the floor. Focus on keeping your head, neck, and buttocks in a straight line. Hold the pose for 20-30 seconds. Breathe evenly.

Move your
shoulders back

Do not let
your abdomen sag

Rest on the center
of your heels

VIRASANA
Hero pose

In this asana, you assume the pose of a seated warrior. *Vira* in Sanskrit means "hero" or "warrior." Regular practice of this asana helps to develop your strength and endurance. The asana stretches the chest and increases your capacity for deep breathing.

● BENEFITS

Relieves gout
Eases stiffness in the shoulders, neck, hip joints, knees, and groin
Alleviates arthritis of the elbows and fingers
Relieves backache
Reduces the pain of broken, deviated, or fused tailbones
Corrects herniated disks
Improves circulation in the feet
Relieves calcaneal spurs

● CAUTIONS

If the ligaments of your knee are injured, use a blanket to support your legs (*see page* 184), or sit on your heels (*see Step* 2). Avoid Steps 4 and 5 if you have a cardiac condition.

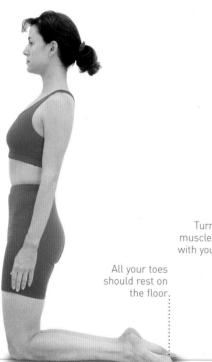

All your toes should rest on the floor.

Turn your calf muscles outward with your thumbs

Widen your chest ....

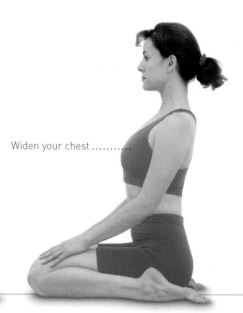

1 Kneel on the floor with your knees together. Spread your feet about 18 in (0.5 m) apart, with your soles facing the ceiling.

INTERMEDIATES Adjust your ankles so that they stretch evenly from the arch to the toes and from the arch to the heels. Feel the energy flow smoothly in both directions.

2 Lean forward and rest your palms on your shins. Lower your buttocks toward the floor. Make sure that the inner side of each calf touches the outer side of each thigh. Turn your calf muscles outward and make sure that you turn your thigh muscles inward.

BEGINNERS If you cannot rest your buttocks on the floor, place one sole on top of the other and rest your buttocks on them. Separate your feet.

3 Rest your buttocks on the floor. Do not sit on your feet. Place both palms on your thighs, close to the knees. Rest your weight on your thighs. Raise your waist and the sides of your torso, and press your shins firmly down on the floor.

BEGINNERS Place your palms on your knees and push your thighs down. Lift your torso from the base of the pelvis.

INTERMEDIATES Imagine that your legs are tied to the floor, then lift your torso. Feel the energy flow upward from the bottom of your chest.

Extend your spine
from the base
of your pelvis

*"Virasana
relieves stiffness
in the joints and
improves the
flexibility of your
whole body."*

4 Raise your arms to shoulder-level. Stretch them forward, parallel to the floor. With your palms facing you (*see inset below*), firmly interlock your fingers. Do not leave any gaps between the base of your fingers and the knuckles. Rotate your wrists and palms outward (*see inset left*), so that your palms face 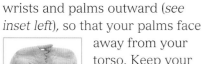 away from your torso. Keep your spine steady.

Make sure that your
arms are perpendicular
to the floor

Lift your
sternum

5 Raise your arms from the armpits until the palms face the ceiling. Keep your neck erect, your chest expanded, and your elbows straight. Make sure that your head does not tilt back, and your body does not lean forward. Breathe evenly, and hold the pose for 1 minute. With practice, increase the length of time spent in the pose to 5 minutes.

Keep your
knees pressed
down firmly

VIRASANA

ADVANCED WORK IN THE POSE **360°** VIEW

The intelligence of the body is energy, while the intelligence of the brain is consciousness. This energy moves with each action. When you stretch your arms upward, it is a physical action. Lifting the arms from the armpits after locking the elbows and deltoids, is an action done by the physiological body (*see page* 62). When you raise your arms, you will feel the energy move to the front of your legs. With every move, the energy in your legs flows to a different position. As the mind moves with this energy, focus on your legs. Imagine you are releasing the energy of your legs into the floor as you stretch your arms up even further. This will calm your mind and free your body of tension.

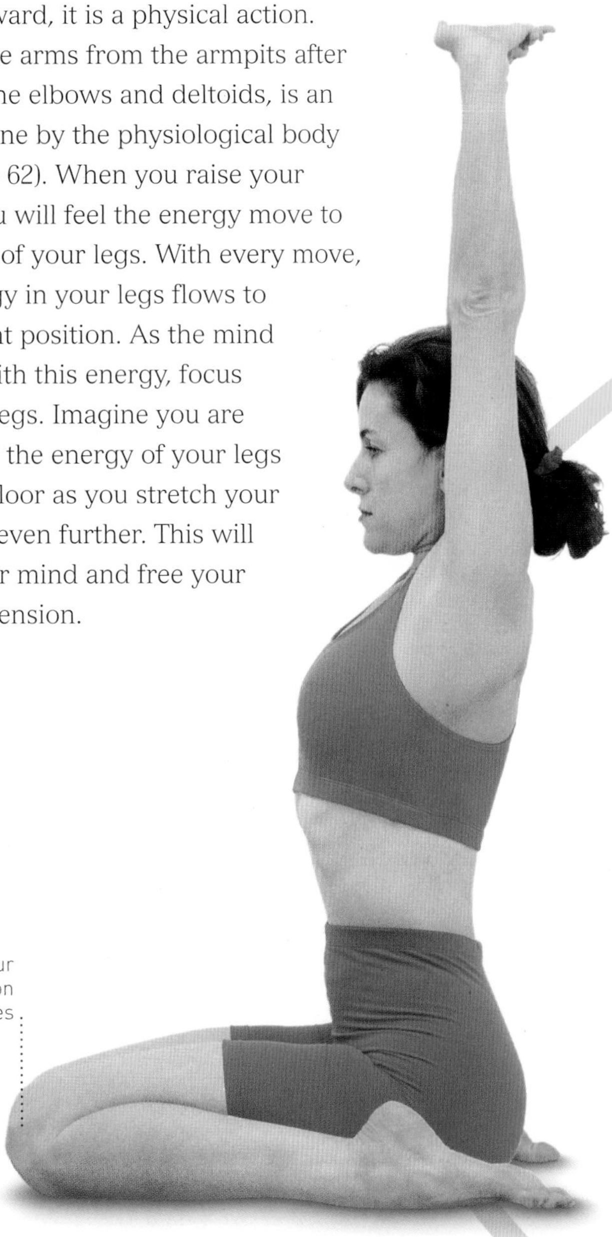

Tuck in your shoulder blades

Stretch and straighten your spine by pressing the outer buttocks downward

Rest your weight on your knees

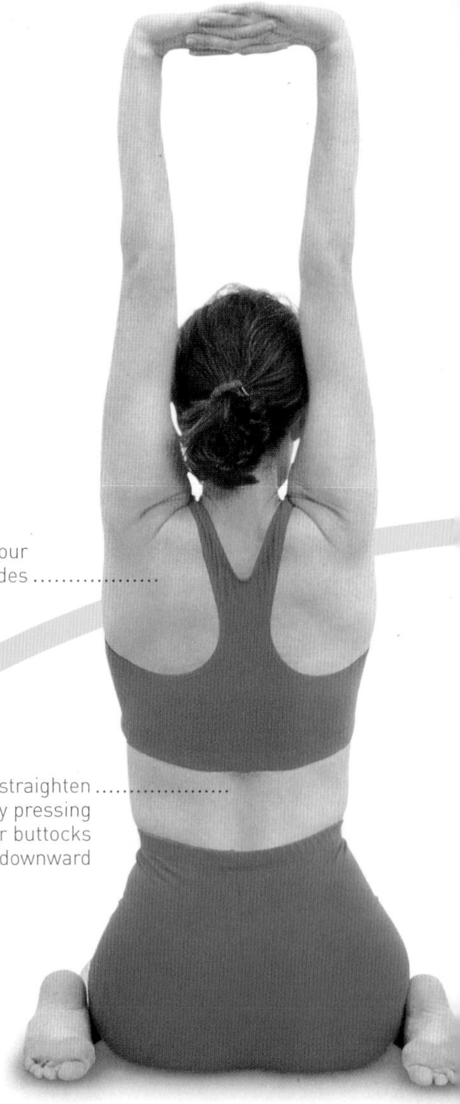

The practice o
change a
attitude in a

COMING OUT OF THE POSE

Bring your arms down to your sides. Place your palms on the floor and raise your buttocks. Kneel, and then straighten your legs, one by one.

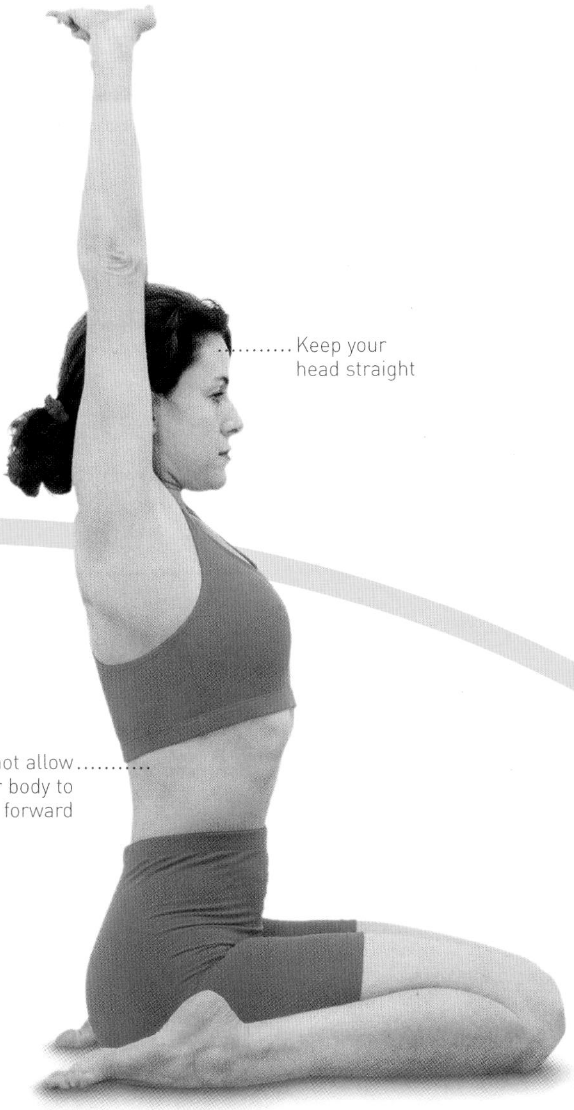

Keep your
head straight

Lock your elbows

Do not allow
your body to
lean forward

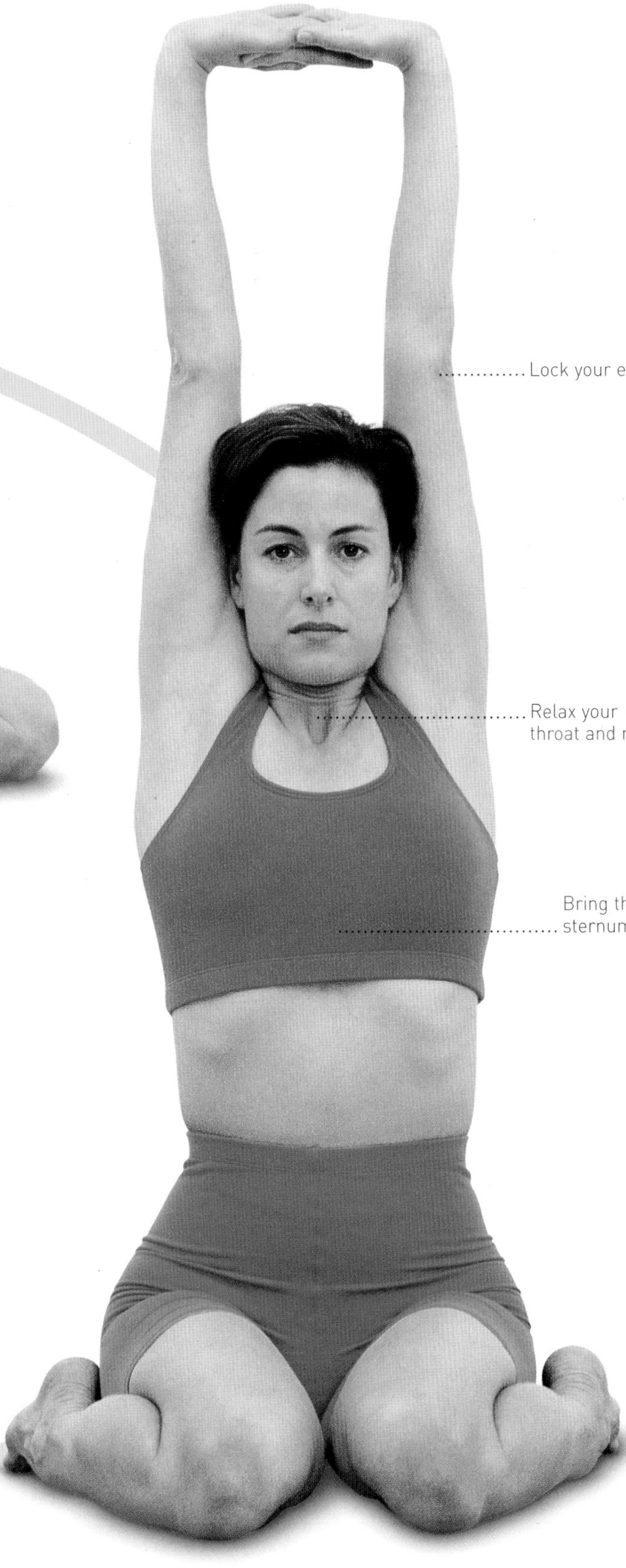

Relax your
throat and neck

Bring the
sternum forward

*yoga **helps***
*person's **mental***
positive way.

BADDHAKONASANA
Fixed angle pose

In Sanskrit, baddha means "bound" or "caught" and *kona* translates as "angle." Regular practice of Baddhakonasana increases the flow of blood to the abdomen, pelvis, and back. It helps to treat arthritis of the knee, hip, and pelvic joints. Pregnant women will experience less pain during labor and will be free of varicose veins if they hold the pose for a few minutes each day.

● BENEFITS

Keeps the kidneys and prostate gland healthy
Helps treat urinary tract disorders
Reduces sciatic pain
Prevents hernia
Relieves heaviness and pain in the testicles, if practiced regularly
Keeps the ovaries healthy
Corrects irregular menstruation
Helps open blocked fallopian tubes and reduces vaginal irritation
Relieves menstrual pain and checks heavy menstruation

● CAUTIONS

Do not practice this asana if you have a displaced or prolapsed uterus.

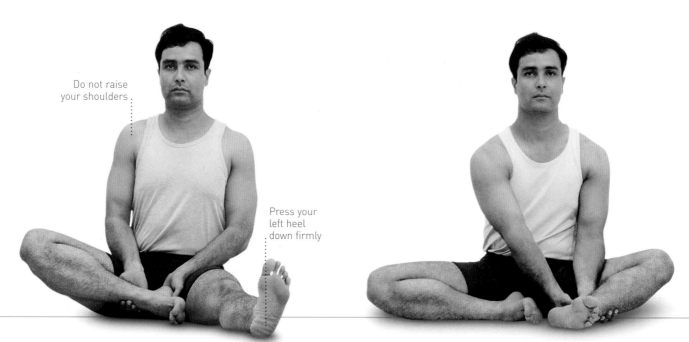

Do not raise your shoulders

Press your left heel down firmly

1 Sit in Dandasana (*see page* 102). Bend your right knee and hold your right ankle and heel with both hands. Draw your right foot toward your groin. Keep your left leg straight and resting on the floor.

2 Bend your left knee the same way as your right knee. Pull your left foot toward your groin, until the soles of both feet touch each other. Make sure that both heels touch the groin. Rest the outer edges of both feet on the floor.

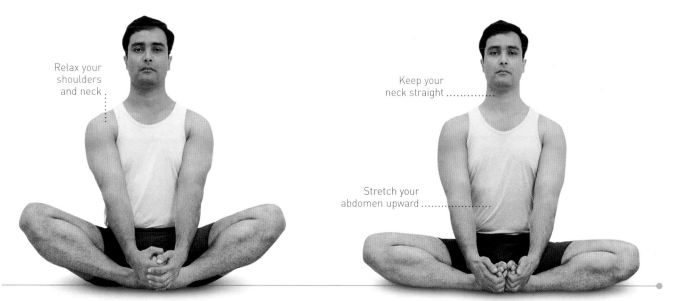

Relax your shoulders and neck

Keep your neck straight

Stretch your abdomen upward

3 Hold your feet firmly near the toes with both hands. Pull your heels even closer to your groin. Stretch your spine upward. Widen your thighs and push your knees down toward the floor. Look straight ahead. Stay in this position for 30-60 seconds.

INTERMEDIATES Maintain your hold on your feet— the firmer your grip, the better the lift of the torso. Stretch out both sides of your chest.

4 Push both your knees down by pressing your thighs firmly down on the floor. Stretch your knees away from the torso (*see inset*). This will also help bring them down to the floor. Then, pull your heels back to the groin and relax your groin. Press your ankles and shins down to the floor and push your soles lightly toward each other. Straighten both your arms by stretching your torso upward even further. Breathe evenly.

BEGINNERS It is difficult, at first, to bring your knees down to the floor. Focus on your groin and consciously relax it.

"You can practice this asana at any time, even just after a meal."

Make sure both sides of your torso are parallel

Press your knees to the floor

5 Take your hands behind your back and place both palms on the floor. Keep your fingers pointing toward your buttocks. Push your shoulders back. Stay in this pose for 30-60 seconds, breathing deeply.

BADDHAKONASANA

ADVANCED WORK IN THE POSE 360° VIEW

Once you are comfortable in the final pose, learn to open your chest, stretching it outward from all sides. Imagine that your legs are tied to the floor, so that you raise your front ribs and lift your torso without disturbing the position of your lower limbs. Then, focus on your kidneys—imagine you are pulling them into your body. Keep your back absolutely straight. Inhale and exhale deeply, feeling your energy flow from the bottom of your chest, over your shoulders and down along the spine into the abdomen in one continuous, cyclical flow. Gradually increase the length of time you stay in this pose to 5 minutes.

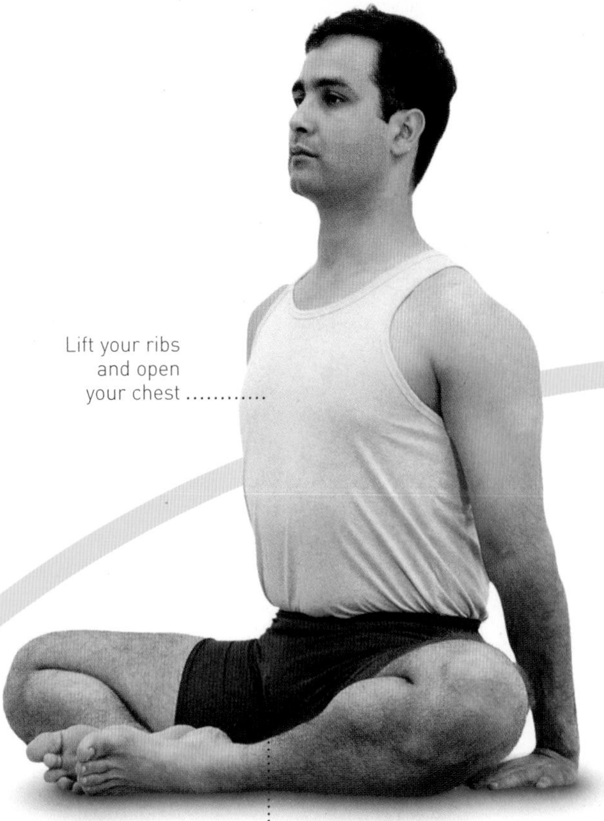

Lift your ribs and open your chest ....

Keep your groin relaxed

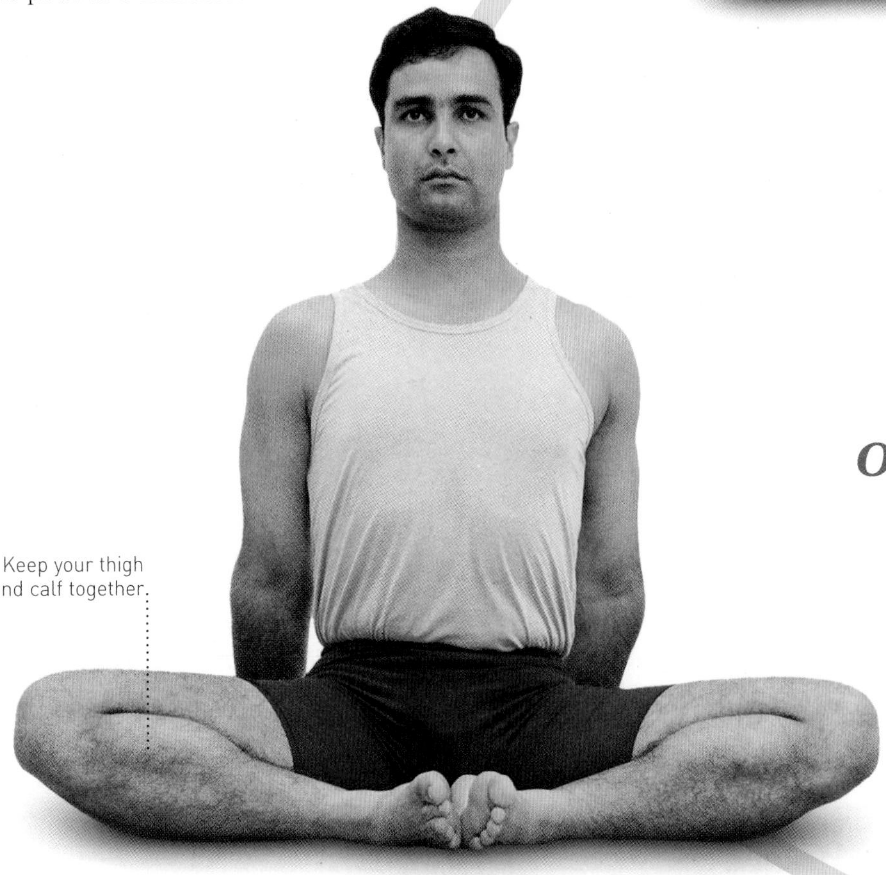

All of us have
of divinity in u.
fanned into

Keep your thigh and calf together.

COMING OUT OF THE POSE

Relax your arms and bring them forward to rest on either side of your body. Raise one knee at a time, then straighten your legs, one by one. Return to Dandasana.

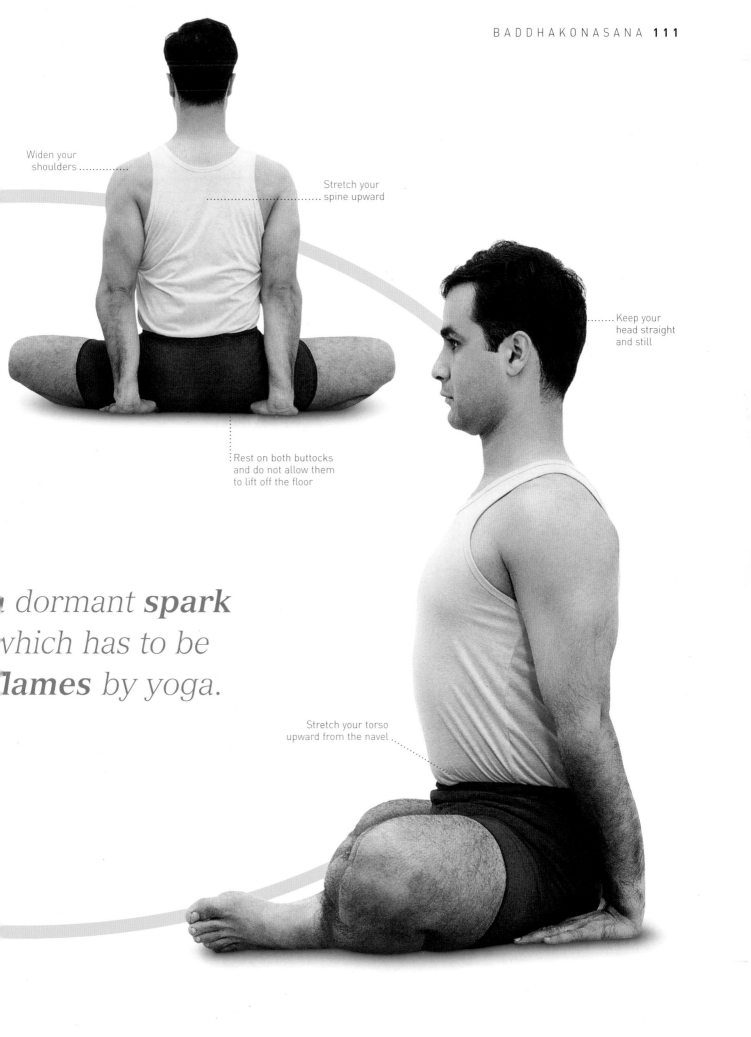

Widen your
shoulders ....

Stretch your
.... spine upward

.... Keep your
head straight
and still

Rest on both buttocks
and do not allow them
to lift off the floor

dormant **spark**
which has to be
lames *by yoga.*

Stretch your torso
upward from the navel ....

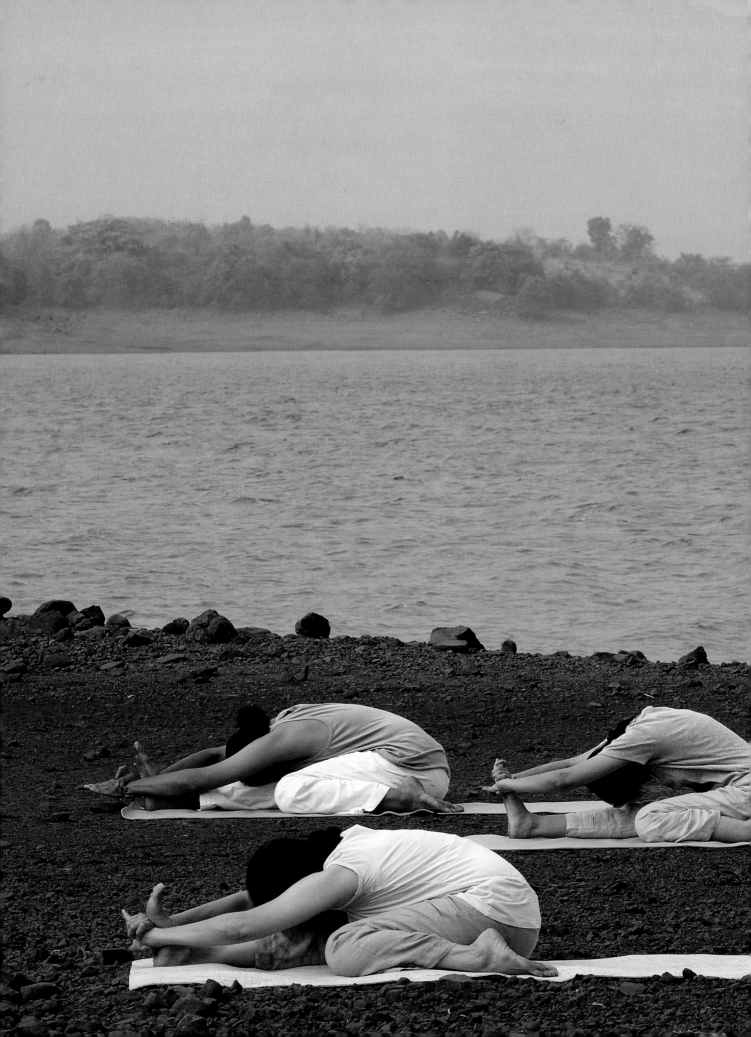

FORWARD BENDS

*"Practice asanas by **creating space** in the **muscles** and **skin**, so that the **fine network** of the **body** fits into the **asana**."*

JANU SIRSASANA
Head on knee pose

In Sanskrit, the word for "knee" is *janu*, while "head" translates as *sirsa*. Practicing this head-on-knee pose has a dynamic impact on the body and has many benefits. It stretches the front of the spine, eases stiffness in the muscles of the legs, and in the hip joints. It increases the flexibility of all the joints of the arms, from the shoulders to the knuckles.

● BENEFITS

Eases the effects of stress on the heart and the mind
Stabilizes blood pressure
Gradually corrects curvature of the spine and rounded shoulders
Eases stiffness in the shoulder, hip, elbow, wrist, and finger joints
Tones the abdominal organs
Relieves stiffness in the legs and strengthens the muscles of the legs

● CAUTIONS

To protect your hamstring muscles from damage, always open out the knee of the outstretched leg completely, extending it evenly on all sides. Do not allow the thigh of the same leg to lift off the floor.

Stretch your arms from the armpits to the fingertips ....

Extend the length of your spine .

1 Sit in Dandasana (*see page* 102). Bend your right knee and move it to the right. Pull your right foot toward your perineum until the big toe touches the inside of your left thigh. Make sure that your bent knee is pressed firmly down to the floor. Push back the bent knee until the angle between your legs is more than 90°. Keep your left leg straight. It should rest on the exact center of the left calf.

2 Stretch your left foot so that it feels as if the sole has widened, but keep your toes pointing straight up. Push the right knee even further away from your body. Then, lift your arms straight up above your head, with the palms facing each other. Stretch your torso up from the hips. Continue the stretch through your shoulders and arms.

3 Exhale, and bend forward from your hips, keeping the lower back flat. For a more effective stretch, push your torso down toward your waist to relax the spinal muscles. Stretch your arms toward your left foot and hold the toes.

BEGINNERS If you cannot reach your toes, stretch as far along the leg as you can, holding on to your knee, shin, or ankle. Gradually, with practice, you will learn to stretch each part of your body separately—the buttocks, the back, the ribs, spine, armpits, elbows, and arms. Focus on keeping your left thigh, knee, and calf on the floor. Always press down on your thigh, not on your calf.

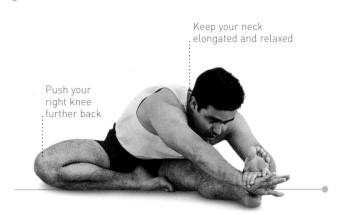

Push your
right knee
further back

Keep your neck
elongated and relaxed

"Forward bends like Janu Sirsasana rest the frontal brain and heart."

4 Now increase the stretch. Exhale and extend your arms beyond your left foot. Hold your right wrist with your left hand. Adjust your position—stretch the spine, press the right knee down to the floor. Keep your arms straight and lift your chest. Hold this position for 15 seconds, breathing evenly.

5 Exhale, and stretch your torso further toward the toes. Bring your forehead to your left knee, or as close to it as possible. Hold the pose for 30–60 seconds.

INTERMEDIATES Try to rest your nose on your knee, then your lips, and finally, rest your chin on your leg, just beyond the kneecap.

CORRECTING YOURSELF

When in the final pose, visualize the shape of your back. If it is rounded, as shown here, only a small part of the spine at the level of the shoulders is being stretched. Lengthen and flatten the lower spine and extend your arms out from your shoulder blades.

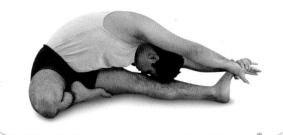

Push your torso
toward your left foot

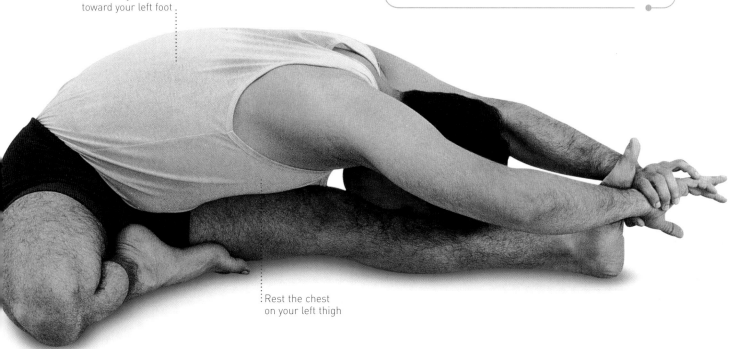

Rest the chest
on your left thigh

JANU SIRSASANA

ADVANCED WORK IN THE POSE 360° VIEW

When you are holding this pose, your sternum and abdomen should rest on the left thigh as though the leg and torso were one. One side of your back and torso might stretch more than the other—this is usually the same side as the outstretched leg. Be conscious of this, and try to equalize the stretch on both sides. Keep your elbows out, widening them to increase the expansion of your chest.

Do not allow the right side of your back to jut upward

Stretch the arms from the armpits

The **intensity** should **increase** from momen

Press your knee to the floor

Hold your wrist firmly and extend the right side of the torso

COMING OUT OF THE POSE

Inhale, then lift your head and torso slightly. After a few seconds, release your hands and sit up. Stretch out your right leg and sit in Dandasana. Now repeat the pose on the other side.

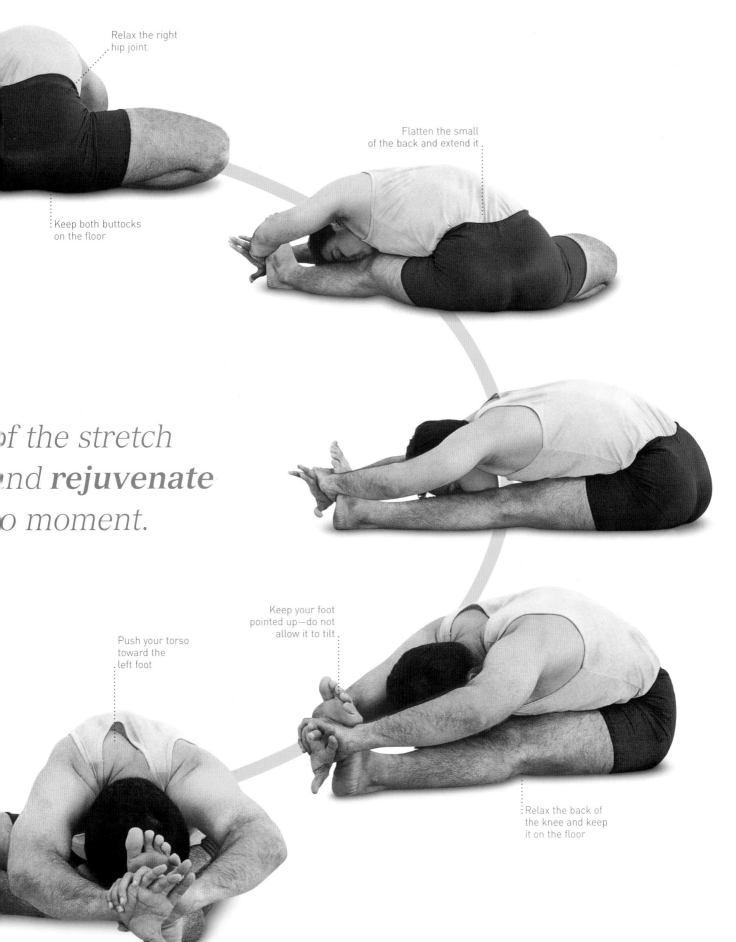

Relax the right
hip joint

Keep both buttocks
on the floor

Flatten the small
of the back and extend it

of the stretch
nd **rejuvenate**
o moment.

Keep your foot
pointed up—do not
allow it to tilt

Push your torso
toward the
left foot

Relax the back of
the knee and keep
it on the floor

TRIANGA MUKHAIKAPADA PASCHIMOTTANASANA
Three parts of the body stretch

In Sanskrit, the literal meaning of *trianga* is "three parts of the body." In this asana, the "three parts" comprise the buttocks, knees, and feet. The back of the body, which is known in Sanskrit as the *paschima* or "west," is stretched over *eka pada* or "one foot," and the *mukha* or "face" rests on the leg. Regular practice of this asana makes the whole body supple and agile.

● BENEFITS
Tones and stimulates the abdominal organs
Assists digestion and counters the effects of excess bile secretion
Reduces flatulence and constipation
Creates flexibility in the knee joints
Corrects dropped arches and flat feet

● CAUTIONS
Avoid this asana if you have diarrhea. Do not twist your torso or allow it to lean toward the outer side of your extended leg, since this could strain your spine or abdominal organs.

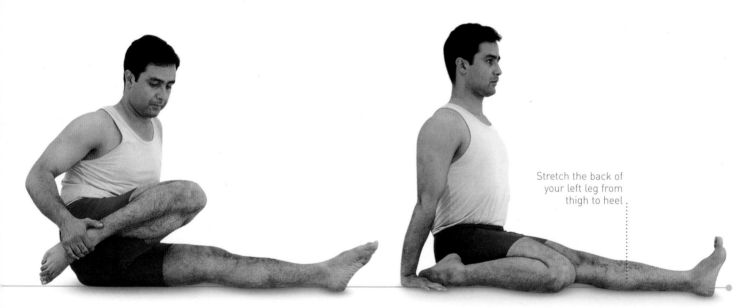

Stretch the back of your left leg from thigh to heel

1 Sit in Dandasana (*see page* 102). Bend your right leg back toward your right hip. Use your right hand to pull the ankle into place. Keep your left leg stretched out, making sure that it rests on the center of your left calf and heel.

2 Keep your thighs together. Press your right knee down on the floor. The inner side of your right calf should touch the outer side of your right thigh. Balance equally on both buttocks. Make sure that your right buttock rests squarely on the floor (*see inset*).

Rest your palms, fingers pointing forward, on the floor beside your hips.

Straighten and stretch your toes

3 Raise your arms up toward the ceiling. Extend your torso upward, and feel the stretch from your waist to your fingertips.

BEGINNERS To maintain your balance, keep the weight of your body on the bent knee. This will make sure that your torso does not tilt toward the left.

Press the shin, ankle, and metatarsals on the floor

4 Exhale, and bend forward from the waist. Stretch both arms beyond your left foot, with the palms facing each other. Ensure your thighs and knees are pressed together. Rest on both buttocks—the essence of the pose is getting this balance right.

INTERMEDIATES While you are getting into the pose, the torso has a tendency to tilt to the left. To guard against this, shift your weight to your right side. This will bring the center of gravity to the middle of your right thigh. Then, equalize your weight on both buttocks.

Push your torso forward

Stretch your arms and lock your elbows

5 Exhale, widen your elbows, and push your torso toward your left foot. Press both your wrists against the sole of your left foot, then hold your right wrist with your left hand. First, touch your forehead to your left knee, then place your nose and lips, and finally, your chin, beyond your left knee. Push your left buttock out and rest on the inside of your left buttock bone. Hold the pose for 30–60 seconds.

BEGINNERS Stretch forward as far as you can. With practice, you will learn to hook your wrists around your foot.

Do not let your torso tilt to the left

Extend your shoulders and keep your neck relaxed

TRIANGA MUKHAIKAPADA PASCHIMOTTANASANA

ADVANCED WORK IN THE POSE 360° VIEW

In the final stretch, make sure that your body weight is distributed evenly over your legs and buttocks. Both arms should be equally stretched forward. Make sure that the weight on the knee of the outstretched leg is equal to the weight borne by the bent knee. Focus on maintaining the center of gravity of this pose at the middle of the right thigh. Extend the right side of your torso from the pelvic rim toward your head. Elongate the right side of your chest and waist, and expand the side of the ribs resting on your bent knee, so that your torso stretches further forward.

Rest your sternum on your thighs

Keep the muscles of your neck soft

A yogi's brain the bottom to the top

Point your toes straight upward

Make sure that your bent knee remains pressed to the floor

COMING OUT OF THE POSE

Inhale, raise your head and torso, and wait for a few seconds. Keep your back concave. Release your hands, then sit up and straighten your right leg. Repeat the pose on the other side. Return to Dandasana.

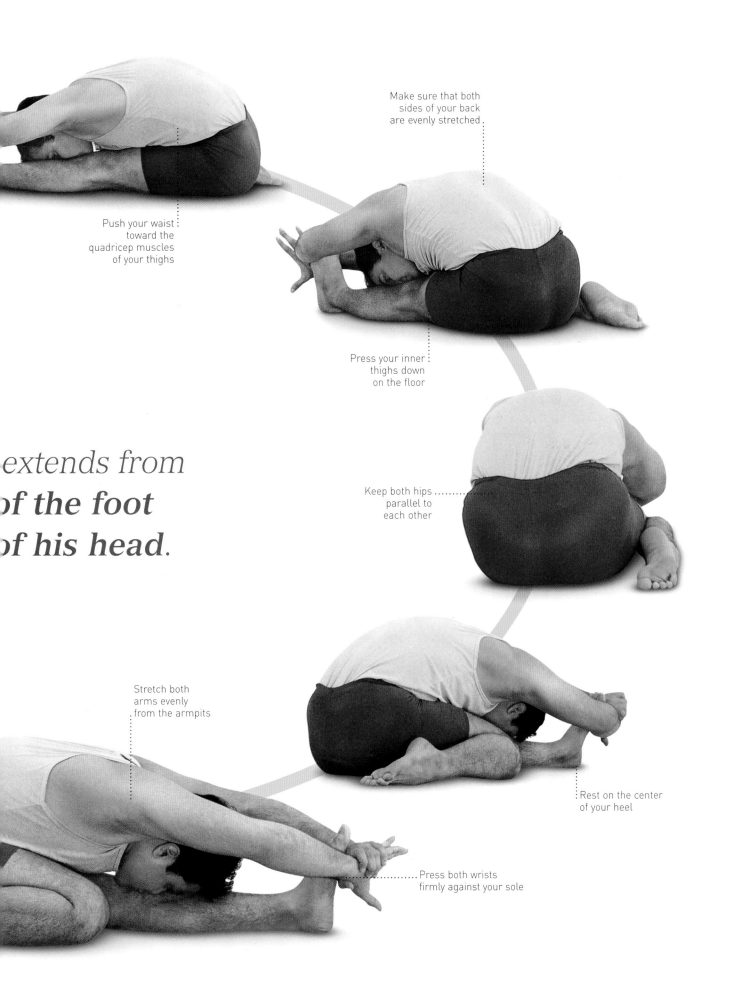

Make sure that both sides of your back are evenly stretched

Push your waist toward the quadricep muscles of your thighs

Press your inner thighs down on the floor

Keep both hips parallel to each other

extends from

of the foot

of his head.

Stretch both arms evenly from the armpits

Rest on the center of your heel

Press both wrists firmly against your sole

PASCHIMOTTANASANA
Intense back stretch

The back of your body, from your heels to your head, is known as *paschim*, which means "west" in Sanskrit. *Ut* indicates "intense," while *tan* means "stretch." This asana stretches the length of your spine, allowing the life-force to flow to every part of your body. Resting your forehead on your knees, calms the active front brain, and keeps the meditative back brain quiet, yet alert.

● BENEFITS

Rests and massages the heart
Soothes the adrenal glands
Tones the kidneys, bladder, and pancreas
Activates a sluggish liver, and improves the digestive system
Helps treat impotence
Stimulates the ovaries, uterus, and the entire reproductive system

● CAUTIONS

Do not practice this asana during, or just after, an asthmatic attack. Avoid this pose if you have diarrhea. Do not allow your thighs to lift off the floor, as the muscles at the back of your knees might rupture.

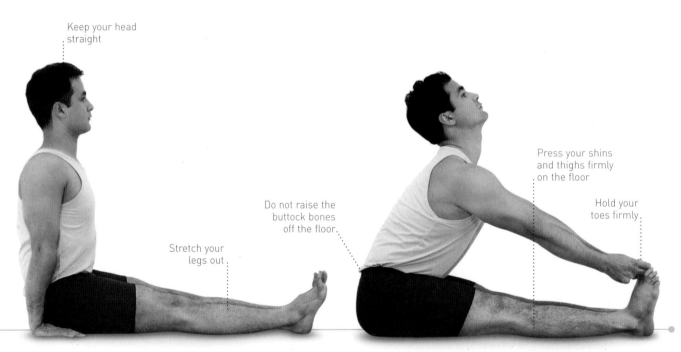

Keep your head straight

Do not raise the buttock bones off the floor.

Stretch your legs out.

Press your shins and thighs firmly on the floor

Hold your toes firmly.

1 Sit in Dandasana (*see page* 102). Keep your legs together. Stretch your heels, making sure that both are evenly pressed down. Put your palms on the floor beside your hips. Take a few deep breaths. Now, stretch your arms above your head (*see inset*), with the palms facing each other. Stretch your spine upward.

2 Exhale, and stretch your arms toward your feet. Grip the big toe of your left foot with the thumb and first two fingers of your left hand. Do the same to your right toe with your right hand (*see inset*). Press your thighs down on the floor. The pressure on your thighs should be greater than that on your calves. This helps you stretch more effectively.

BEGINNERS Focus on keeping your thighs flat on the floor. You must not allow them to lift off the floor. This is more important than holding your toes.

THE GURU'S ADVICE

"Stretch from the seat of the buttocks and feel the lightness in your buttocks. This is the heart of the perfect pose."

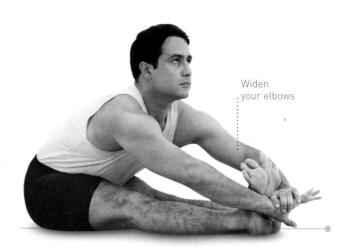

Widen your elbows

3 Make sure that you are sitting on your inner buttock bones and that your weight is distributed equally on them. Do not allow either buttock to rise off the floor. Then, hold your right wrist with your left hand.

INTERMEDIATES Hold the soles of your feet with the interlocked fingers of both hands. Breathe evenly.

4 Exhale, and lift your torso. Bend forward from your lower back, keeping your spine concave. Stretch forward from both sides of the waist. First, place your forehead firmly on your knees, and then push it toward your shins. Widen and lift your elbows. Do not allow them to rest on the floor. Hold the pose for 1 minute.

BEGINNERS Rest your forehead on a folded blanket placed on your shins.

Stretch your arms from your shoulder blades

PASCHIMOTTANASANA

ADVANCED WORK IN THE POSE **360° VIEW**

As you bend, keep your diaphragm as soft as dough. For a more effective stretch, bring your diaphragm closer to your chest as you lower your head. The front of your chest is the "brain" of this pose (*see page* 65). Bring it close to your thighs. Check that both sides of your chest are evenly stretched, so that there is a symmetry in the final pose. Press your forehead on your shins. Consciously descend your mind into the pose. Focus on your back—extend the skin of your back toward your head. Descend your spine completely. This will bring lightness and calm to the brain. Rejuvenate the stretch constantly. With practice, increase the duration of the pose to 5 minutes.

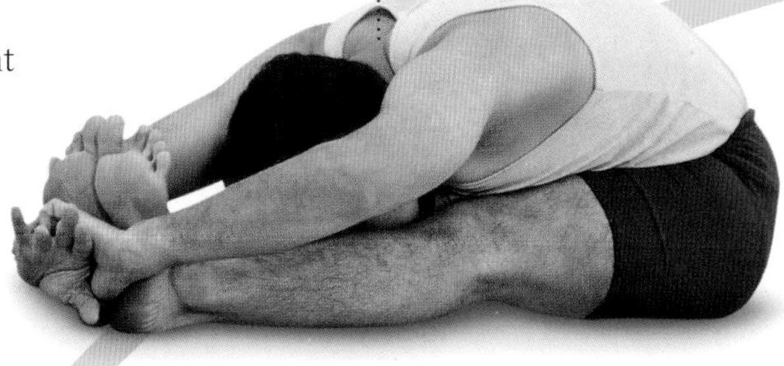

Keep the muscles of your neck passive

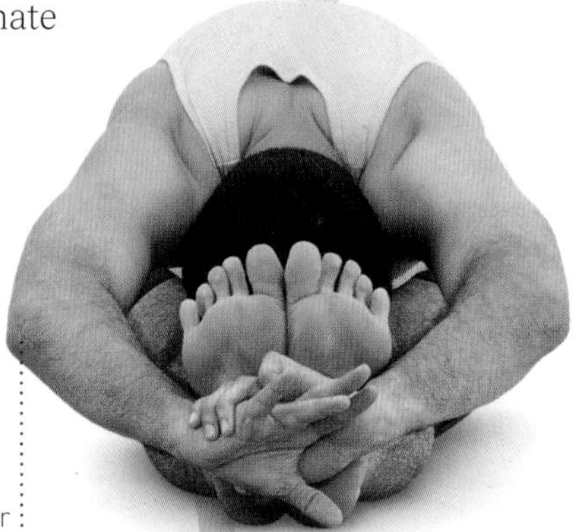

Do not let your elbows move down

The movemen
intelligence o
synchronize and

Push your feet and hands against each other

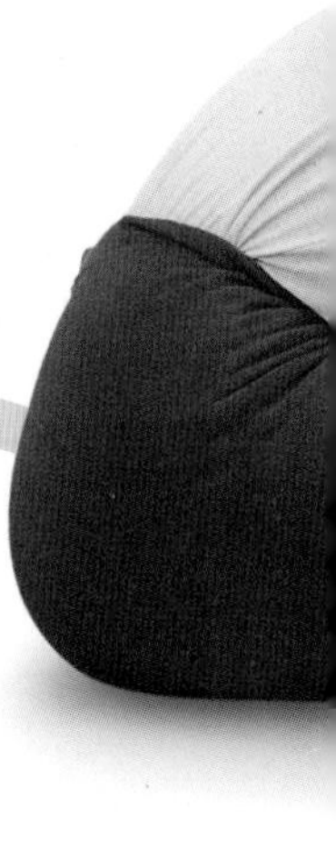

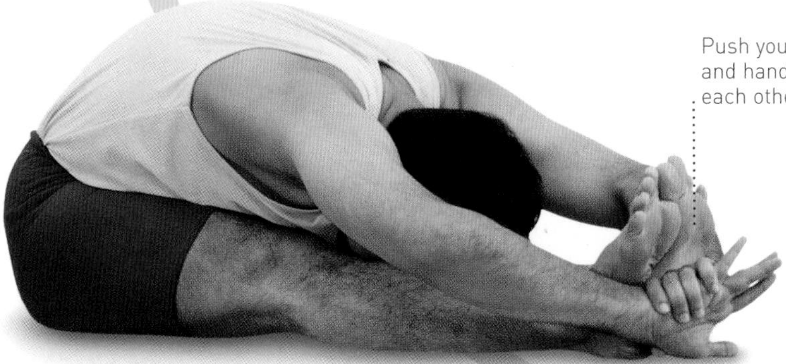

COMING OUT OF THE POSE

Inhale, then raise your head and torso, keeping your back concave. Wait for a few seconds, then release your hands. Sit up and come back to Dandasana.

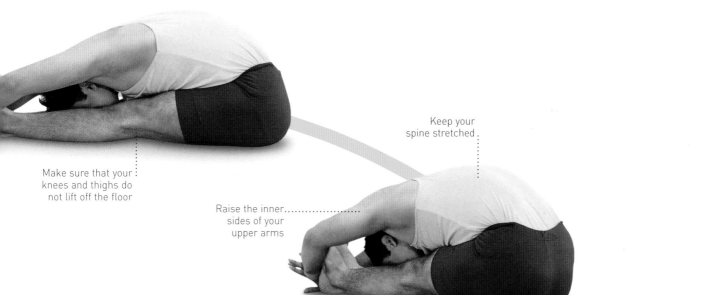

Keep your
spine stretched

Make sure that your
knees and thighs do
not lift off the floor

Raise the inner
sides of your
upper arms

of the body and the
he brain should
eep pace with each other.

Compress your hips and
keep them parallel
to each other

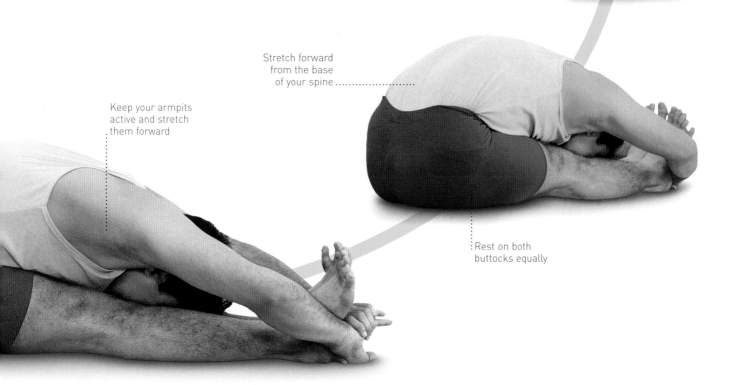

Stretch forward
from the base
of your spine

Keep your armpits
active and stretch
them forward

Rest on both
buttocks equally

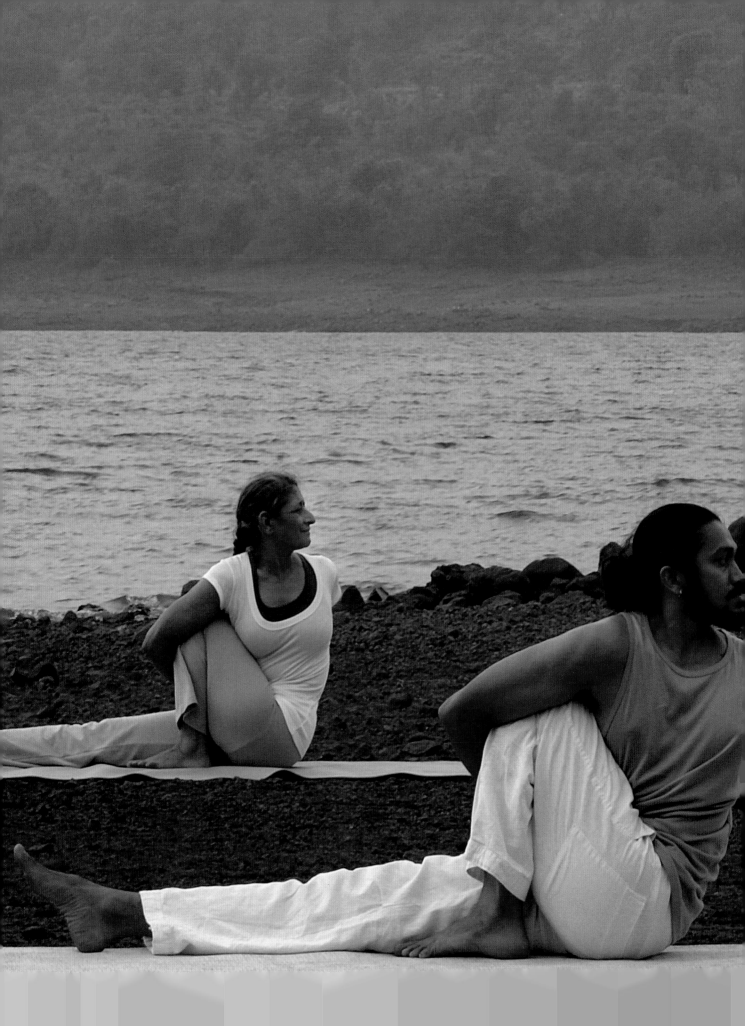

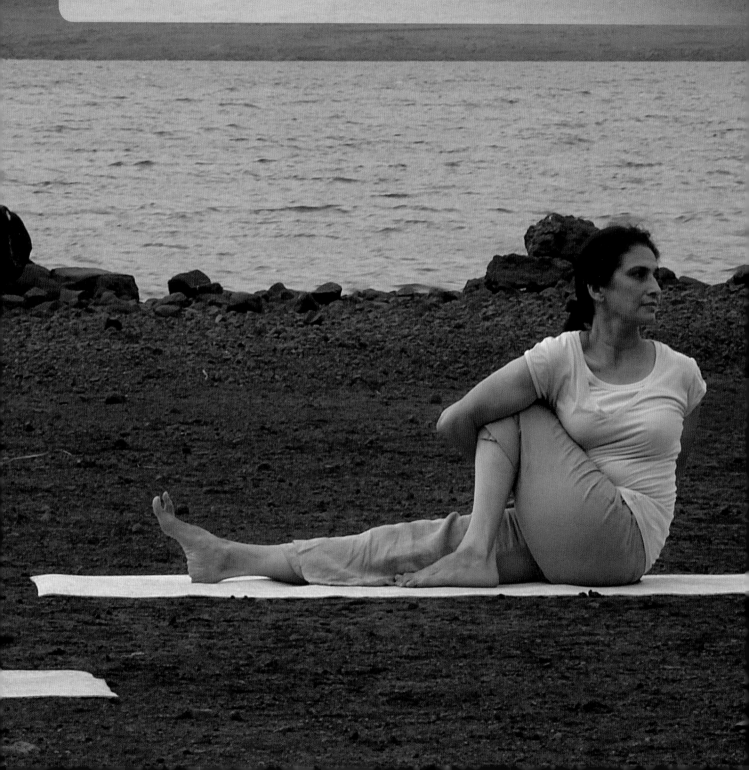

TWISTS

*"If you **practice yoga** every day with **perseverance**, you will be able to face the turmoil of **life** with **steadiness** and **maturity**."*

BHARADVAJASANA
Lateral twist of the spine

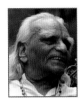

This asana is named after the ancient sage Bharadvaja, who was the father of the great warrior Dronacharya. Both are major characters in the Indian epic, *Mahabharata*. Regular practice of this asana teaches you to rotate your spinal column effectively, which increases the flexibility of your back and torso, and prepares you for the more advanced twists.

● BENEFITS

Relieves pain in the neck, shoulders, and back
Helps keep the spine and shoulders supple
Eases a painful, stiff, sprained, or fused lumbar spine
Reduces discomfort in the dorsal spine area
Increases the flexibility of the back and hips

● CAUTIONS

Do not practice this asana if you have eye strain, a stress-related headache, or a migraine. The asana should not be attempted if you have diarrhea or dysentery.

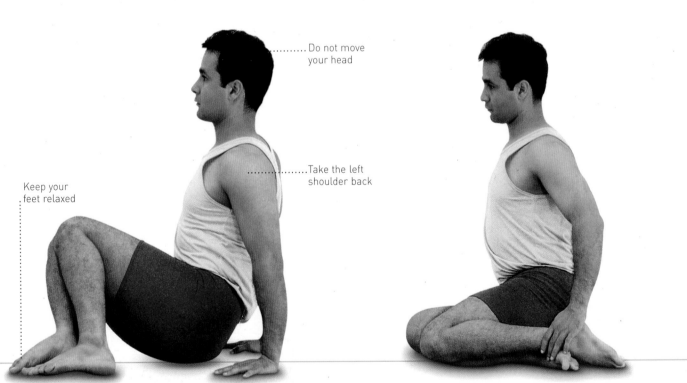

Do not move your head

Take the left shoulder back

Keep your feet relaxed

1 Sit in Dandasana (*see page* 102). Place your palms flat on the floor behind your buttocks, with your fingers pointing forward. Bend your knees, and with your legs together, move your shins to the left. Make sure that your thighs and knees are facing forward. Breathe evenly.

2 Hold your ankles and bring your shins further to the left, until both feet are beside your left hip. The front of your left ankle should rest on the arch of your right foot (*see inset*). Extend the toes of your left foot and keep your right ankle pressed down to the floor. Rest your buttocks on the floor,

not on your feet. Lift your torso, so that your spine is fully stretched upward. Pause for a few breaths.

3 Exhale, then turn your chest and abdomen to the right, so that your left shoulder moves forward to the right, and your right shoulder moves back. Place your left palm on your right knee and rest your right palm on the floor. Revolve your right shoulder blade to the back and tuck in your left shoulder blade. Take one or two breaths.

"Bharadvajasana also massages, tones, and rejuvenates your abdominal organs.

Turn your head to the right

Expand your chest fully

4 Press your right shin to the floor. This will help to lift your torso and turn it even further to the right. Rotate, until the left side of your body is in line with your right thigh. Turn your head and neck to the right. Inhale, and holding your breath, firmly press the fingertips of your right hand down on the floor. Then, exhale, and simultaneously raise and rotate your spine even more strongly to the right. Look over your right shoulder. Hold the pose for 30–60 seconds.

Keep your arm extended and lock your elbow

Press your fingertips to the floor

BHARADVAJASANA

ADVANCED WORK IN THE POSE **360° VIEW**

Once you have turned your neck and head to the right and rotated your torso, tuck in both your shoulders. Lift your sternum, keeping the spine erect as it turns on its axis. Do not change the position of your knees while turning, since they tend to move with the body. Make sure that your body does not lean back. Maintain the turn of your head and neck to the right. Keep the left hip and the left shoulder in line when you revolve your torso. Twist the spine strongly, turning it as far to the right as you can. Focus on the skin of your back. Try, consciously, to push your skin down from your neck, and pull the skin up from your lower back. Breathe evenly.

Keep both sides of your rib cage parallel

Make sure that your spine remains erect

Rest your left foot on the arch of the right foot

Keep your left shoulder in line with your right thigh

Press and lift the spine up

COMING OUT OF THE POSE
Release your hands and bring your torso to the front. Straighten your legs. Repeat the pose on the other side. Come back to Dandasana.

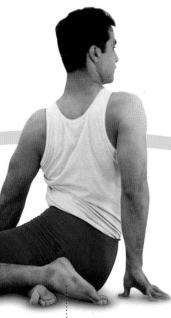

Relax the
muscles of
your neck ....

Tuck in your right
shoulder blade

Rest both feet
on the floor

Do not allow
your torso to
lean back ....

Press your knees
down and keep
them facing forward .

Look over your................
right shoulder

.... Keep both sides of
the chest level

MARICHYASANA
Torso and leg stretch

This asana is dedicated to the sage, Marichi. His father was Brahma, creator of the universe, and his grandson was the sun god, Surya, the giver of life. Regular practice of the asana stretches your entire body and rejuvenates it. Marichyasana increases your levels of energy.

● BENEFITS

Increases energy levels
Tones and massages the abdominal organs
Improves the functioning of the liver, spleen, pancreas, kidneys, and intestines
Reduces fat around the waistline
Alleviates backache
Relieves lumbago

● CAUTIONS

Do not practice this asana if you have diarrhea or dysentery. Avoid this pose if you have a headache, migraine, insomnia, or when you are feeling fatigued. Do not practice during menstruation.

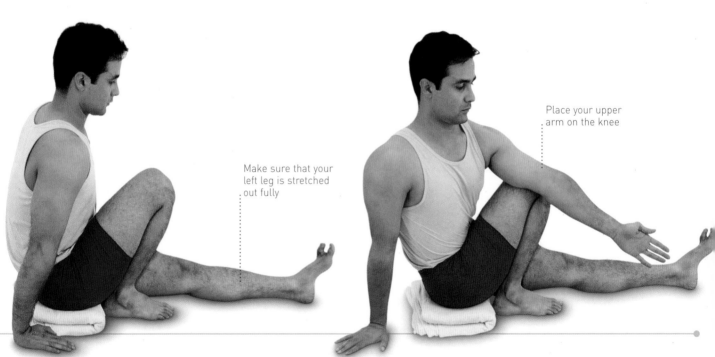

Make sure that your left leg is stretched out fully

Place your upper arm on the knee

1 Sit on a folded blanket (*see page* 185) in Dandasana (*see page* 102). Bend your right knee, and pull your right foot toward its own thigh so that your right heel touches your right buttock. Keep the toes pointing forward and press the foot down on the floor. Place your palms on the floor, beside your buttocks, fingers pointing forward.

2 Exhale, and lift your spine. Turn your torso 90° to the right. Bend the left arm and, moving your left shoulder forward, stretch it out against your right thigh. Extend this arm from the armpit to the elbow—this is crucial to the final stretch. Do not allow your left leg to tilt to the left. Your weight should not fall on your right palm.

3 Press your right ankle down on the floor and turn your torso further to the right. Push your left armpit against the outer side of the right knee. This will help you rotate your torso more effectively. Make sure that you turn from your waist first, and then the chest. Exhale, and encircle your right knee with your left arm.

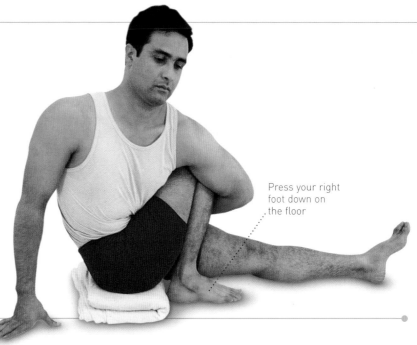

Press your right foot down on the floor

"The asana also massages and tones your abdominal organs."

There should be no gap between your armpit and thigh

4 Exhale, and lift your right palm off the floor. Take your right arm behind your back. Bend it, and bring it toward the left hand. First hold the fingers, then the palm, and finally the wrist, of the left hand with your right hand (*see inset*). Lift your torso and rotate further to the right. Turn your head to the left and look

over your shoulder. Hold the pose for 20–30 seconds, breathing evenly.

Intensify the stretch of your left leg

MARICHYASANA

ADVANCED WORK IN THE POSE **360° VIEW**

This asana requires spinal action. Do not turn from your arms, but from your spine. The torso has a tendency to lean to the right in this pose, so consciously keep the left side of your body higher than the right. Stretch and lift the front of your spine. Bring your waist—and not just your chest—close to the middle of your right thigh. The entire length of the left side of your torso should be in contact with your right thigh. Bring your arms closer to each other and intensify your grip. The upper part of your right arm is the "brain" of the pose (*see page* 65), so keep it completely stable.

Push your right shoulder blade into your spine

Keep intensifying the grip of your fingers

Move your whole body closer to the bent knee

Keep the muscles of your neck relaxed

Your chest should touch the length of your right thigh

COMING OUT OF THE POSE

Inhale, and holding your breath, rotate your spine to straighten it. Turn your head to face the front. Release your hands and straighten your leg. Repeat the pose on the other side. Return to Dandasana.

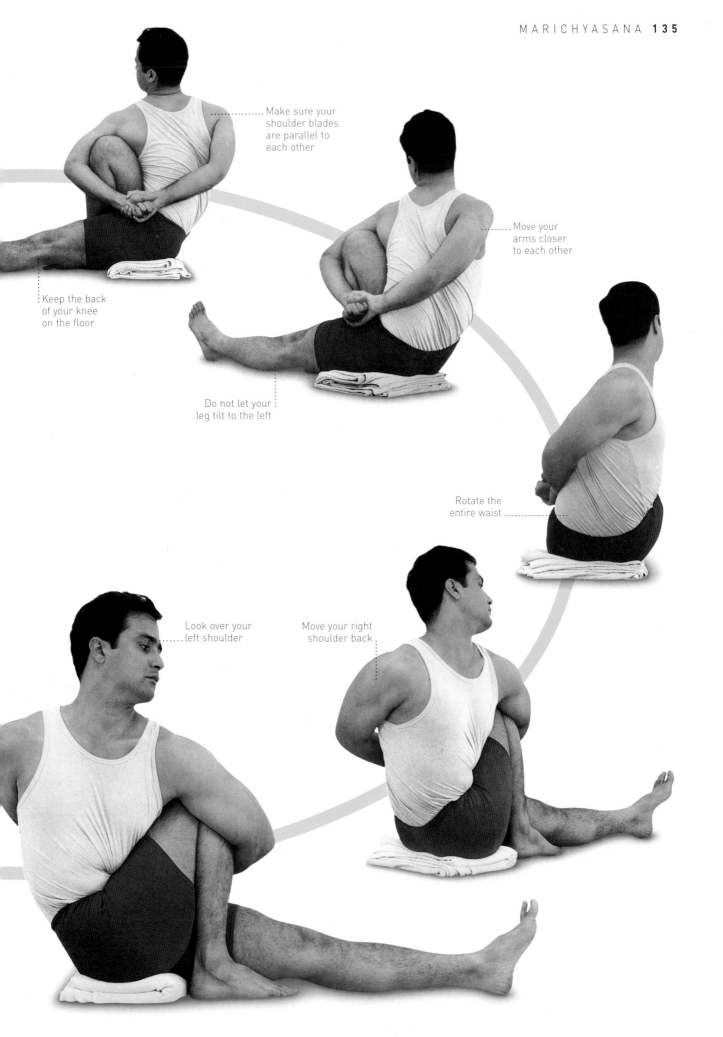

Make sure your shoulder blades are parallel to each other

Keep the back of your knee on the floor

Move your arms closer to each other

Do not let your leg tilt to the left

Rotate the entire waist

Look over your left shoulder

Move your right shoulder back

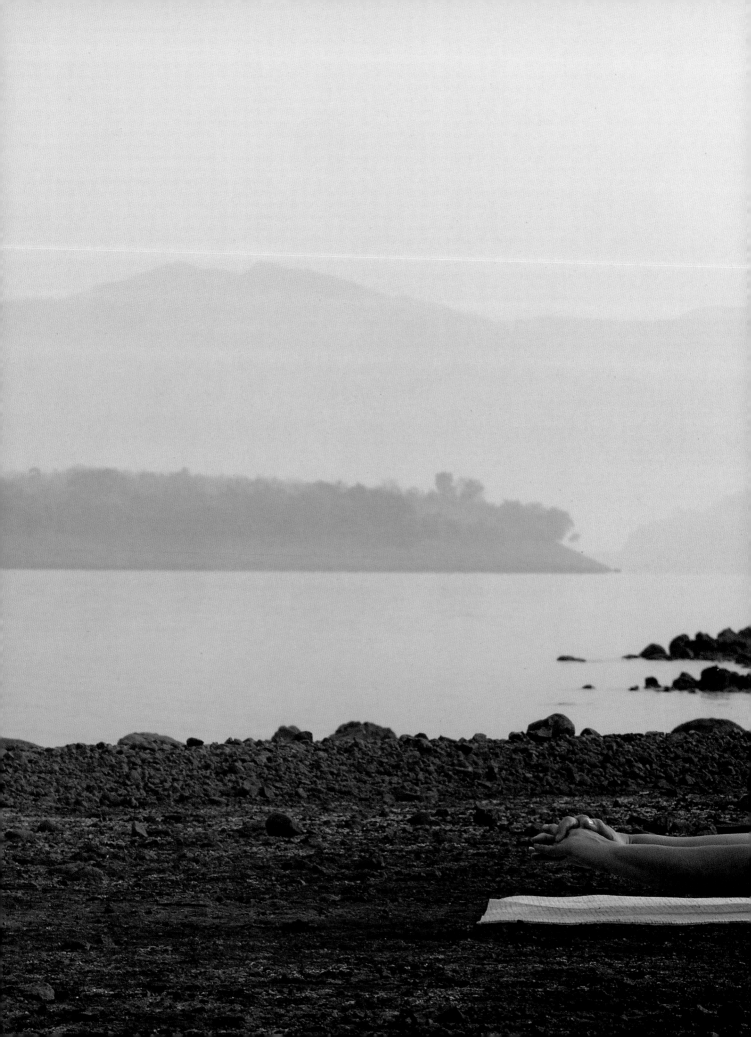

INVERSIONS

*"The practice of asanas **purges** the body of its impurities, bringing **strength**, firmness, **calm**, and **clarity** of **mind**."*

SALAMBA SIRSASANA
Headstand

The headstand is one of the most important yogic asanas. The inversion in the final pose brings a rejuvenating supply of blood to the brain cells. Regular practice of this asana widens your spiritual horizons. It enhances clarity of thought, increases your concentration span, and sharpens memory. This asana helps those who get mentally exhausted easily. In Sanskrit, *salamba* means "supported" and *sirsa* translates as "head."

● BENEFITS

Builds stamina
Alleviates insomnia
Reduces the occurrence of heart palpitations
Helps cure halitosis
Strengthens the lungs
Improves the function of the pituitary and pineal glands
Increases the hemoglobin content in the blood
Relieves the symptoms of colds, coughs, and tonsillitis
Brings relief from digestive and eliminatory problems, when practiced in conjunction with Salamba Sarvangasana

● CAUTIONS

Do not practice this asana if you have high blood pressure, cervical spondylosis, a backache, headache, or a migraine. Do not start your yoga session with this pose if you have low blood pressure. Perform the asana only once in a session and do not repeat it—your body should not be overworked. Do not practice this asana during menstruation.

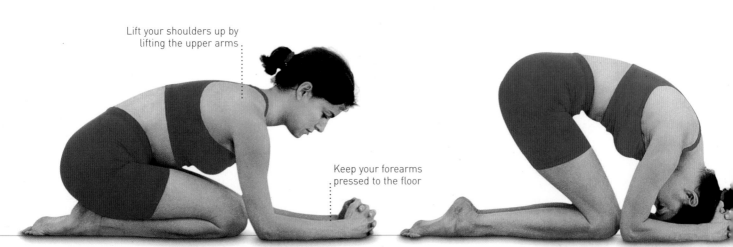

Lift your shoulders up by lifting the upper arms

Keep your forearms pressed to the floor

1 Kneel on the floor in Virasana (*see page* 104). Clasp the inside of your left elbow with your right hand and the inside of your right elbow with your left hand. Now lean forward and place your elbows on the floor. Make sure that the distance between your elbows is not wider than the breadth of the shoulders. Release your hands and interlock your fingers to form a cup with your hands (*see inset*). Keep your fingers firmly locked, but not rigid. Place your joined hands on the floor.

2 Place the crown of your head on the floor, so that the back of the head touches your cupped palms. Check that only the crown is resting on the floor, not the forehead, or the back of the head. In the final pose, your weight must rest exactly on the center, not the back or front, otherwise, the pressure will fall on your neck or eyes, causing your spine to bend. Make sure that your little fingers touch the back of the head, but are not underneath it. Hold this position for a few seconds, breathing evenly.

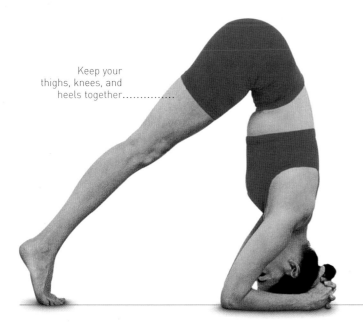

Keep your thighs, knees, and heels together..............

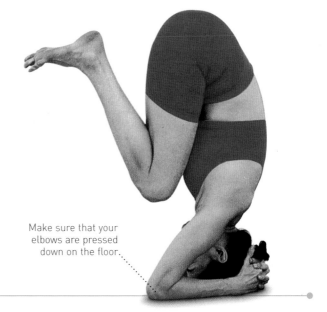

Make sure that your elbows are pressed down on the floor...

3 Push up on the balls of your feet and straighten your knees. Keep your heels raised off the floor. To ensure that your torso is perpendicular to the floor, walk your feet toward your head, until the back of your body forms a vertical line from your head to the back of the waist.

4 Exhale, and bring your knees toward the chest. Then, press your toes down on the floor, and push your legs upward, off the floor. This action resembles a hop and gives you the thrust to raise your legs. Bring your heels close to your buttocks.

BEGINNERS Practice this asana against a wall (*see box below*).

SALAMBA SIRSASANA AGAINST A WALL

BEGINNERS Practice against a wall. Place a folded blanket against the corner. Then follow Steps 1–3 (*see left and above*). Make sure that your cupped hands are placed not more than 2–3 in (5–8 cm) from the wall. If not, your weight will fall on your elbows, causing your spine to bend and your eyes to protrude. Follow Steps 4, 5, and 6 shown here. Initially, ask someone to help you raise your legs off the floor. To come out of the pose, follow the instructions on page 142 or reverse Steps 4–6.

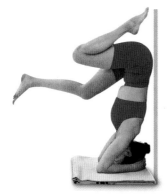

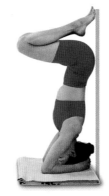

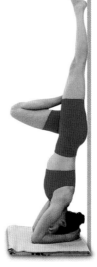

4 Once your torso is positioned perpendicular to the floor, rest your hips against the wall. Now bend your knees and raise your right foot off the floor with a swing. The swing should be such that the thigh and knee are at buttock level. Repeat this swing with the left leg.

5 In this position, your hips and the balls of your feet rest against the wall. Adjust your body in the pose—press your elbows to the floor and stretch your upper arms. Follow the stretch through the armpits and along the torso to the waist.

6 Straighten your legs, one by one, until your hips, legs, and heels rest against the wall. With practice, bring your hips away from the wall and let your head, arms, and torso bear your weight. Constant support of the wall will bend your spine.

SALAMBA SIRSASANA

"This asana helps those who get mentally exhausted easily."

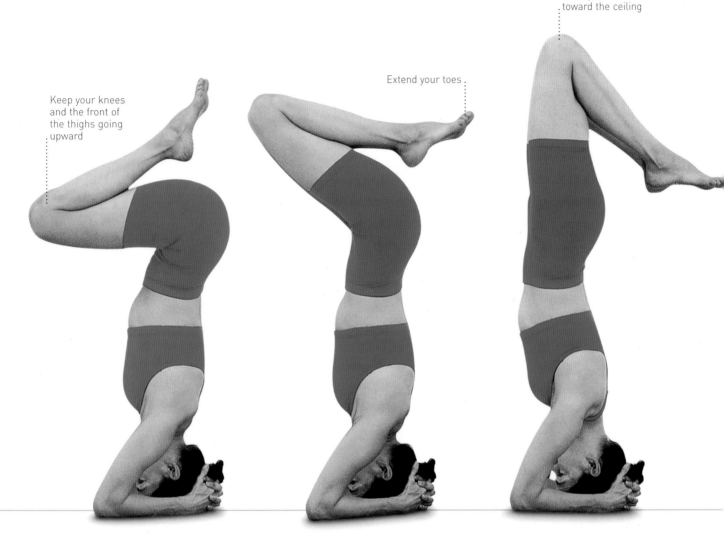

Keep your knees and the front of the thighs going upward

Extend your toes

Point your knees toward the ceiling

5 Press your elbows to the floor and lift your shoulders up, away from the floor (*see inset*). Exhale, and gently swing your knees upward in a smooth arc, until both your thighs are parallel to the floor. In this position, the entire upper body, from the head to the waist and hips, should be perpendicular to the floor. Do not

 move your elbows until you come out of the final pose.

6 Continue to move the knees upward, slowly bringing them to point to the ceiling. Keep the heels close to the buttocks. Focus on your balance and do not allow your torso to move during this action. Steps 5, 6, and 7 constitute a gentle, continuous movement, as you raise your legs toward the ceiling.

7 Once your knees are pointing to the ceiling, hold the pose for a few breaths. Make sure that the spine is straight. Tighten the buttocks. Make sure that your thighs are positioned perpendicular to the floor, your lower legs bent toward your back. Check that your shoulders do not tilt. Pause and get used to the feel of the position.

.... Stretch the backs
of your knees
and thighs

Tighten the
quadricep
muscles ....

Expand
your chest ....

CORRECTING YOURSELF

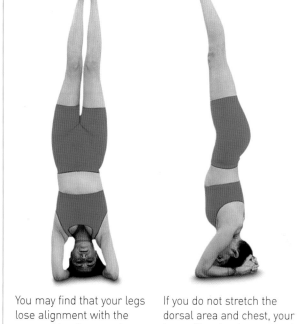

You may find that your legs
lose alignment with the
torso, either by wavering to
the right or left. Check the
position of your elbows and
tighten your knees.

If you do not stretch the
dorsal area and chest, your
legs will swing forward and
your buttocks jut back,
When this happens, your
weight falls on your
elbows, not your head.

8 Straighten your knees to bring the lower legs in
line with the thighs, so that your body forms a
vertical line. Point your toes toward the ceiling.
Tighten both knees, as in Tadasana (*see page 68*),
and keep your thighs, knees, and toes together. The
entire body should be balanced on the crown, not
on the forearms and hands, which should simply
support the balance in the pose. Stretch your upper
arms, torso, and waist upward, along the legs to
the toes, ensuring that your torso does not tilt.
Steadiness and a constant lift of the shoulders
ensure stability in the posture. Hold the pose for 5
minutes, breathing evenly.

SALAMBA SIRSASANA

ADVANCED WORK IN THE POSE **360° VIEW**

As you hold the pose, stretch your whole body, from the upper arms to the toes. Lift and widen the sternum so that your chest expands equally on all sides. Tighten your knees and bring your legs to the median plane. This will ensure that they are perpendicular to the floor. Pull the abdominal muscles in and toward the waist to extend the lower spine. You must practice this asana from the spine, not the brain. Balance is the key to this asana, not strength. You must develop the skill to balance effortlessly on the small surface area of the crown. This brings a feeling of lightness to the brain and complete relaxation to each part of the body.

Extend the backs of the knees and stretch your shins

Stretch the biceps and deltoids up

Lengthen the spine from the neck to the tailbone

Elongate the inner sides of your legs

Relax the fingers but keep them firmly locked

COMING OUT OF THE POSE

Keep your legs straight and close together. Lower them until your toes rest on the floor. Bend the knees, kneel, and sit on your calves. Rest your forehead on the floor. Stay in this position for a few seconds before sitting up in Virasana.

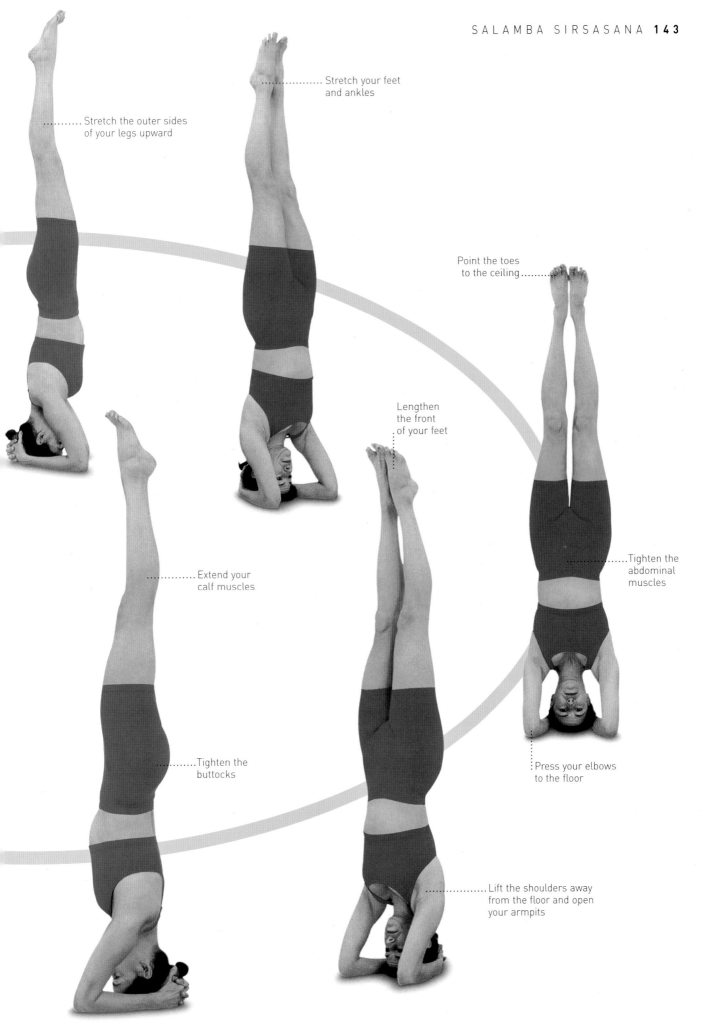

Stretch the outer sides of your legs upward

Stretch your feet and ankles

Point the toes to the ceiling

Lengthen the front of your feet

Extend your calf muscles

Tighten the abdominal muscles

Tighten the buttocks

Lift the shoulders away from the floor and open your armpits

Press your elbows to the floor

SALAMBA SARVANGASANA
Shoulderstand

Practicing this asana integrates your mind with your body and soul. Your brain feels bright yet calm, your body feels light and infused with radiance. The inverted pose allows fresh, healthy blood to circulate around your neck and chest. This alleviates bronchial disorders and stimulates the thyroid and parathyroid glands.

● BENEFITS

Alleviates hypertension
Relieves insomnia and soothes the nerves
Improves the functioning of the thyroid and parathyroid glands
Alleviates asthma, bronchitis, and throat ailments
Relieves breathlessness and palpitations
Helps treat colds and sinus blockages
Improves bowel movements and relieves colitis
Helps treat hemorrhoids
Alleviates urinary disorders
Helps treat hernia
Helps treat a prolapsed uterus and reduces uterine fibroids
Relieves congestion and heaviness in the ovaries, and helps treat ovarian cysts
Reduces menstrual cramps and helps regulate menstrual flow, if done regularly between two menstrual periods

1 Place a mat on 3 folded blankets, one on top of the other, (*see page* 184) on the floor. Lie down with your neck, shoulders, and back on the blankets. Rest your head on the floor. Stretch your legs and tighten your knees. Push the inner sides of your legs toward your heels. Press the outer sides of your shoulders down on the blankets. Raise your upper spine, but push your lower spine down on the blankets. Stretch your arms out close to your body, palms facing the ceiling. Make sure that your wrists touch your body. Raise and expand your sternum without moving your head.

Lift your sternum

Rest on the back of your head

Keep your toes, heels, and ankles together

2 Roll your shoulders back and pull in your shoulder blades. Turn your upper arms out slightly and stretch the inner sides of your arms toward the little fingers of each hand. Exhale, and bend your knees.

Relax the muscles of your face

● CAUTIONS
Do not practice this pose during menstruation. People with high blood pressure should only attempt this asana immediately after holding the pose of Halasana (*see page* 150) for at least 3 minutes.

3 Without moving the upper part of your body, exhale and raise your hips and buttocks off the floor. Bring your knees over your chest.

BEGINNERS If you find it difficult, at first, to raise your hips off the floor, ask a helper to hold your ankles and push your bent legs toward your head. At the same time, lift your hips and back off the floor and come to the final pose. Keep your body firm, and rest your back against your helper's knees. Alternatively, once you have been helped to raise your legs off the floor, follow Steps 5, 6, and 7 on the next page.

.... Keep your knees together

"Salamba means "propped up" in Sanskrit, while sarvanga indicates "all the limbs" of the body."

Tighten your buttocks .

.... Keep your shins pressed together

4 Place your palms on your hips and keep your elbows pressed firmly down on the blankets. Lift your torso until your buttocks are perpendicular to the floor. Bring your knees toward your head.

SALAMBA SARVANGASANA

CORRECTING YOURSELF

If your legs tilt to the right or left in the final pose, bend your knees and move your waist so that it aligns with your chest. Then, straighten your legs again.

If your torso tilts forward, you will feel a heaviness in your chest and find it difficult to breathe. Push up your waist, thighs, and hips, and do not allow your buttocks to drop.

.... Stretch and open the soles of your feet

Press your fingers into your back ....

5 Now, slide your hands down to the middle of your back, so that your palms cover your kidneys (*see inset*). Point your thumbs toward the front of your body and your fingers toward the spine. Exhale, and raise your torso, hips, and knees, until your chest touches your chin. Breathe evenly.

6 Raise your feet toward the ceiling. Only the back of your neck, shoulders, and upper arms should rest on the blankets. Make sure that your body is perpendicular to the floor, from the shoulders to the knees.

THE GURU'S ADVICE

"Do not throw the legs back, but raise them slowly. Turn the inner calves outward and extend the skin of the outer legs up toward the heels."

Stretch your legs from your groin to your toes

Pull up your pelvic rim

Keep your palms close to your shoulder blades

Rest your elbows squarely on the blankets

Keep your eyes on your chest

7 Press both palms into your back and straighten and stretch your body from the armpits to the toes. Your spine must be absolutely straight. Keep both elbows close to your body, as this keeps your chest expanded. To raise your torso further, release your palms, then press them into your back again. This will push your chest up further. Lift your body from the back of your neck, and not your throat. Push both shoulders back, to relax and stretch your neck. Extend your inner and outer legs toward the ceiling. Do not allow your legs to waver back and forth. Hold the pose for 2–3 minutes. Continue to breathe evenly.

SALAMBA SARVANGASANA

ADVANCED WORK IN THE POSE **360° VIEW**

Create life in your spine. The energy in your spine should flow into your body through your fingers. Keep your eyes on your sternum, as this reinforces your will power and steadies your mind. Press your thumbs into the muscles of your back to push them toward the spine. This compresses the back. In the asana, your back should be narrow and your chest broad. Do not allow your elbows to spread outward. Bring them together, since too wide a distance between them makes your chest concave. Keep the bridge of your nose aligned with the middle of your sternum. Move your shoulders back. Focus on your inner legs, and stretch them toward the ceiling. This is a subtle and difficult action, but can be achieved over time. With practice, increase the duration of the pose to 5 minutes. Breathe evenly.

Contract your kneecaps evenly from all sides ....

Keep your shoulders back—away from your head ....

.... Keep your sternum straight

COMING OUT OF THE POSE

Exhale, and bend your legs at the knees. Bring your thighs toward the stomach, then gently lower your buttocks and back toward the floor. Release the hands and bring them to your sides. Lie on the floor and relax your whole body.

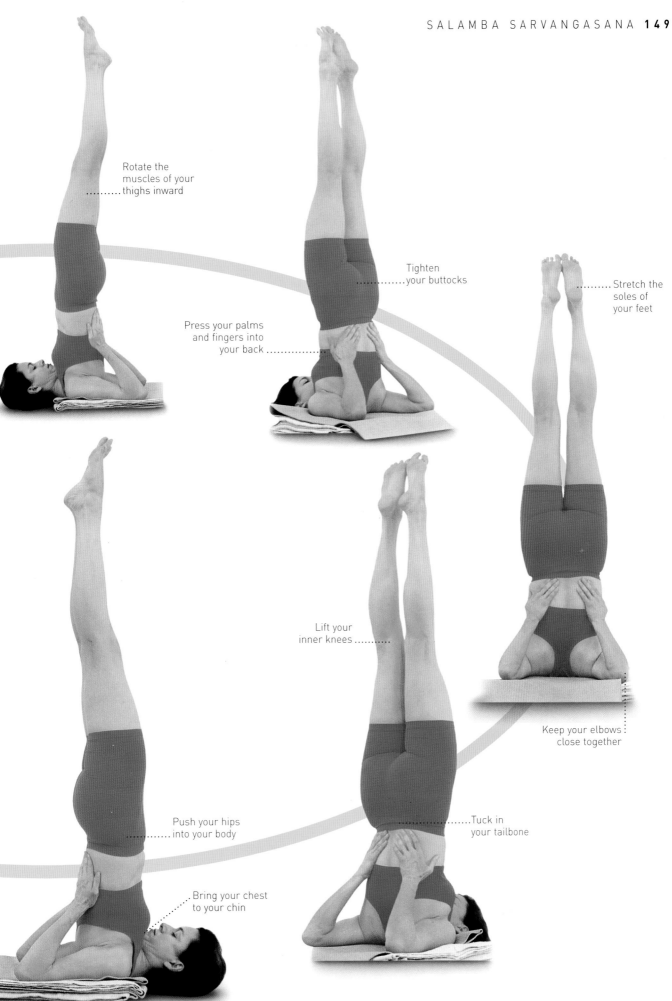

Rotate the
muscles of your
thighs inward

Press your palms
and fingers into
your back

Tighten
your buttocks

Stretch the
soles of
your feet

Keep your elbows
close together

Lift your
inner knees

Tuck in
your tailbone

Push your hips
into your body

Bring your chest
to your chin

HALASANA
Plough pose

In this asana, your body takes the shape of a plough—*hala* is the Sanskrit word for "plough." Practicing Halasana regularly helps to increase your self-confidence and energy. The asana helps to restore calm and clarity of mind after a long illness. Halasana alleviates the effects of stress and strain by resting and relaxing your eyes and brain.

● BENEFITS

Relieves fatigue and boosts energy levels
Controls hypertension
Rejuvenates the abdominal organs and improves digestion
Lengthens the spine, and improves its alignment
Helps treat hernia and hemorrhoids, if practiced with legs separated
Relieves pain or cramps in the fingers, hands, wrists, elbows, and shoulders, if practiced with arms and interlocked fingers extended toward the legs

1 Place two folded blankets, covered by a mat (*see page* 184), on the floor. Lie down with your back, neck, and shoulders resting on the blankets. Keep your legs stretched out and tightened at the knees. Focus on your inner legs and stretch from your thighs to your heels. Place your arms by your sides, with your palms flat on the floor.

Rest your head on the floor

● CAUTIONS

Do not practice this asana if you have ischemia, cervical spondylosis, or diarrhea. Avoid this pose during menstruation. If you are prone to headaches, migraines, asthma, breathing difficulties, high blood pressure, physical and mental fatigue, or are overweight, practice Halasana with props (*see page* 232) and with your eyes closed.

Keep your knees together

2 Exhale, lift your buttocks off the floor, and bring your knees to your chest. Keep your arms straight and press your fingers firmly down on the floor. Push your shoulders back and broaden your chest.

Interlock your fingers firmly

Straighten and stretch your arms

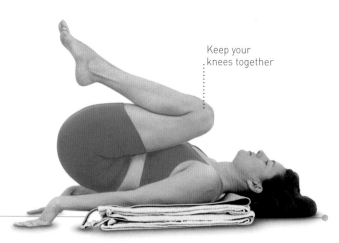

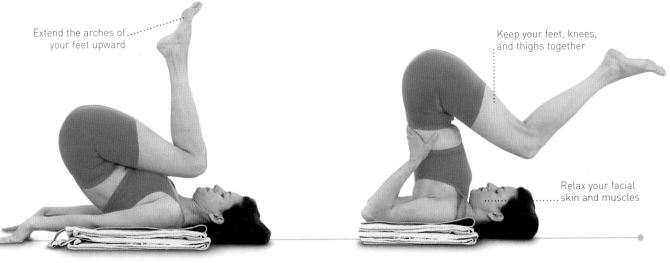

Extend the arches of your feet upward

Keep your feet, knees, and thighs together

Relax your facial skin and muscles

3 Raise your hips and buttocks toward the ceiling in a smooth, rolling action. Bring your knees close to your chin and raise your lower legs, until your shins are perpendicular to the floor.

BEGINNERS Once you have raised your buttocks off the floor, ask a helper to hold your ankles and push your legs toward your head.

4 Bend your elbows. Place your hands on the small of your back (*see inset*). Raise your hips and buttocks even further, until your torso is perpendicular to the floor and your thighs are positioned above your face. Bring your bent knees over your forehead, before you lower your legs to the floor. Breathe evenly.

Tighten your buttocks

5 Swing your hips and buttocks over your head, until they are perpendicular to the floor and in line with your shoulders. Slowly straighten your legs, and lower them until your toes rest on the floor. Raise your chest, bringing your sternum to touch your chin. Stretch your arms out behind your back on the blankets. Then interlock your fingers firmly at the knuckles, rotating your wrists until your hands point toward the ceiling. Stay in the pose for 1–5 minutes. Breathe evenly.

BEGINNERS Initially, stretch your arms out toward your feet. Once you are comfortable in this pose, stretch your arms out behind your back.

Open both sides of the chest

Do not bend your knees

Press your toes down on the floor

HALASANA

ADVANCED WORK IN THE POSE **360° VIEW**

As you hold this pose, make sure that your brain is not tense. Consciously relax the skin and muscles of your face. Keep your gaze on your chest—do not look up. Drop your eyes down in their sockets, since this helps relax the facial muscles. Your neck should be completely soft, since this rests the brain. Remember that your throat is the site of the Vishuddhi chakra (*see page 57*). If it tightens, your brain will become tense. Lift your sternum and chest to relax your throat and ensure smooth and effortless breathing. Increase the space between your navel and diaphragm.

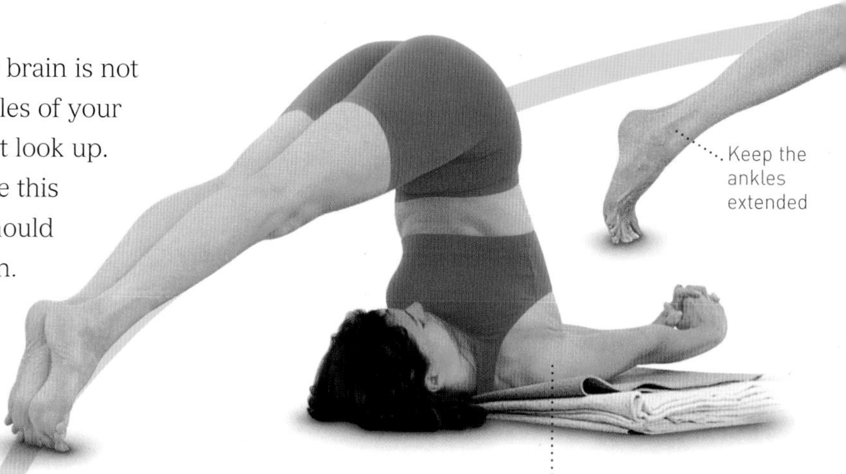

Keep the ankles extended

Push your shoulders into your body

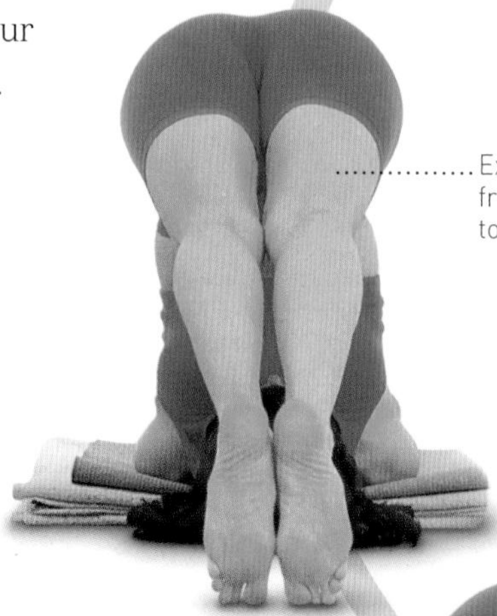

Extend your legs from the buttocks to the heels

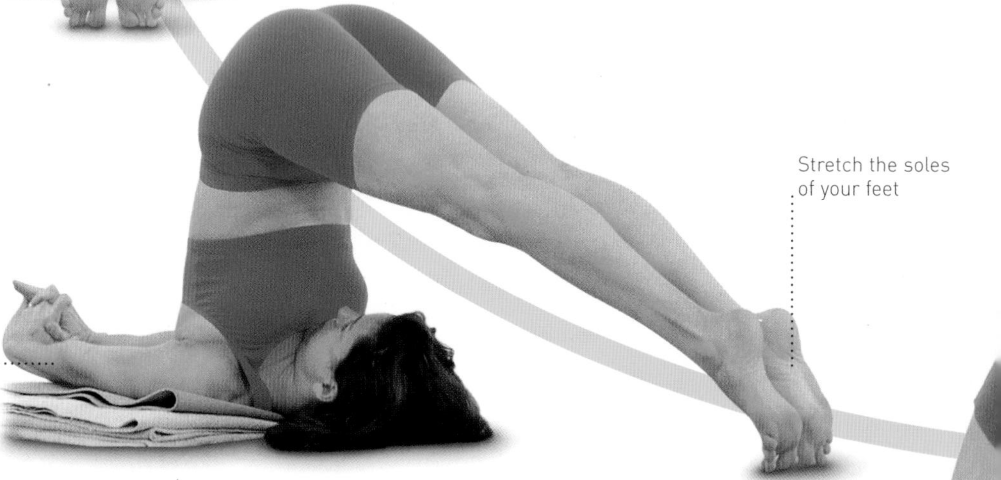

Stretch the soles of your feet

Press the arms downward

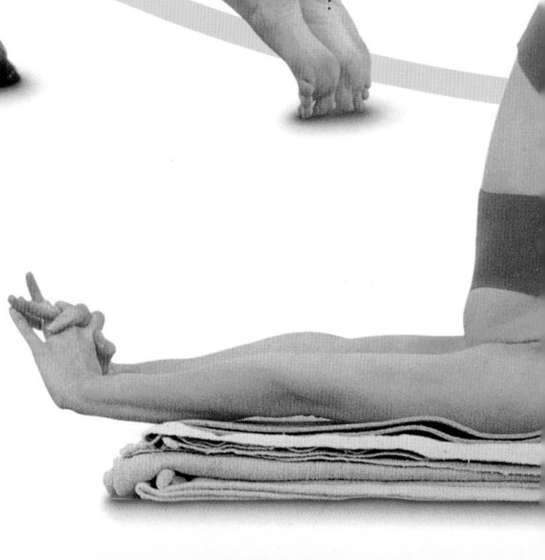

COMING OUT OF THE POSE

Slowly, and with control, lift your legs off the floor. Bring your thighs and knees toward your stomach. Push your buttocks back and lower them to the floor. Flatten your back and relax your entire body, breathing deeply.

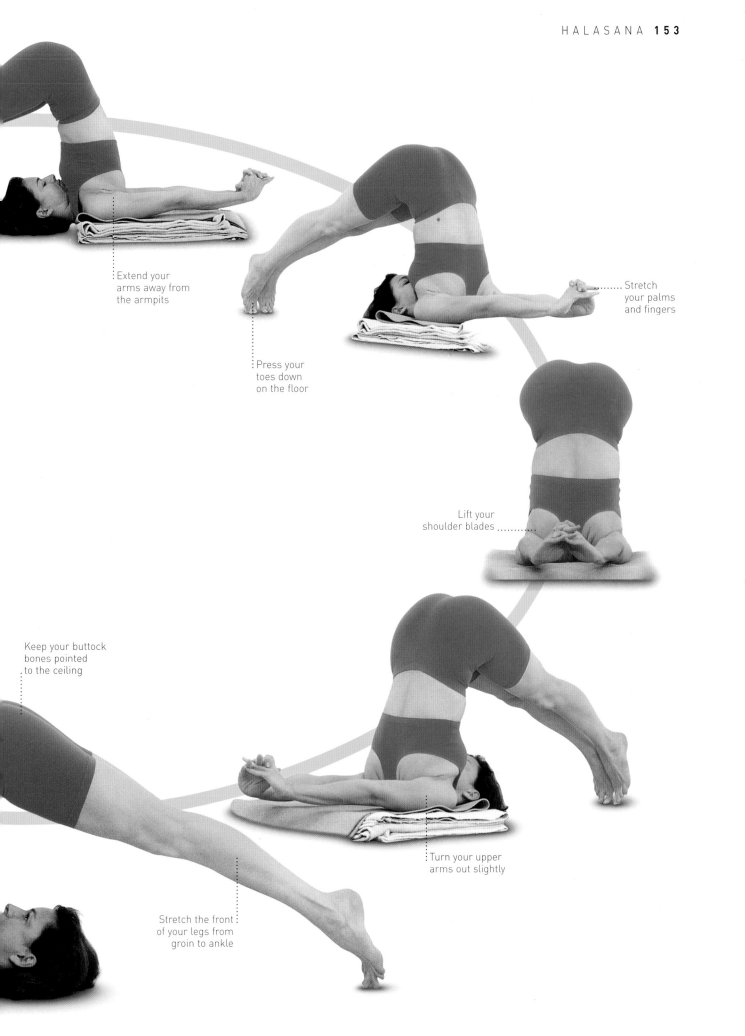

Extend your arms away from the armpits

Press your toes down on the floor

Stretch your palms and fingers

Lift your shoulder blades

Keep your buttock bones pointed to the ceiling

Turn your upper arms out slightly

Stretch the front of your legs from groin to ankle

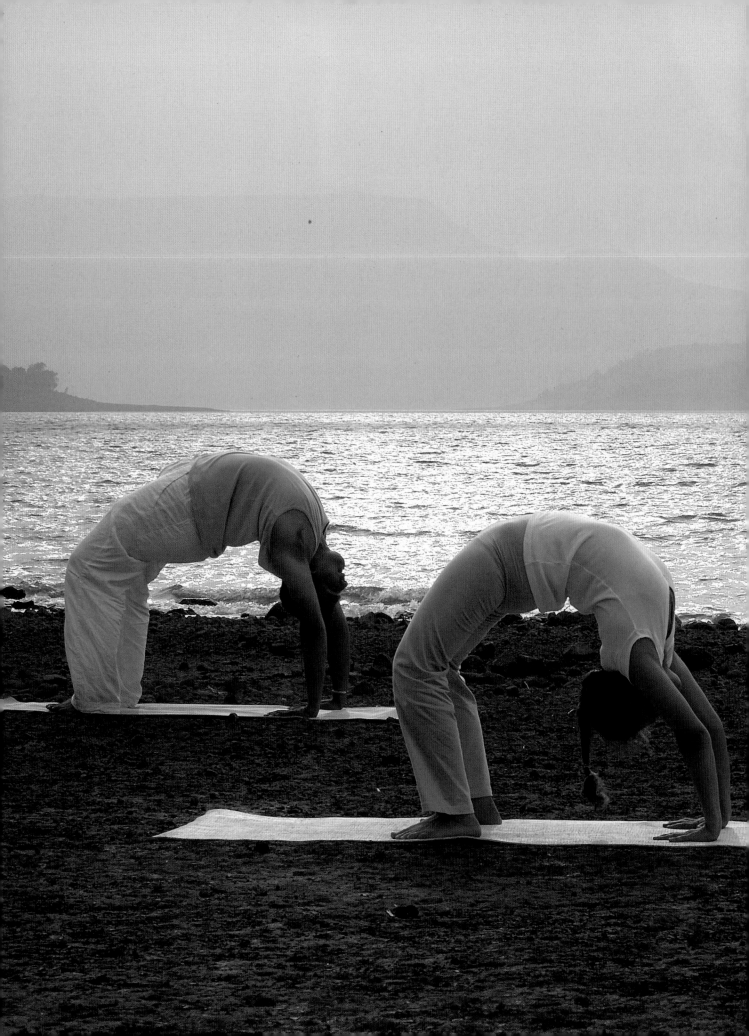

BACK BENDS

*"Asanas **penetrate** deep into each **layer** of the **body** and ultimately into the **consciousness** itself."*

USTRASANA
Camel pose

In this asana, you bend back until the shape of your body resembles that of a camel—*ustra* means "camel" in Sanskrit. Ustrasana is recommended for beginners, as well as for the elderly, because the balance of the final pose is relatively easy to attain. The asana also helps people in sedentary occupations, whose work entails bending forward for long periods.

● BENEFITS

Helps correct posture
Increases lung capacity
Improves blood circulation to all the organs of the body
Tones the muscles of the back and spine
Removes stiffness in the shoulders, back, and ankles
Relieves abdominal cramps
Regulates menstrual flow

● CAUTIONS

Do not practice this asana if you have severe constipation, diarrhea, headaches, migraines, or hypertension. For a heart attack, practice Ustrasana with props (*see page* 240).

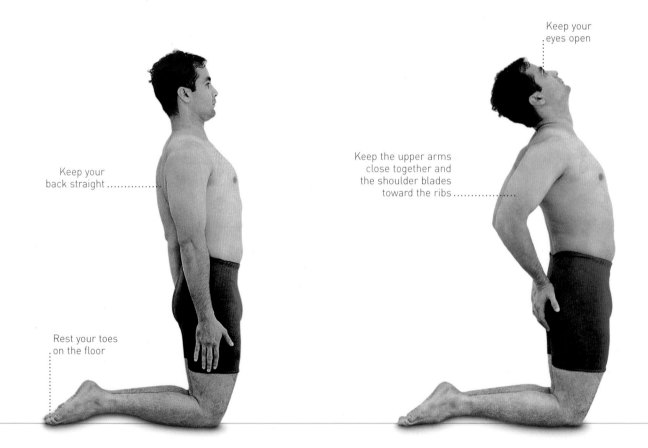

Keep your back straight

Rest your toes on the floor

Keep your eyes open

Keep the upper arms close together and the shoulder blades toward the ribs

1 Kneel on the floor with your arms by your sides. Keep your thighs, knees, and feet together. Rest on the front of your feet, with the toes pointing to the back. Keep your torso upright and breathe evenly.

BEGINNERS If keeping your knees together leads to a feeling of strain in your thighs, practice with your knees slightly apart. This also allows for a freer movement of the spine.

2 Exhale, and place your palms on your buttocks. Push your thighs forward slightly and then pull them up toward your groin. Push your spine into your body. Then, gradually bend your back, and lower it toward the floor. Simultaneously, extend your rib cage and broaden your chest. Continue to breathe evenly.

3 Push your shoulders back and stretch your arms from your shoulders toward your feet. Inhale, throw your head back, and hold both heels with your hands. Make sure that your thighs are perpendicular to the floor. Push your spine down toward your legs and breathe evenly.

BEGINNERS Initially, hold one heel at a time by tilting each shoulder individually.

Expand your chest

"Practicing the asana regularly will relieve stiffness in the back, shoulders, and ankles."

Lift your sternum

4 Push your feet down on the floor. At the same time, press down on your soles with your palms. Your fingers should point toward your toes (*see inset*). Tighten your buttocks and pull in your tailbone. Push your shoulder blades back. Take your head as far back as possible, but be careful not to strain your throat. Stay in the pose for 30 seconds.

Pull your spine into your body

Do not tilt your head too far back

Slide your hands over the heels to cover your soles fully

Keep your quadricep muscles stretched

USTRASANA

ADVANCED WORK IN THE POSE 360° **VIEW**

Push your shins down on the floor, and press your palms down on your soles. Lift and stretch the length of your spine, so that your body forms an arch. Your chest, armpits, and back should coil inward, as this will support the back of your chest. Consciously suck in your back ribs, and feel your kidneys being drawn in and squeezed. Try to create a space first between the dome of the diaphragm and the navel; and second, between the navel and the groin. By doing this, you will be extending your abdominal and pelvic organs, as well as your intestines. Roll the inner sides of your upper arms to the front and the outer sides of your upper arms to the back. Keep your elbow joints locked. Breathe evenly.

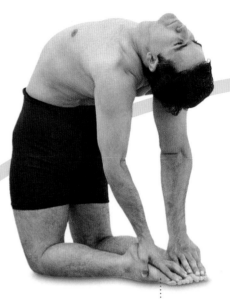

Keep the front of your feet on the floor

Lock your elbows

Do not strain your throat

Press the palms on your feet and extend the arms toward their sockets

COMING OUT OF THE POSE

Exhale, and lessen the pressure of your palms on the feet. Raise your torso, keeping your arms by your sides. The impetus for the upward movement should come from the thighs and chest. If you cannot raise both your arms together, lift them, one by one.

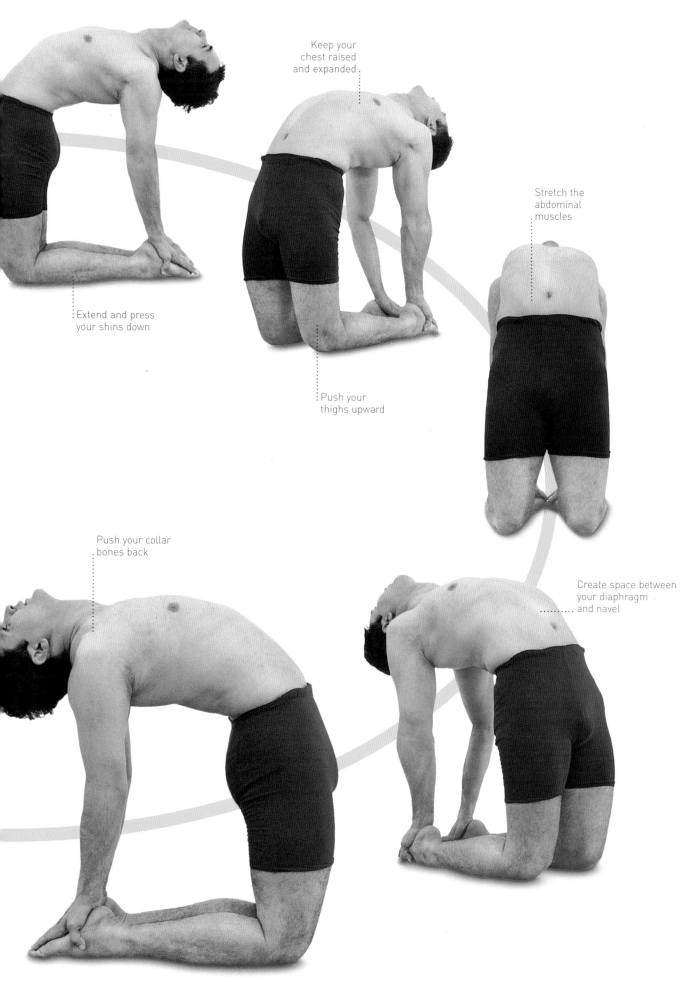

Keep your
chest raised
and expanded

Stretch the
abdominal
muscles

Extend and press
your shins down

Push your
thighs upward

Push your collar
bones back

Create space between
your diaphragm
and navel

URDHVA DHANURASANA
Bow pose

Your body arches back to form an extended bow in this asana. *Urdhva* means "upward" in Sanskrit, while *dhanur* translates as "bow." Regular practice of Urdhva Dhanurasana keeps your body supple, and creates a feeling of vitality and lightness. The asana stimulates the adrenal glands, strengthening your will power, and increasing your capacity to bear stress.

● BENEFITS

Prevents the arteries of the heart from thickening, and ensures healthy blood circulation throughout the body
Tones the spine
Strengthens the abdominal and pelvic organs
Stimulates the pituitary, pineal, and thyroid glands
Prevents prolapse of the uterus
Helps prevent excess menstrual flow and eases menstrual cramps

● CAUTIONS

Do not practice this asana if your blood pressure is too high or too low. Avoid this pose if you have constipation or diarrhea, or when you are feeling tired. Do not practice during a migraine or a severe headache. If you have a cardiac condition or ischemia, practice Viparita Dandasana (*see page* 238) instead of this pose.

1 Lie on your back on the floor. Bend both knees and pull your heels to your buttocks. Spread your feet, so that they align with your hips. Bend your elbows and bring them over your head. Place your palms on the floor, on either side of your head. Your fingers should point toward your shoulders.

BEGINNERS At first, you may find it difficult to bring your heels close to your buttocks. Use your hands to pull the feet into position.

Press your thighs and calves together

Press the palms and keep the elbows pointed upward

Make sure that your elbows are shoulder-width apart

Keep your shoulders on the floor.

2 Focus on your palms and feet, since you are going to use them to launch your pose. Pull your shoulder blades up and pull the muscles of your back into your body. Exhale, then lift your torso and buttocks off the floor. Breathe evenly.

THE GURU'S ADVICE

"Do not merely push your chest forward, as this alone will not prevent the arch of the torso from collapsing. Look at how I am lifting the sides of my student's lower rib cage. You must lift both sides of your chest up toward the ceiling."

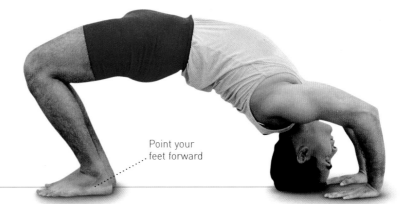

Point your
feet forward

3 Lift your chest and place the crown of your head on the floor. Take two breaths. Exhale sharply, and suck in your back and buttocks. Shift your weight from your palms to the front of your feet, and push up your torso in one single movement. Adjust your pose until your weight is equally distributed on your arms and legs.

Do not take your
head too far back

4 Push your body further upward. Press both palms and soles down on the floor and lift your head off the floor. Exhale, then pull your spine into your body. Straighten your arms and lock your elbows, sucking in the outer arms at the elbows. Now, take your head back without straining your throat. Hold the pose for 5–10 seconds.

Keep your wrists
firm and steady

INTERMEDIATES For a more effective stretch, exhale, pull the muscles of your thighs upward, and lift your heels off the floor (*see inset*). Extend your chest and push up your lower spine, until your abdomen is as taut as a drum. Maintain the

Spread your fingers and
stretch your palms

height of your body, and stretch all your joints. Then bring your heels back to the floor.

URDHVA DHANURASANA

ADVANCED WORK IN THE POSE **360° VIEW**

In the final pose, your body stretches in two directions: one from the palms, and the other from the feet. The meeting point is at the base of the spine. Try to raise this point higher and higher. Open up the spaces between the ribs, especially at the bottom of your chest. Broaden your diaphragm. Suck in your shoulder blades and back ribs—imagine you are squeezing your kidneys. Make sure your weight is evenly distributed on your hands and feet. Make sure your arms and legs are extended (pulled up) toward the ceiling. Initially, hold the pose for 5-10 seconds, breathing evenly. With practice, repeat the asana 3 to 5 times. This will bring greater freedom of movement to your body and improve the effectiveness of your stretch.

Press the outer edges of your feet down on the floor

Open out your armpits

Stretch your arms from the wrists to the armpits

Move your chest toward the ceiling

Pull your shins up toward your thighs

COMING OUT OF THE POSE

Exhale, and bend your elbows and knees. Lower your torso, then bring the crown of your head down to the floor. Lower your back and buttocks to the floor. Lie on your back and take a few breaths.

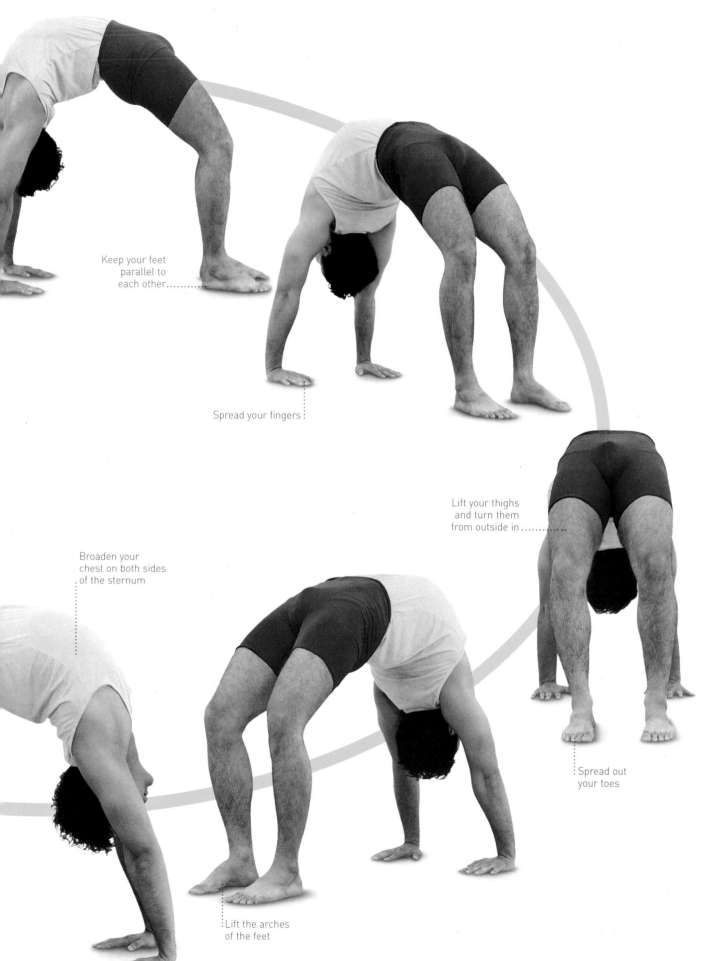

Keep your feet parallel to each other..........

Spread your fingers

Lift your thighs and turn them from outside in ....

Broaden your chest on both sides of the sternum

Spread out your toes

Lift the arches of the feet

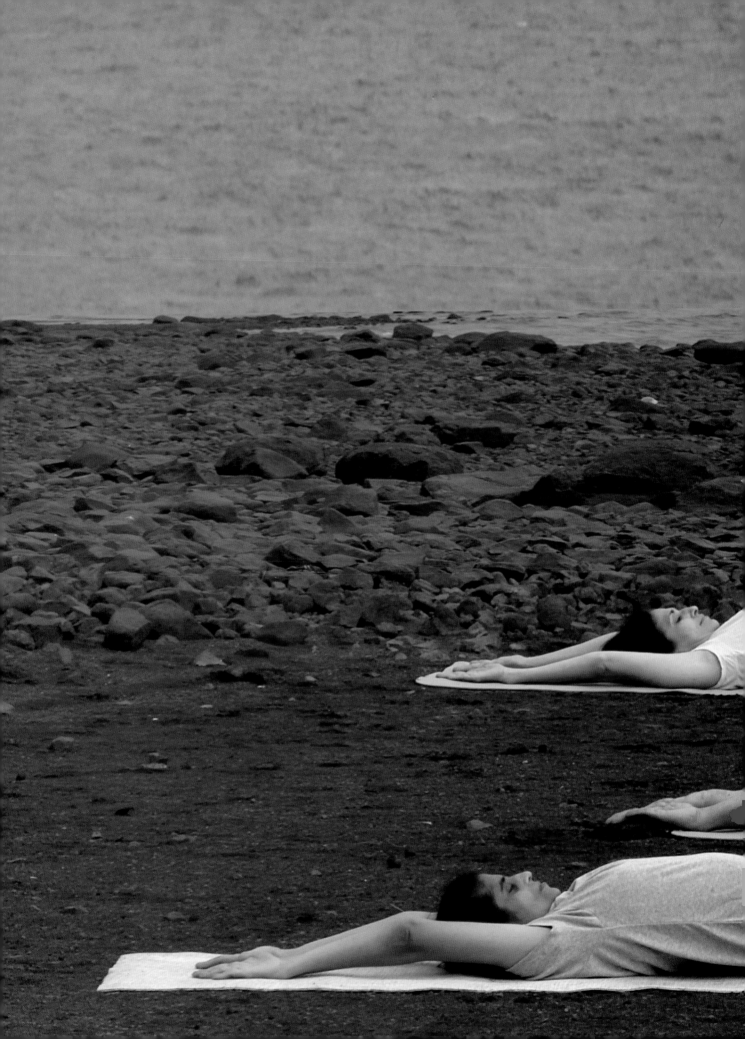

RECLINING ASANAS

*"Feel the **inner mind** touching your entire **body**—even the **remotest** parts where the **mind** does not normally **reach**."*

SUPTA VIRASANA
Reclining hero stretch

This is a variation of the sitting pose, Virasana (*see page* 104). In this asana, you rest your torso on the floor. *Supta* means "lying down" in Sanskrit, while *vira* translates as "hero" or "champion." Athletes, and all those who are on their feet for long periods, will find this asana helpful, since the legs receive an intense and invigorating stretch. If you practice this pose last thing at night, your legs will feel rested and rejuvenated in the morning.

● BENEFITS

Helps reduce cardiac disorders
Stretches the abdomen, back, and waist
Relieves rheumatism and pain in the upper, middle, and lower back
Eases gout and osteoarthritis of the knees
Aids digestion after a heavy meal
Soothes acidity and stomach ulcers
Relieves the symptoms of asthma
Reduces menstrual pain, and helps treat disorders of the ovaries

● CAUTIONS

Those with arthritis of the ankles, or spinal disk disorders should practice this asana with props (*see page* 246). Women should place a bolster under the back during menstruation (*see page* 246).

.... Expand your chest

Press the forearms down and extend your torso ....

Make sure that your knees remain together.

1 Sit in Virasana (*see page* 104). Keep both knees together and spread your feet about 18 in (0.5 m) apart, until they rest beside your hips. To avoid strain, make sure that the inner side of each calf touches the outer side of each thigh. Turn your soles toward the ceiling. Each of your toes should rest on the floor. Stretch your ankles fully and extend the soles toward the toes. Let the energy flow in both directions through your feet.

2 Adjust your legs by turning in your thighs and turning out your calves. Exhale, and lower your back gradually toward the floor. Rest your elbows, one by one, on the floor. Keep your palms on your soles. Breathe evenly.

Turn the thighs in and press them down.

3 Place the crown of your head on the floor. Now, lower your shoulders and upper torso to rest your head, and then your back, on the floor. Stretch your arms along your sides. Press your wrists against your soles.

THE GURU'S ADVICE

"Do not push your buttocks toward the spine, since this causes your lumbar spine to arch. Look at how I am pushing my student's waist and buttocks toward her knees. You must lengthen your buttock muscles and allow the lumbar spine to extend. Then rest the spine on the floor."

4 Move your elbows out to the sides and lie flat on the floor, until the spine is fully extended. Bring your head down and spread your shoulders away from your neck. Rest your shoulder blades and knees on the floor.

Turn the heels out by holding them with your palms

5 Take your arms over your head and stretch them out behind you on the floor, with your palms facing the ceiling. Make sure that both shoulder blades remain flat on the floor and do not let your buttocks or knees lift off the floor. Release your back and allow it to descend completely to the floor. If your back arches, it causes stress to the lower back. Press your thighs together, being careful not to jerk your knees. Breathe evenly and stay in the pose for 30–60 seconds.

Expand your chest evenly on either side of the sternum

Straighten your arms and keep them flat on the floor

Rotate the outer edges of the feet toward the floor

SUPTA VIRASANA

ADVANCED WORK IN THE POSE **360°** VIEW

In the final pose, the stretch of your arms pulls your thighs and abdomen toward your chest—massaging them in the process. Move both shoulder blades in, and open your chest fully. Press your shoulders down, ensuring that your knees and buttocks remain on the floor. The front and the back of your body should be evenly elongated and your armpits fully stretched. Push your pelvis toward the knees and press it down on the floor. Focus on your ribs. Consciously extend them toward your head. Gradually, increase the time spent in the pose to 5–7 minutes.

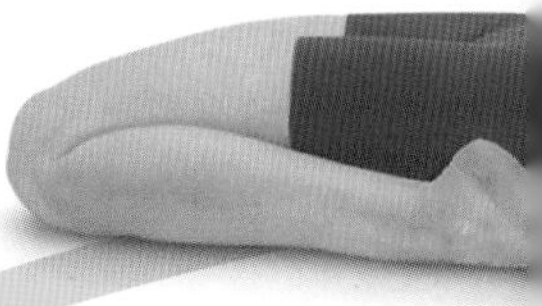

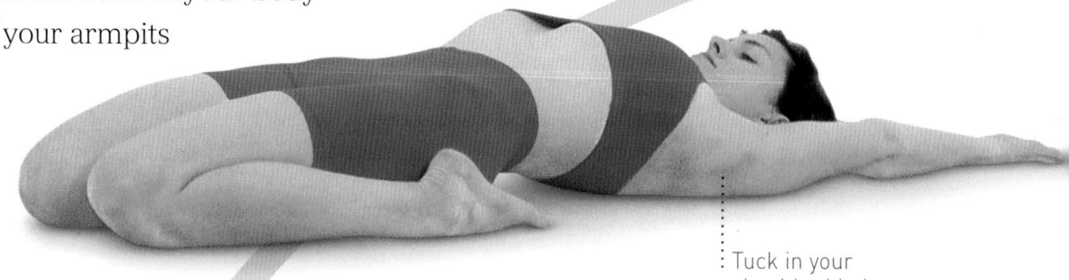

Tuck in your shoulder blades

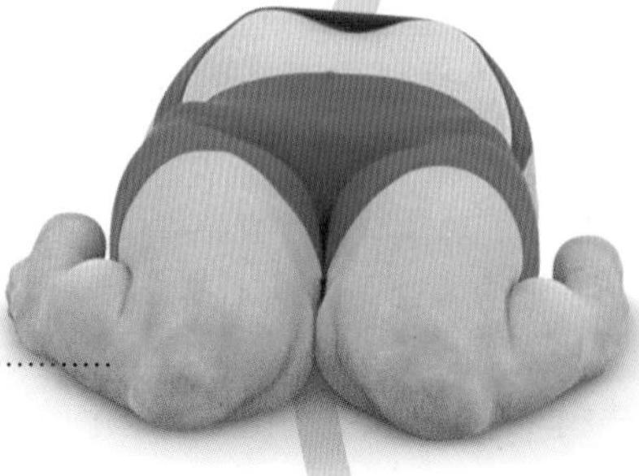

Press your shins down on the floor

When th
and ***still****, wha*

Push your thighs together

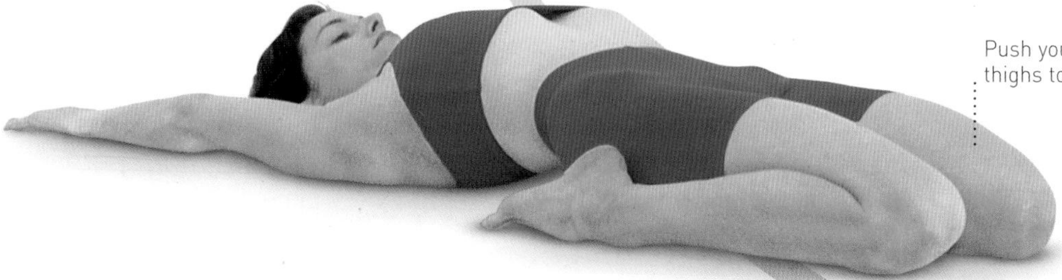

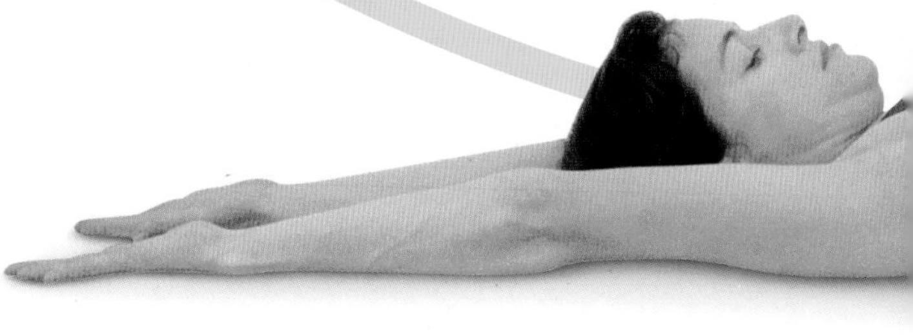

COMING OUT OF THE POSE

Bring your hands over your head and hold your ankles. Lift your head and torso off the floor, supporting yourself on your elbows. Sit up in Virasana. Exhale and straighten your legs, one at a time. Sit in Dandasana.

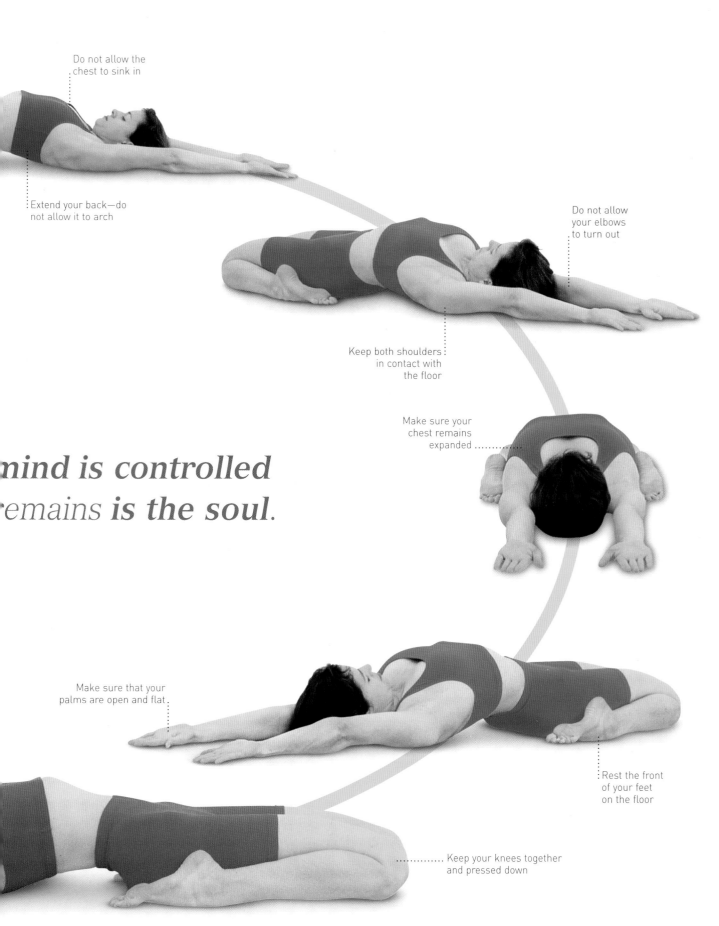

Do not allow the chest to sink in

Extend your back—do not allow it to arch

Do not allow your elbows to turn out

Keep both shoulders in contact with the floor

Make sure your chest remains expanded

mind is controlled
*remains **is the soul**.*

Make sure that your palms are open and flat

Rest the front of your feet on the floor

Keep your knees together and pressed down

SAVASANA
Corpse pose

In this asana, the body is kept as motionless as a corpse and the mind is alert, yet calm. The word *sava* means "corpse" in Sanskrit. When you practice this asana, your organs of perception—the eyes, ears, and tongue—withdraw from the outside world. The body and the mind become one, and you experience inner silence. This asana is the first step in the practice of meditation.

● BENEFITS

Helps alleviate nervous tension, migraines, insomnia, and chronic fatigue syndrome
Relaxes the body and eases breathing
Soothes the nervous system and brings peace of mind
Enhances recovery from all long-term or serious illnesses

● CAUTIONS

If you are pregnant, have a respiratory ailment, or experience anxiety, practice Savasana with your head and chest raised on a bolster (*see page* 256). If you have a backache, lie with your back on the floor, and rest your calves on the seat of a chair, with your thighs perpendicular to the floor. Do not practice Savasana between other asanas.

Make sure that your back is straight ....

Press the backs of your knees to the floor

1 Sit in Dandasana (*see page* 102). Push the flesh of your buttocks out to the sides, so that your weight is equally distributed on both buttock bones. Breathe evenly.

2 Bend your knees and bring your heels closer to the buttocks. Hold the tops of your shins and press your buttock bones down on the floor. Check that your back is straight.

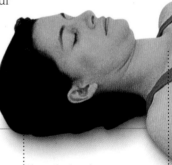

Keep the head straight—do not tilt it to one side

Spread the collar bones out to the sides

3 To lower your torso toward the floor, place your forearms and palms on the floor and lean back on your elbows. Do not move your feet, knees, or buttocks.

4 Lower your torso to the floor, vertebra by vertebra, until the back of your head rests on the floor. Turn your palms to face the ceiling. Close your eyes, then straighten your legs, one by one.

INTERMEDIATES Stretch your torso away from your hips to straighten the spine. Extend the spine fully and keep it flat on the floor. Make sure that the stretch along the legs and the torso is equal on both sides of the body.

"Savasana removes fatigue and soothes the mind. Each part of the body is positioned properly to achieve total relaxation."

Keep the torso still as you straighten the legs

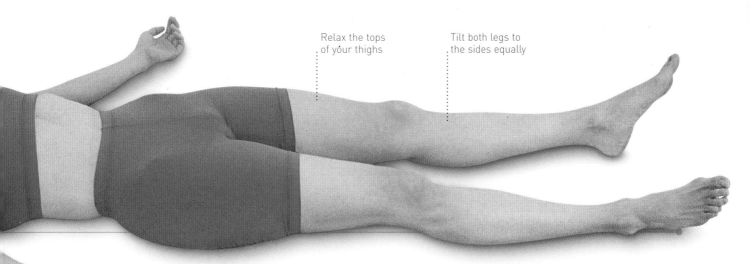

Relax the tops of your thighs

Tilt both legs to the sides equally

Relax the fingers and the centers of the palms

5 Relax your legs, allowing them to drop gently to the sides. Make sure that your kneecaps drop to the sides equally. Move your arms away from your torso without raising your shoulders off the floor. Push your collar bones out to the sides. Keep your eyes closed and focus on your breathing. Stay in this pose for 5–7 minutes.

INTERMEDIATES Visualize your spine. Rest the outer edge of your spine comfortably on the floor. Expand your chest out to the sides and relax your sternum. Focus on your diaphragm— it should be absolutely free of tension. As you push your collar bones out to the sides, allow your neck to dip to the floor. Relax the muscles of your neck.

SAVASANA

ADVANCED WORK IN THE POSE 360° VIEW

As your neck dips to the floor (*see Step 4, page* 171), you will feel a soothing sensation in the back of your brain. When this area of the brain relaxes, move on to the front of the brain. From the crown of the head, the energy should descend in a spiral action toward the bridge of the nose, and down to a point located at the sternum. When the energy reaches this point, the three layers and five sheaths that comprise your body (*see page* 46) come together and are integrated into a single, harmonious whole. This is the ultimate aim of Savasana.

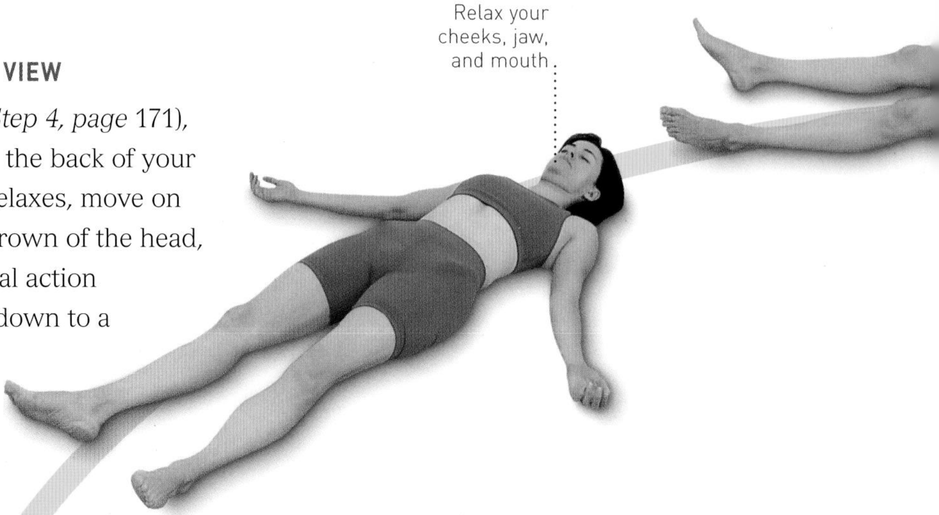

Relax your cheeks, jaw, and mouth

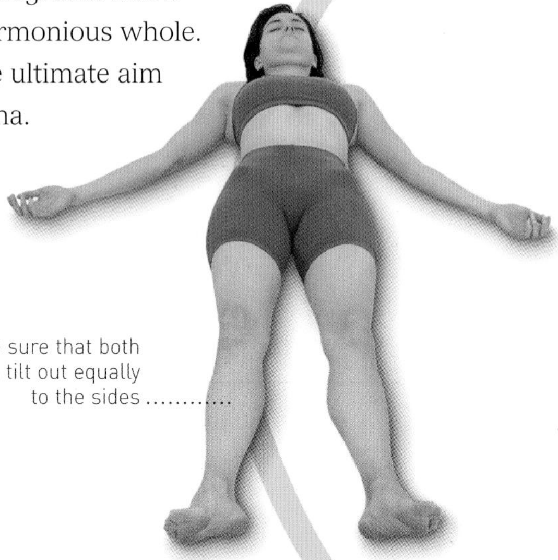

*Relaxation begins
layer of the
the **deep layers**

Make sure that both legs tilt out equally to the sides ....

Keep the lumbar area extended downward

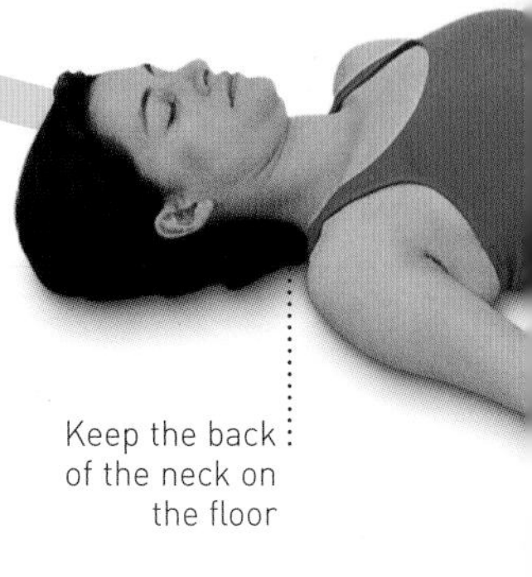

Keep the back of the neck on the floor

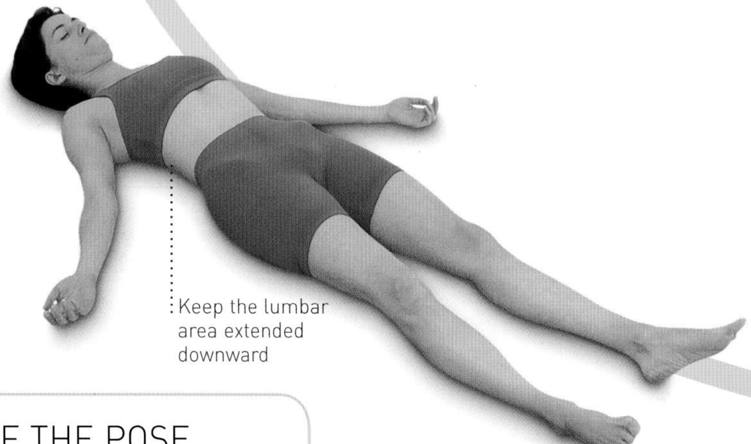

COMING OUT OF THE POSE

Slowly bring your awareness back into contact with your surroundings. Open your eyes. Bend your right knee and roll on to your right side. Push yourself up on your right arm and come to a cross-legged sitting position.

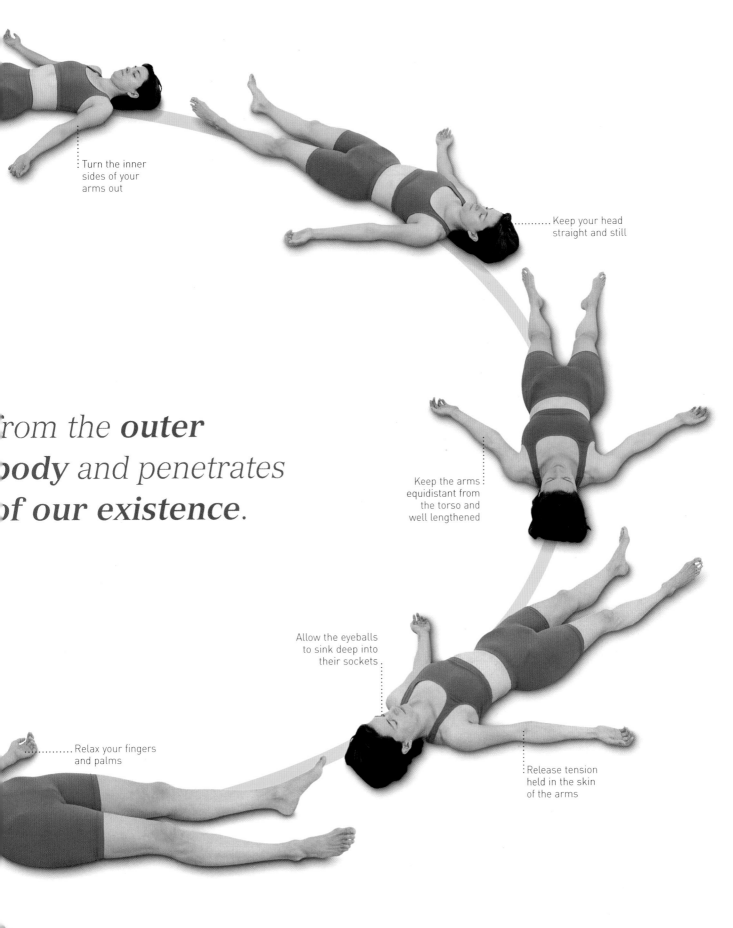

Turn the inner
sides of your
arms out

Keep your head
straight and still

from the **outer**
body and penetrates
of our existence.

Keep the arms
equidistant from
the torso and
well lengthened

Allow the eyeballs
to sink deep into
their sockets

Release tension
held in the skin
of the arms

Relax your fingers
and palms

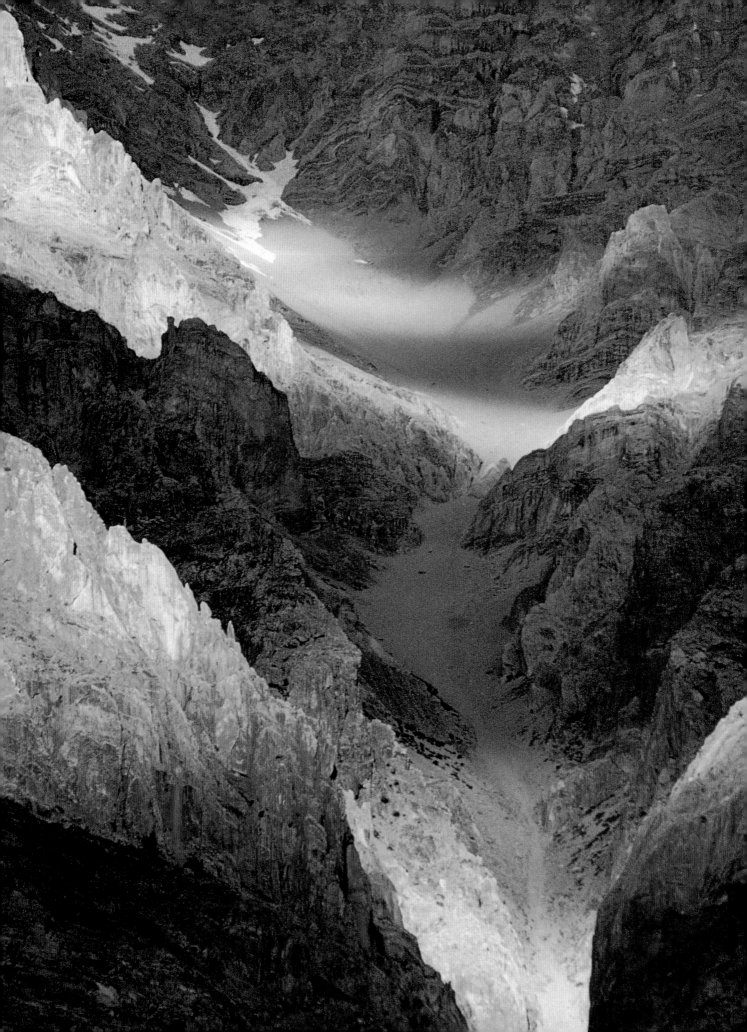

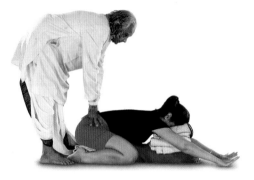

CHAPTER 5

YOGA FOR STRESS

*"An intellectual **mind** that is unconnected to the **heart** is an **uncultivated** mind."*

The practice of asanas and pranayama is not only the most effective, but also the most natural therapy for stress. Practiced together, they generate enormous amounts of energy in the body, stimulating the cells and relaxing tense muscles. The effect on the mind takes longer to register because yoga deals with the causes, and not just the symptoms of stress. With regular practice, the senses that divert the mind to the external environment are drawn inward, calming the restless mind. When your stress levels are high, it is sometimes hard to achieve the final pose effectively. In this case, practicing with the recommended props helps you to attain the benefits of the asanas in a relaxed manner.

Understanding Stress

Stress is as old as civilization itself. The ancient sages understood the impact on the mind and body of the turmoil of daily life. Yoga helps to detach the mind from this turmoil and allows you to face the effects of stress with equilibrium.

We experience stress from the moment of birth, and spend our lives adjusting to it. Some of us manage better than others for a variety of reasons. It could be because of one's personality, environment, or one's physical condition. But everyone has to deal with the effects of stress at some time or another, and in order to do so, he or she has to cultivate and discipline the mind, the physical body, psychological body, and spiritual body. We all evolve ways of coping with stress, checking and minimizing its effects with varying degrees of success. Yoga provides one of the most comprehensive and effective solutions to this problem.

Stress is not a modern phenomenon; it has always been with us. Our ancestors may not have had to deal with the same pressures that those of us who live in modern, technologically advanced cultures do, but even the ordinary events of daily life can cause inner turmoil. People have sought solutions for stress ever since civilization began.

Patanjali's understanding of stress led him to begin the *Yoga Sutras* with the phrase, "*Chittavritti niruddha.*" This translates as "controlling the thought waves or mental fluctuations which bring about stress." He goes on to describe how the path of yoga can help to cope with stressful situations.

The causes of stress

All of us seek refuge in momentary and transient pleasures. Our desires, needs, or demands are ceaseless. We are often pulled in two opposite directions. On the one hand, our mind is attracted by the external world and our attention irresistibly drawn toward it. On the other, we yearn to look inward, to discover the core of our being and our inner self. This conflict entangles us in a web of desire, dissatisfaction, and anger, and manifests itself in feelings of anguish, exhaustion, and breathlessness.

Controlling the senses

The senses are directly controlled by the mind. To control the senses, therefore, you must control the mind. By relaxing our senses and turning them inward, we can detach them from the mind. When a person is calm, and his or her state of mind is meditative, the senses are under control. At this point, external events cease to cause stress. It is only then that one can reflect on the emotional forces controlling one's life and analyze what should be discarded, what should change. The practice of yoga harmonizes your body and mind. The steady pace and rhythm of breath relaxes the body and detaches the mind from the worries of the external world. This healing effect can then be felt in your daily life when routine activities are performed efficiently and well.

A relaxed person possesses dynamic energy that does not dissipate. In this state of being, none of the common symptoms of stress, such as migraines, fatigue, or hypertension occur. Whatever the external environment may be, the mind remains cool and collected, and the body remains free from disease.

*"We can **rise** above our **limitations**, **only** once we **recognize them**."*

The Modern World

The technological and scientific advances of the modern world do not automatically bring happiness. If anything, modern life has led to greater levels of stress, as people are unthinkingly caught up in the pursuit of wealth, success, and worldly pleasures.

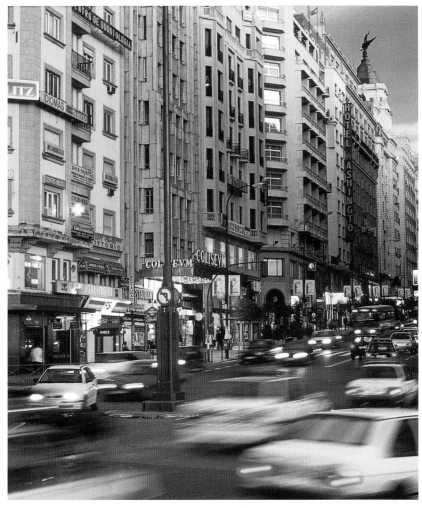

In frantic haste
The speed of modern life causes stress

The information explosion has allowed access to more knowledge than ever before. Paradoxically, such scientific and technological advances have increased, rather than reduced stress levels. The pressures of financial security, the need for recognition and success, the desire for worldly pleasures, all push us into a spiral of anxiety and haste. Inevitably, our spiritual life, peace of mind, and our health suffer.

If you are caught up in the maelstrom of constant challenge and competition, you lose your ability to perceive reality clearly. You may unknowingly twist the truth to suit your own personal goals and fail to recognize friendliness, honesty, and compassion, and instead perceive deceit, dishonesty, or pride.

An intellectual mind, if unconnected with the heart, is an uncultivated mind. The intelligence of the head must be controlled to allow the emotional center to awaken. It is only when the head and the heart are in harmony, that peace of mind, stability, and happiness can be achieved. Egoism and pride cause an individual to lose contact with his or her emotional center. In order to achieve a fully integrated personality, you must develop emotionally as well as intellectually. Only then will you be able to control the stresses and strains which knock you off balance from time to time. As long as your heart and your mind remain separate, stress will manifest itself physically and emotionally through contracted body muscles, tense facial expressions, and undesirable behavioral patterns.

Food and Nourishment

The food we eat and the surroundings we inhabit must be conducive to stress-free living. If we increase our intake of fruit and vegetables, and nourish our senses with calming scents, sounds, and sights, we will be on the way to a healthier lifestyle.

The *Upanishads*, ancient Indian scriptures compiled between 300 and 400 BC, divide food into 16 categories: 10 parts are classified as wastage, 5 parts affect the energy of the mind, and one part is vital for the intelligence. In this system, food can have positive or negative effects, depending on the immediate environment, the geographical and climatic conditions, and a person's constitution. Yogic science recognizes three different qualities of food: *sattva, rajas*, and *tamas*. *Sattva* means "pure essence," and represents the well-balanced and meditative aspect; *rajas* is the energy which seeks to accomplish, achieve, or create; and *tamas* indicates inertia and decay.

Sattvic food, which includes fruit and vegetables, is pure, wholesome, and fresh. *Rajasic* food, such as onions, garlic, and pungent spices, are stimulants. *Tamasic* substances, such as alcohol and meats, are considered to be heavy and enervating. Junk food is a relatively new term, but its properties would certainly be categorized as *tamasic*.

Every activity in our modern world is fast, and this includes activities related to food and the way we eat it. Junk food and food out of cans and packages has a tremendously negative impact on the body. The mind is as alert after a meal of *sattvic* food as it was before the food was eaten, but after meals which are largely *rajasic* or *tamasic* in nature, the mind becomes dull and sluggish. It is equally important to keep the mind healthy and the body well-nourished.

The five organs of perception, the eyes, ears, nose, tongue, and skin, are the gateways to the mind. For better control of the mind, the senses need appropriate nourishment. Soothing music for the ears, soft, natural light, or beautiful, peaceful scenery for the eyes, and fresh pure air and the scent of flowers for the nose, all help to nourish the mind. The tongue needs nutritious, delicately flavored foods. The skin should be kept clean, soft, and supple. Finally, the mind must be nurtured by developing clarity of thought.

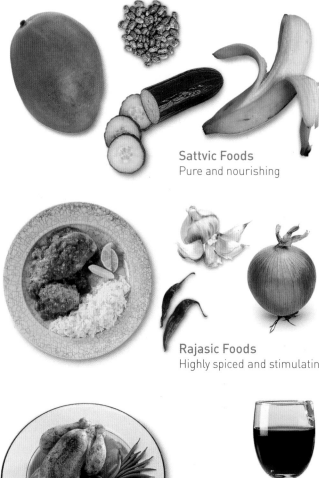

Sattvic Foods
Pure and nourishing

Rajasic Foods
Highly spiced and stimulating

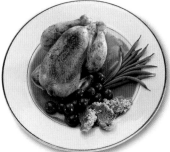

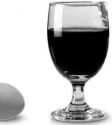

Tamasic Foods
Lead to heaviness and inertia

Positive and Negative Stress

Stress can motivate an individual to develop creativity and to strive for achievement. This is positive stress. Negative stress can lead to ill health, depression, and inertia. Yoga teaches you to transform negative stress into positive stress.

The cumulative effects of stress can damage your health and undermine your emotional stability. There is a growing awareness today that stress is a health hazard. It can paralyze, and make you feel fragmented and off balance. However, stress can also trigger the motivation to create and achieve. This type of stress can be positive and constructive.

Types of stress

We must distinguish clearly between positive and negative stress. Negative stress leads to the inability to adjust to illness or feelings of uncertainty. Like some diseases, it can remain dormant, but may have physical symptoms such as tremors or labored breathing. Though positive and negative stress are two sides of the same coin, one type usually predominates.

Every person must find a way to transform negative stress into positive energy, so that it can be harnessed to build a healthy mind and body. The mind, body, and emotions are affected by physical, physiological, intellectual, emotional, and spiritual stress. The result may be tense or stiff muscles and joints, atrophying of skeletal bones, slowing down of body systems, or sluggishness in the vital organs. Emotional and muscular tension are closely related—continuous stress causes muscular contraction, severe muscle and joint pain, and tightness in the jaw or facial muscles. If you suffer from stress, you may experience indigestion, irritable bowel syndrome, headaches, migraines, a feeling of constriction in the diaphragm, breathlessness, or insomnia.

Reactions to stress

Different people respond to the same stressful situation with different levels of intensity. Some may become angry, others confused or depressed; ultimately stress leads to disease, premature aging, or even fatal illness. The science of psycho-neuro-immunology has established the connection between the body, mind, and emotions, but the ancient yogis recognized this a millennium ago. According to yogic science, the health of the psyche is reflected in the body. Psychological pressures stress all the systems of the body.

Alleviating stress

To reduce stress, the body and mind must be treated as one. The tension associated with stress is stored mainly in the muscles, the diaphragm, and the nervous system. If these areas are relaxed, stress is reduced. The organs of perception and the central nervous system also react physically to stress. Yogic methods of deep relaxation have a profound effect on all the body systems. When a part of the body is tense, blood flow to that area decreases, reducing immunity. Yoga works on that area to relieve tension and improve blood flow to the entire body, stabilizing the heart rate and blood pressure. Rapid, shallow breathing becomes deep and slow, allowing a higher intake of oxygen, and removing stress from the body and the mind.

Positive action
Stress can be harnessed to have a positive effect

Asanas and Stress

The practice of asanas and pranayama is the most natural therapy for stress. Practicing asanas with props builds up your stamina and allows you to benefit from the pose without unnecessary strain.

Many people respond to stress by resorting to tranquilizers, alcohol, nicotine, or comfort eating. These may bring momentary relief, but as we know all too well, they are only temporary solutions and are, in fact, counterproductive. They also have dangerous side effects that actually increase stress levels. Simple relaxation techniques can alleviate stress levels for a short time, but cannot tackle the causes of stress comprehensively.

The yogis and sages of the past have emphasized that emotional turmoil or anxiety have to be faced with calmness and stability. Yoga can help you to internalize those positive attitudes which allow you to face stressful situations with equanimity.

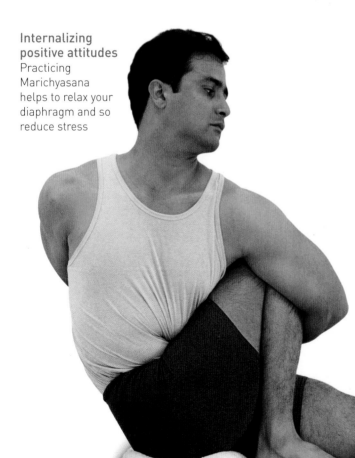

Internalizing positive attitudes Practicing Marichyasana helps to relax your diaphragm and so reduce stress

Learning to deal with stress

Every individual has the power to discriminate between good habits and bad, and to develop his or her sense of ethical behavior. By adopting good habits, such as regular yoga practice, you can check the stress that depletes the body's bio-energy. The practice of asanas and pranayama is not just the most effective, but also the most natural therapy for stress, and unlike many other therapies, there is no danger of harmful side effects. Mere relaxation is not sufficient in itself to counter the negative effects of stress. The regular practice of yoga, along with a healthy diet and lifestyle, helps to generate enormous amounts of energy in the body, stimulating the cells and relaxing tensed muscles.

While the effect of asanas and pranayama on the mind takes longer to be felt, with patience and dedication, you will soon discover a feeling of mental poise and well-being during and after your practice. While practicing asanas and pranayama, the five senses of perception that divert the mind to the external environment are drawn inward. When the restlessness of the mind is stilled, your entire being becomes calm and steady. The impact of negative stress is reduced, while the benefits of positive stress are enhanced, building up the resilience and flexibility of the nerves, organs, senses, mind, and intelligence to create a healthy mind and body. Clarity, firmness of purpose, self-discipline, and ethical and moral sensibility follow naturally, enabling you to live a tranquil life, free of stress, and in harmony with your environment.

"The **brain** *must be* **calm***, the* **body active***."*

Active and passive practice

There are many different types of stress which we deal with every day—physical, psychological, and physiological. The only way to effectively combat the negative effects of these is through a balanced combination of active and passive practice. I use the term "passive practice" when talking of yoga with props, since this helps to promote calmness of the mind, patience, and endurance. "Active practice," as the term suggests, is more vigorous, and generally refers to classical poses without the use of props. These poses, especially the standing poses and those involving back bends, help to build stamina, vitality, and flexibility. The balance between active and passive poses will vary from individual to individual, and even from season to season. Reclining asanas, inversions, and resting asanas, for example, are particularly beneficial on a hot day. These asanas slow the metabolism, and conserve energy. During the winter months, standing, back bends, and inverted asanas stimulate the body's systems, and help fight off common ailments such as colds, coughs, congestion in the chest, and sinusitis.

Sequencing and timing

Sequencing is the method of practicing asanas in a particular order so as to maximize their effectiveness. Too much active practice may result in egoism and exhaust the body's systems. On the other hand, too much passive practice may lead to depression, lethargy, and feelings of restlessness and irritability. As you gradually discover more and more about yoga and about your own body, you will be able to adjust the sequences of your practice, to achieve the ideal blend of active and passive poses. As your stamina and flexibility increase, you will also be able to hold poses for longer periods. The effect of an asana cannot take place in seconds, and timing is dependent on energy, intelligence, and awareness.

Asanas with props

If you are experiencing high levels of stress, or if you have a minor injury, or are fatigued in any way, it is best for you to practice yoga using props.

Minimizing strain
Using simple props lessens strain and enables you to hold the pose for a longer period

Asanas with Props

The ancient yogis used logs of wood, stones, and ropes to help them to practice asanas effectively. Extending this principle, Yogacharya Iyengar invented props which allow asanas to be held easily and for a longer duration, without strain.

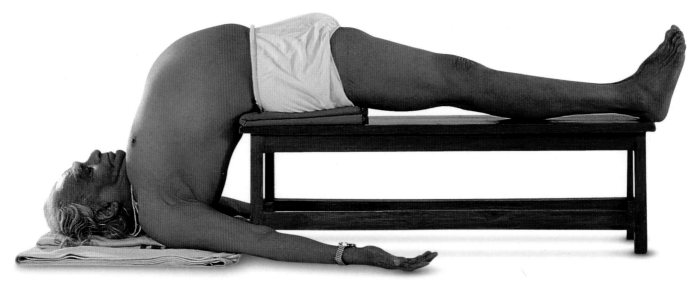

Yogacharya Iyengar in Setubandha Sarvangasana
This version of the pose requires considerable strength in the neck, shoulders, and back, requiring years of practice to achieve. It should not be attempted without supervision.

Yoga asanas involve extension, exertion, as well as relaxation of the body. More importantly, the aim of the movements is to align the body correctly. This also includes mental alignment, in which the mind touches each and every part of the body evenly.

The practice of yoga requires you to be in good mental and physical condition. Yet, during my long years of teaching yoga, I have found that even those in good condition occasionally find some poses difficult to sustain for the required length of time. Some asanas, too, entail body movements that are initially too complicated for even the healthiest students to attempt without help. It is for this reason that I developed the use of props in yoga. With these props, the practice of asanas has never been easier, less tiring, or more enjoyable, making

each asana equally accessible to all yoga students, whether they are weak or strong, young or old, beginners or advanced students, or those who wish to conserve their energy because of fatigue or injury.

How props help

A yoga prop is any object that helps to stretch, strengthen, relax, or improve the alignment of the body. It helps to sustain the practice of asanas for a longer duration, and conserves energy. These props allow asanas to be practiced in a relaxed way, balancing the body and mind actively as well as passively. At first, I would use my own body to support my students during their practice, but found that this exhausted my own reserves of energy. I then began experimenting with ordinary, everyday objects such as walls, chairs, stools, blocks, bolsters, blankets, and belts to help my students achieve the final pose. As I worked with people who were affected by illness or disease, I came to realize the value of props. I discovered that props helped to retain key movements and subtle adjustments of the body by providing more height, weight, or support. I also found that the use of props improved blood circulation and breathing capacity. This inspired me to create props adjusted to suit individual needs.

The yoga asana practiced with props is unique in that it is the only form of exercise which allows both action and relaxation simultaneously. It activates the muscles, tones the body's organs, and relieves undue mental and physical stress or strain. Props help to increase flexibility and stamina and, at the same time, relax slack and tired muscles. They help to rejuvenate the entire body, without increasing physical fatigue.

Students of yoga find the practice of asanas with props a very encouraging exercise. It gives them the confidence to attempt difficult asanas, and ensures correct practice. Props provide a sense of direction and alignment, and help to increase and enhance the understanding of each asana. They serve as silent instructors.

Props and therapy
When the body is lethargic, sluggish, and fatigued, practice with props works wonders. The nervous system relaxes, the brain is calmed, and the mind soothed. Asanas with props build up emotional stability and will power. As stress is reduced, anxiety, fears, and depression also disappear, helping those under emotional strain to cope better with all aspects of their lives. Blood circulation increases, and the heart, as well as the respiratory, abdominal, and pelvic organs are rested and rejuvenated. For instance, Setubandha Sarvangasana (*see page* 236) practiced on a broad wooden bench increases coronary blood supply by resting and energizing the heart without any bodily strain. This makes it ideal for cardiac patients.

Asanas practiced with the help of bolsters, blocks, stools, or chairs help to relieve many common ailments. They regulate blood pressure, ease breathlessness and asthma, and remove stiffness in the back, hips, knees, and feet, alleviating rheumatism and arthritis. Yoga with props frees you from attachment to the body and liberates the spirit. It helps to improve posture and maintain balance, allowing you to stretch, and experience a state of relaxation during practice.

Ultimately, yoga with props creates a feeling of peace and tranquillity, culminating in a fresh perspective and renewed strength. Some of the props shown on the following pages have been specifically developed for your practice. Others are objects that you will find in your own homes.

Practice against a wall
The support of a wall helps to maintain balance and a sense of alignment, particularly in standing and inverted asanas. It gives you the confidence to practice without fear of injury or strain. The wall is invaluable in the practice of Tadasana (*see page* 186). Make sure that you practice standing asanas on an even, smooth surface. To avoid slipping, do not practice on a mat or blanket, and do not wear socks. Always practice Tadasana and its variations with bare feet, as shoes restrict movement, cramp the toes, and reduce sensitivity in the soles, impairing your ability to sense all the adjustments in the pose.

A wall gives you alignment
Yogacharya Iyengar adjusts the position of the student's arms in Tadasana Urdhva Hastasana

Props

The props shown on these pages can be found in your home or can be bought at the addresses listed on page 432. When you practice with props, use them in the way that you find most suitable. I have provided some basic guidelines, but the most important point is that you should feel comfortable and relaxed when practicing an asana.

Invaluable support
Yogacharya Iyengar in Ustrasana with one stool

The props shown below support the entire body when you practice the asana, giving you the height to coordinate your movements more effectively, and allowing better balance in the pose.

CHAIR

This folding metal chair has an open back rest which allows you to place your legs through it. This makes for an easier, yet still effective rotation of the torso in seated twists, such as Bharadvajasana. Holding the sides of the back rest steadies you when getting into the pose in Salamba Sarvangasana and Halasana. It provides support to the torso in back bends, such as Viparita Dandasana. Make sure that the chair is completely stable and rests firmly on the ground.

WOODEN BENCH

This bench should be broad enough to support your torso comfortably, and should be approximately 2 ft (60 cm) high. It must rest firmly on the ground. Cardiac patients or those with migraines or respiratory disorders will benefit from the use of this bench in their practice of Setubandha Sarvangasana.

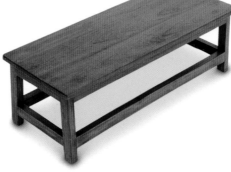

HALF-HALASANA STOOL

This stool should be approximately 1–1.5 ft (30–45 cm) high to support the back and feet in Paripurna Navasana, and the back in Ustrasana. This stool helps in the practice of asanas requiring flexibility and strength in the back, abdomen, arms, and legs.

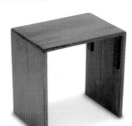

LOW, OPEN STOOL

A stool with open sides helps support the body in back bends, such as Ustrasana, helping to lift and arch the torso easily. The stool should not be more than 1.5 ft (45 cm) high, and should rest firmly on the ground.

HIGH STOOL

This stool, of mid-thigh height, helps in the practice of standing twists, such as Utthita Marichyasana. The stool allows you to rotate the spine and torso effectively without strain. Make sure that the stool rests firmly on the ground and that it has a top wide enough to rest your entire foot on comfortably.

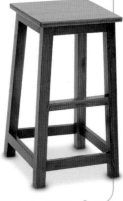

The props below support specific parts of the body and allow asanas to be held without strain and for a longer duration. Beginners, people with stiff joints or muscles, or those who have high blood pressure and need support for the head in forward bends, will find these of use.

BOLSTER

Bolsters support your body while enabling you to relax and stretch effectively without strain. The bolster should weigh about 7 lbs (3 kg) and be stuffed with dense cotton. The bolster should be about 2 ft (60 cm) long, with a diameter of 9 in (23 cm). It should preferably have a removable cotton cover.

WOODEN BLOCK

The support of wooden blocks is often used in all types of asanas. In sitting and standing asanas they support the legs, knees, or palms, and give height to seated twists. In Ujjayi Pranayama, a block supports the back and helps to open the chest. In forward bends, such as Uttanasana, blocks provide support to the head and to the hands. The measurements of the block should be about 9 in (23 cm) x 4.5 in (12 cm) x 3 in (7 cm). It can be placed on its short side (a); on its long side (b); and on its broad side (c); according to your requirement. While a height has been suggested for many asanas in this chapter, you should place the block at the height you find most comfortable.

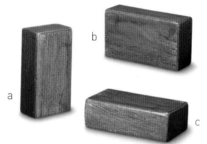

FOLDED BLANKET

Folded blankets are used to support the back, to open the chest in reclining asanas and pranayama, and to support the head and shoulders in inversions, such as Salamba Sarvangasana. They provide height in seated asanas, helping keep the torso and spine erect and also correct poor structural posture. Cotton blankets, measuring about 6.5 ft (2 m) x 4 ft (1.2 m), are most suitable. Fold one in half three times when using it to cushion the impact of a chair or a bench on the body. Fold in half four or five times to give added height for sitting asanas and seated twists.

FOAM BLOCK

A foam block is placed under stacked wooden blocks to support the head in forward bends and the back in pranayama. Its dimensions are about 1 ft (30 cm) x 7 in (18 cm) x 2 in (5 cm).

ROUNDED WOODEN BLOCK

A small block is used to give added height in the standing twist, Utthita Marichyasana. It helps you rotate your body more effectively and without strain. It is about 2 in (5 cm) high and 4 in (10 cm) long.

ROLLED BLANKET

This is used to support the neck in reclining asanas and back bends, and the small of the back in back bends, such as Viparita Dandasana. It helps relieve strain on the chest and on the thighs and ankles in Virasana and Adhomukha Virasana. Fold a cotton blanket in half four times, and then roll it up tightly (*see above*).

These two props increase the effectiveness of some asanas. The belt prevents muscle or joint strain, and enhances the stretch. The bandage helps you relax completely by making it easier to turn your thoughts inward.

YOGA BELT

The belt helps provide the required tension without strain in the final stretch of Supta Padangusthasana, Urdhvamukha Janu Sirsasana, and Paripurna Navasana. The belt is about 2 ft (60 cm) long, made of strong woven material, with a buckle at either end.

CREPE BANDAGE

The blindfold, 8–10 ft (2.5–3 m) long and 4 in (10 cm) broad, helps the eyeballs recede into their sockets. This cools the brain, and relaxes the facial muscles and nervous system in Savasana and pranayama.

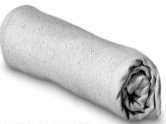

TADASANA SAMASTHITHI
Steady and firm mountain pose

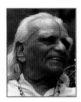

This pose, the starting point of all standing asanas, lifts the sternum, which is the site of the anahata or "heart" chakra (*see page 57*). This helps reduce stress and boost your self-confidence, while the perfect balance of the final pose increases your alertness. In Sanskrit, *tadasana* means "mountain pose" while *samasthithi* indicates an "upright and steady state."

PROPS (SEE PAGE 182)
A WALL helps you align your body correctly. It also makes adjustments in the pose easier, and gives stability to the final pose.

.... Relax your facial muscles

.... Keep your shoulders level with each other

.... Lengthen both sides of your waist evenly

● BENEFITS
Helps treat depression
Improves incorrect posture
Strengthens the knee joints
Revitalizes the feet and corrects flat feet
Reduces sciatic pain
Prevents hemorrhoids
Improves bladder control
Tones and lifts the pelvis and abdomen

● CAUTIONS
Do not practice this asana if you have stress-related headaches, migraines, eye strain, low blood pressure, osteoarthritis of the knees, bulimia, diarrhea, insomnia, or leukorrhea. If you have a problem with balance, practice this asana with your feet about 10 in (25 cm) apart.

1 Stand in your bare feet on a smooth and even surface. Keep your feet together, with your heels touching the wall. Beginners may find it easier to keep their feet 2 in (5 cm) apart.

2 Stretch your arms along your sides, with the palms facing your thighs, and your fingers pointing to the floor. Stretch your neck upward, keeping the muscles soft and passive.

3 Distribute your weight evenly on the inner and outer edges of your feet, and on your toes and heels. Tighten your kneecaps and open the back of each knee. Turn in the front of your thighs. Tighten your buttocks. Pull in your lower abdomen, and lift your chest.

4 Keep your head erect and look straight ahead. Breathe evenly and with awareness. Experience your body and mind as an integrated whole and feel the surge of energy. Stay in the pose for 30–60 seconds.

TADASANA URDHVA HASTASANA
Mountain pose with arms stretched up

This is a variation of the mountain pose, with the arms extended upward. *Urdhva* translates as "upward" in Sanskrit, while *hasta* means "hands." This is recommended for people in sedentary occupations, since it exercises the arms, and the joints of the shoulders, wrists, knuckles, and fingers.

PROPS (SEE PAGE 182)
A WALL helps you align your body correctly, makes adjustments in the pose easier, and gives stability to the final pose.

● BENEFITS
Helps treat depression, and boosts self-confidence
Tones and stimulates the abdomen, pelvis, torso, and back
Relieves arthritis
Reduces sciatic pain
Strengthens the knee joints
Stretches the hamstring muscles
Corrects flat feet

● CAUTIONS
Do not practice this asana if you have stress-related headaches, migraines, eye strain, low blood pressure, osteoarthritis of the knees, bulimia, diarrhea, insomnia, or leukorrhea. If you have high blood pressure, do not hold the pose for more than 15 seconds. If you have a slipped disk, keep the feet apart. If you have a prolapsed uterus, keep the tips of the toes together and heels apart.

Keep the muscles of your neck soft

Lift your sternum and rib cage

Tighten your kneecaps

1 Stand in your bare feet in Tadasana (*see page* 68) on an even, uncovered surface. Exhale, and stretching from your waist, lift your arms in front of you, to shoulder level. Keep your palms open and facing each other.

2 Raise your arms above your head, perpendicular to the floor. Stretch your arms and fingers. Push your shoulder blades into your body.

3 Stretch your arms further up from your shoulders, keeping them parallel to each other. Extend your wrists, palms, and fingers toward the ceiling. Feel the stretch along both sides of your body.

4 Pull in your lower abdomen. Turn your wrists so that the palms face front. Hold the pose for 20–30 seconds. Breathe evenly.

TADASANA URDHVA BADDHANGULIYASANA
Mountain pose with fingers interlocked

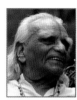

This is a variation of Tadasana, the "mountain pose." *Urdhva* means "upward" in Sanskrit, *baddha* indicates "caught" or "bound," while *anguli* translates as "fingers." In this pose, the brain is relaxed but alert, and you are aware of the intense stretch of your whole body, from your feet to your interlocked fingers. Feel the energy flow upward from your feet to your knuckles.

● BENEFITS
Boosts confidence and helps treat depression
Relieves arthritis
Stretches the shoulders, arms, wrists, and fingers
Helps to treat spinal disorders
Tones and activates the torso, back, abdomen, and pelvis
Strengthens the knee joints
Reduces sciatic pain
Corrects flat feet

● CAUTIONS
Do not practice this asana if you have a cardiac condition, stress-related headaches, migraines, low blood pressure, insomnia, osteoarthritis of the knees, bulimia, diarrhea, or leukorrhea. If you have high blood pressure, do not hold the pose for more than 15 seconds. If you have had polio, are knock-kneed, or have a problem with your balance, keep your feet 8 in (20 cm) apart. If you are prone to backaches, have a slipped disk, or a prolapsed uterus, keep the tips of the big toes together and keep your heels apart.

PROPS (SEE PAGE 182)
A WALL helps you to align your body correctly, makes adjustments in the pose easier, and gives stability to the final pose.

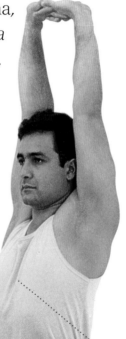

Lift your sternum

Pull up your quadriceps

Extend the mounds of your toes away from your heels

1 Stand in your bare feet in Tadasana (*see page* 68) against a wall, on an even, uncovered surface. Bring your arms toward your chest, with your palms facing the chest. Interlock your fingers firmly, from the base of the knuckles, with the little finger of your left hand lower than the little finger of the right hand (*see inset above*).

2 Turn your interlocked palms inside out (*see inset below*). Exhale, and stretch your arms out in front of you at shoulder level. Then inhale, and raise your arms above your head until they are perpendicular to the floor. Extend your arms fully and lock your elbows. Feel the stretch in your palms. Hold the pose for 30–60 seconds.

PASCHIMA BADDHA HASTASANA

Mountain pose with the arms folded behind the back

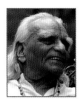

The Sanskrit words *paschima baddha hastasana mean* "hands folded at the back." *Baddha* means "bound" or "caught." This asana is an easier version of Tadasana Paschima Namaskarasana (*see page* 190), and helps to prepare you for the regular pose, which calls for greater flexibility and extension of the back and arms.

● BENEFITS

Boosts confidence and helps reduce depression
Helps in the treatment of cervical spondylosis
Relieves arthritis of the shoulders, arms, wrists, and fingers
Strengthens the knee joints and reduces sciatic pain
Corrects flat feet

● CAUTIONS

Do not practice this asana if you have angina, stress-related headaches, migraines, eye strain, insomnia, low blood pressure, osteoarthritis of the knees, leukorrhea, or bulimia. If you have a slipped disk, keep your feet apart. If you have a displaced uterus, keep the tips of your big toes together and your heels apart. If you have had polio, or have any problems with your balance, keep your feet at least 10 in (25 cm) apart.

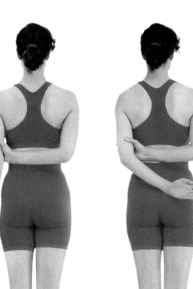

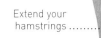

Keep your back erect

Tighten your buttock muscles

Extend your hamstrings

Rest your weight equally on both feet

2 Hold your right arm just above the elbow with your left hand. Your grip should be firm but not tight. Keep your forearms pressed to your back. Turn in your upper arms slightly. Push your elbows back, but do not allow them to lift. Initially, hold the pose for 20–30 seconds. With practice, increase the duration to 1 minute. You should breathe evenly throughout.

1 Stand in your bare feet in Tadasana (*see page* 68) on an even, uncovered surface. Take your right arm behind your back, and hold your left arm just above the elbow. Bend your left arm and take it behind your back. Stretch both legs and imagine you are pulling the skin, muscles, and bones of your legs up to your waist.

TADASANA PASCHIMA NAMASKARASANA
Mountain pose with hands folded behind the back

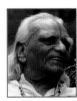

In this standing asana, the hands are folded at the back in the Indian salutation of *namaskar* or "greeting." This stretch requires considerable flexibility in the upper body and arms. Practice Paschima Baddha Hastasana (*see page* 189) until your shoulder, elbow, and wrist joints are sufficiently supple to perform this asana easily.

● BENEFITS
Reduces depression
Relieves cervical spondylosis
Increases the flexibility of the upper body, arms, elbows, and wrists
Strengthens the knee joints
Reduces sciatic pain
Corrects flat feet

● CAUTIONS
Do not practice this asana if you have stress-related headaches, migraines, low blood pressure, insomnia, osteoarthritis of the knees, bulimia, diarrhea, or leukorrhea. If you have high blood pressure, do not hold the pose for more than 15 seconds. If you have had polio, or are knock-kneed, or have a problem with your balance, keep your feet 8 in (20 cm) apart. If you are prone to backaches, have a slipped disk or a prolapsed uterus, keep your feet together and knees apart.

.... Move your elbows back and down

2 Press your palms together, and move them up your back until they are between your shoulder blades. Keep your palms joined from the base to the fingertips. Push your elbows down, to stretch your upper arms and chest. Focus on keeping your chest and armpits open. Keep your neck and shoulders relaxed. Hold the pose for 30–60 seconds. Breathe evenly.

.. Open out the backs of your knees

1 Stand in your bare feet in Tadasana (*see page* 68) on an even, uncovered surface. Gently turn your arms in and out a few times. Take them behind you and join your fingertips, pointing them to the floor. Rest your thumbs on your lower back. Move your elbows back and rotate your wrists, so that your fingertips turn and point first toward your back, and then upward.

Stretch your toes
.... away from your heels

TADASANA GOMUKHASANA

Mountain pose with hands held in the shape of a cow's face

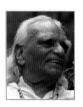

The interlinked hands in the final pose of this asana take the shape of *gomukha*, which means "a cow's face" in Sanskrit. The asana is a variation of Tadasana, the mountain pose. It activates the muscles of the shoulders and back. The stretch in the arms helps relieve arthritis in the shoulders, elbows, wrists, and fingers.

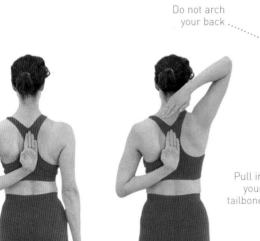

Do not arch your back

Pull in your tailbone

Keep your legs stretched upward

2 Place your right palm on your left palm and interlink the fingers of both hands. If this proves difficult, touch the fingertips of both hands to each other. Do not force your arms to bend—give yourself time to adjust to the action. Consciously relax your arms. Open your right armpit to create space between your chest and your upper right arm. Keep your right elbow pointed up and back, and your right forearm close to your head. Lower your left elbow further. Then place the back of your left wrist on your back. Hold the pose for 20–30 seconds. Repeat the pose on the other side.

1 Stand in your bare feet in Tadasana (*see page* 68) on an even, uncovered surface. Take your left arm behind you and place the back of your left palm on the middle of your back. Raise your right arm. Bend your right elbow and move your hand down, with your palm facing your body.

UTTHITA TRIKONASANA
Extended triangle pose

This asana is a variation of the classic pose (*see page* 70). Regular practice of this asana taps energy stored in the tailbone, which is an important source of vitality and strength. This helps those who require more energy to function efficiently when under stress. The pose activates the spine, keeping it supple and well-aligned. It relieves backaches, and reduces stiffness in the neck, shoulders, and knees.

● BENEFITS

Tones the abdominal organs
Stimulates digestion, relieving gastritis, acidity, and flatulence
Tones the pelvic organs, correcting the effects of a sedentary lifestyle or faulty posture
Alleviates backaches
Reduces stiffness in the neck, shoulders, and knees
Tones the ligaments of the arms and legs
Helps relieve menstrual disorders

● CAUTIONS

Do not practice this asana if you have stress-related headaches, migraines, eye strain, diarrhea, low blood pressure, varicose veins, or if you are depressed, or extremely fatigued. Patients of rheumatoid arthritis who have fever should avoid this asana. Do not practice during menstruation. If you have high blood pressure, do not look up at the raised arm in the pose. If you have cervical spondylosis, do not look up for too long.

PROPS (SEE PAGE 182)
A WALL AND A BLOCK
Practice against a wall supports the body, reduces strain, and helps to align the body correctly. The mat prevents your feet from slipping, helping to maintain the final balance in the pose. The block helps those with stiff backs to reach the floor, and allows for greater extension of the spine, neck, and shoulders.

.... Look straight ahead

Keep your elbows straight and firm

Press the heel and big toe to the floor.

Pull the inner sides of your legs up

1 Spread a mat against a wall. Place a wooden block on its long side on the right edge of the mat. Stand in Tadasana (*see page* 68) on the center of the mat. Inhale, then spread your feet about 3.5 ft (1 m) apart. Your heels and buttocks should touch the wall. Raise your arms out to your sides until they are in line with your shoulders.

2 Now, turn the right foot out to the right until it is parallel to the wall. Turn your left foot in slightly to the right. Your left heel and buttocks should touch the wall. Keep your left leg straight. Stretch your arms away from your body, keeping them parallel to the floor, with your palms facing down.

THE GURU'S ADVICE

"You must keep your arms fully stretched out in this asana. Look at how I am straightening and extending the student's arm, wrist, and fingers."

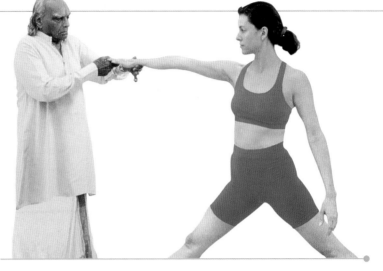

Do not tilt your head

Open your armpits

3 Bend to the right and extend your right arm toward the floor. Place your right palm on the block. Pull the tailbone into your body, keeping your left buttock and shoulders firmly pressed to the wall. Raise the left arm up toward the ceiling. Turn your head and look at your left thumb. Rest your weight on both heels, and not on your right palm. Breathe evenly, not deeply. Hold the pose for 20–30 seconds. Repeat the pose on the other side.

Push your right shoulder into your body

Lift your kneecap by contracting your quadricep muscles

Extend and relax the tips of your toes

UTTHITA PARSVAKONASANA
Intense side stretch

This asana is a variation of the classic pose (*see page* 80) and is practiced against a wall, with a block under the lowered hand. There is often a tendency to sink down on the bent leg in the final pose of this asana. Using the recommended props guards against this, and gives greater freedom for adjustments in the pose, without strain or injury.

BENEFITS

Corrects misalignment of the shoulders and shoulder blades
Relieves backaches and neck sprains
Makes the hip joint and spinal column supple
Strengthens the legs and knees, particularly the hamstring muscles
Stretches and tones the abdominal and pelvic organs
Stimulates digestion by relieving gastritis, acidity, and flatulence
Helps relieve menstrual disorders

PROPS (SEE PAGE 200)

A WALL AND A WOODEN BLOCK
The support of the wall reduces fatigue, helps you hold the pose longer, and aligns your neck and head correctly. A wooden block is placed at an appropriate height under the lowered hand. This helps those who have a stiff spine or who find it difficult to reach the floor. It also helps to maintain steadiness in the pose.

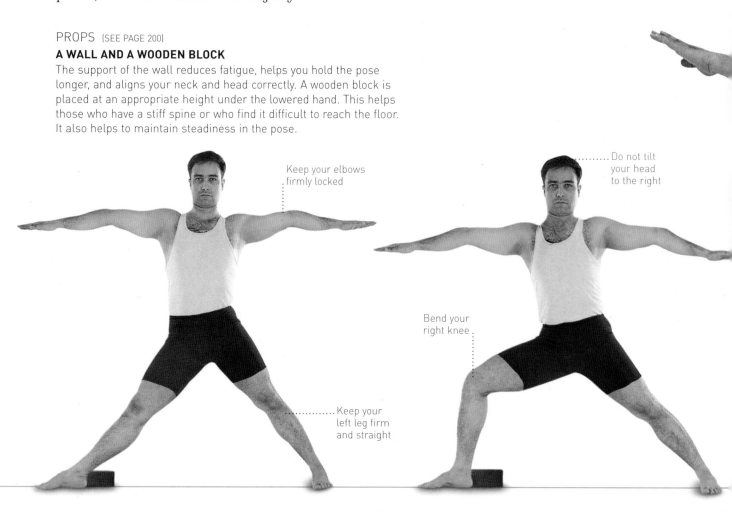

Keep your elbows firmly locked

Keep your left leg firm and straight

Do not tilt your head to the right

Bend your right knee

1 Stand in Tadasana (*see page* 68) against a wall, with your heels and your buttocks touching it. Place the block on the floor behind your right foot. Inhale, and spread your feet 3.5 ft (1 m) apart. Turn your right foot out to the right, until it is parallel to the wall.

2 Turn your left foot in slightly to the right. Press the outer edge of your left foot firmly on the floor, and bend the right knee, pushing your thigh down until your calf is at right angles to the floor. Stretch your left arm away from your left shoulder.

THE GURU'S ADVICE

"Look at how I am supporting the student's right side, in the region of his floating ribs. I rotate his bottom ribs and floating ribs from right toward the left so that it does not remain back. This improves his rotational action and balance by drawing in his left buttock and rotating the left side of his torso up toward the ceiling."

● CAUTIONS

Do not practice this asana if you have stress-related headaches, migraines, osteoarthritis of the knees, rheumatic fever, varicose veins, low blood pressure, chronic fatigue syndrome, diarrhea, psoriasis, insomnia, depression, or bulimia. Avoid the pose during menstruation, premenstrual stress, or leukorrhea. Do practice if you have heavy or irregular periods during the rest of the month, avoiding the days of menstruation. If you have cervical spondylosis, look up briefly in the final pose. Those with hypertension should look at the floor.

Open your armpit

Turn your left hip back to touch the wall

3 Bend to the right, and place your right palm on the block. Stretch the left arm up, with the palm facing forward. Now rotate the arm and bring it toward your left ear. Your left thumb should touch the wall. Turn your head and look at your left arm. Maintain a continuous stretch from the left ankle to the left wrist. Press your outer left foot into the floor. Move your shoulder blades into your body, and extend your spine toward your head. Hold the pose for 30 seconds. Repeat the pose on the other side.

Lift your kneecap

Do not rest your weight on your palm

Keep your toes stretched and relaxed

ARDHA CHANDRASANA
Half moon pose

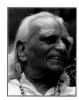

In Sanskrit, *ardha* means "half," while *chandra* translates as "moon." In this asana, your body takes the shape of a half moon. Regular practice enhances your span of concentration. It also improves coordination and motor reflexes. The intense stretch it gives to the spine, strengthens the paraspinal muscles, keeping the spine supple and well-aligned.

● BENEFITS

Rotates and flexes the vertebral joints, keeping the spinal muscles supple
Tones the lumbar and sacral spine, relieving backache
Corrects misalignment of the shoulders
Helps relieve sciatica
Improves circulation in the feet
Relieves gastritis and acidity
Corrects a prolapsed uterus
This is the only standing asana that removes fatigue, provided it is done against a wall

● CAUTIONS

Do not practice this asana if you have stress-related headaches, migraines, eye strain, varicose veins, diarrhea, or insomnia.
If you have hypertension, do not look up at your raised arm. Look straight ahead.

PROPS (SEE PAGE 182)
A WALL AND A WOODEN BLOCK
The wall gives stability and helps to align the head and neck. The wooden block makes the pose easier for those who have stiff backs and cannot reach the floor.

........Point your fingers toward the ceiling

Keep the left hip pressed to the wall .

Extend your left leg away from your torso .

.... Keep your arms straight

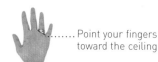

1 Stand in Tadasana (*see page* 68). Place a block on its short side against the wall. Inhale, spread your feet 3.5 ft (1 m) apart. Raise your arms to shoulder level.

2 Turn your right foot out to the right, parallel to the wall, and turn your left foot in, slightly to the right. Bend your right knee, and place the right palm on the block. Raise your left arm.

3 Straighten your right leg. Raise your left leg, until it is parallel to the floor. Keep your left arm stretched up, in line with the right arm. The back of your left hand should touch the wall.

4 Look up at your left thumb. Keep your right foot, thigh, and hip aligned. Balance on the right leg and not on your right arm. Hold the pose for 20 seconds. Repeat the pose on the other side.

UTTANASANA
Intense forward stretch

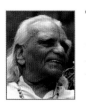

This is a less strenuous version of the classic pose (*see page 92*) that helps beginners and those with stiff backs to achieve the final forward stretch. There are five variations of the final pose. Practice the one you find most comfortable, and which suits your needs the best. This is both a calming and recuperative asana, which rests and energizes the heart and lungs.

PROPS (SEE PAGE 182)
A FOAM BLOCK AND FIVE WOODEN BLOCKS
Stack three wooden blocks on top of the foam block. Place a wooden block on either side of the stacked blocks.

SPECIFIC BENEFIT
Soothes and calms the body and brain.

SPECIFIC CAUTION
Until your back muscles become more flexible, use props to support your head.

● BENEFITS
Reduces depression if practiced regularly
Cures insomnia and relieves fatigue
Increases blood flow to the brain, soothing the brain cells and sympathetic nervous system
Regulates blood pressure
Relieves migraines and stress-related headaches
Tones the abdominal organs
Relieves stomachaches by neutralizing acidity
Strengthens and stretches the hamstring muscles
Increases the flexibility of the hip joint
Strengthens the knee joint and its surrounding tissue and muscles

● CAUTIONS
Do not practice this asana if you have osteoarthritis of the knees, or diarrhea. Patients of rheumatoid arthritis who have fever should avoid this asana. If you have low blood pressure, come out of the pose gradually to avoid dizziness.

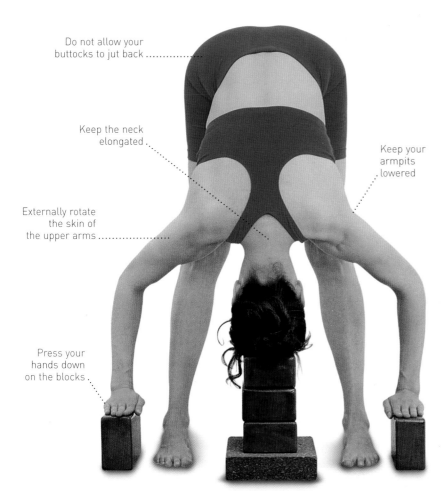

Do not allow your buttocks to jut back
Keep the neck elongated
Externally rotate the skin of the upper arms
Press your hands down on the blocks
Keep your armpits lowered

1 Stand in Tadasana (*see page* 68). Separate your legs to a distance of 1ft (30cm). Keep your feet parallel to each other, with the toes pointing forward. Pull up your kneecaps.

2 Inhale and raise your arms toward the ceiling, your palms facing forward. Extend your spine up.

3 Bend from the waist toward the floor. Press your heels on the floor to increase the stretch of your spine. This is vital for correct practice. Elongate the sides of your torso downward.

4 Rest the crown of your head on the blocks in front of you, and place your palms on the blocks beside your feet. Pull in your kneecaps. Extend your hamstrings and pull your inner legs upward. Feel one single stretch from the heels to the crown of your head. Hold the pose for 1 minute.

UTTANASANA
Variations

VARIATION 1 HANDS ON ELBOWS

PROPS (SEE PAGE 182)

A FOAM BLOCK AND THREE WOODEN BLOCKS
This variation is easier for beginners and for those who are too stiff to place their palms on the floor or on blocks.

VARIATION 2 HANDS ON ANKLES

PROPS (SEE PAGE 182)

A FOAM BLOCK AND THREE WOODEN BLOCKS
The blocks support the head and make the forward bend easier.

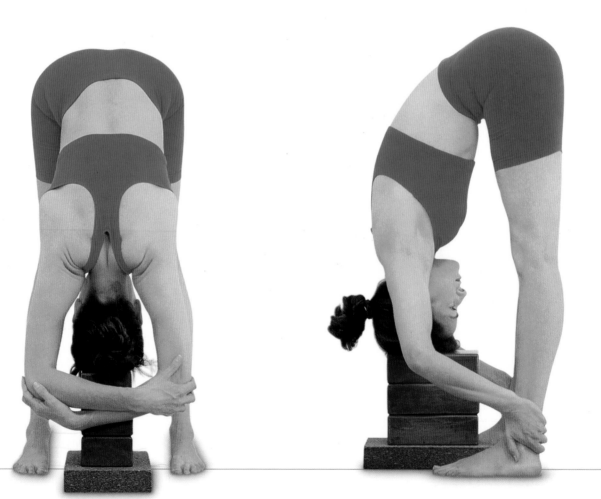

GETTING INTO THE POSE

Place the foam block on the floor and stack the 3 wooden blocks on it. Follow Steps 1, 2, and 3 of the main asana. Place the crown of your head on the blocks. Clasp your left elbow with your right hand and the right elbow with your left hand. Gravitate the folded arms downward. Hold the pose for 1 minute.

GETTING INTO THE POSE

Place the foam block on the floor and stack the 3 wooden blocks on it. Then follow Steps 1, 2, and 3 of the main asana. Exhale, and place the crown of your head on the blocks. Hold your ankles with your hands. Breathe evenly, and stay in the pose for 1 minute. Holding the ankles provides a better balance and firmness, enabling you to bend further.

"The regular, persevering, and alert practice of yoga is the foundation for stabilizing the consciousness."

VARIATION 3 PALMS ON FLOOR

PROPS (SEE PAGE 182)
A FOAM BLOCK AND THREE WOODEN BLOCKS
Once the muscles of your back feel flexible enough, do not use blocks to support your hands. Instead, place your palms flat on the floor in the final pose.

VARIATION 4 PALMS ON BLOCKS

PROPS (SEE PAGE 182)
TWO WOODEN BLOCKS
Practice this variation only when you feel your back muscles are sufficiently flexible to hold the forward bend, without the support of blocks for your head. Variations 1–4 are progressively advanced steps.

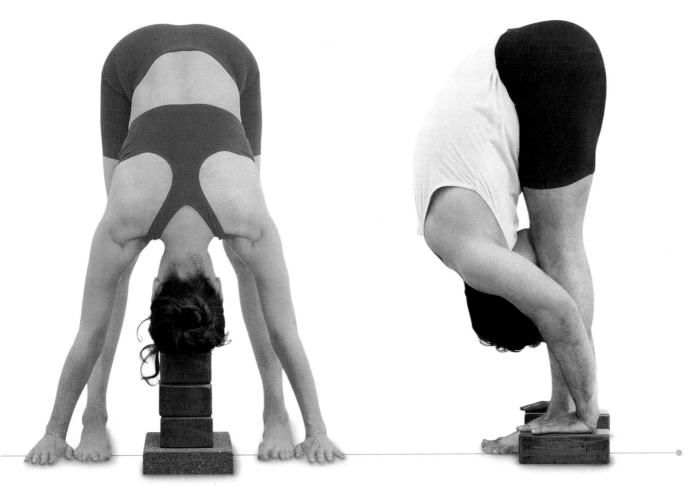

GETTING INTO THE POSE
Place the blocks as given for Variation 2. Then follow Steps 1, 2, and 3 of the main asana. Rest the crown of your head on the blocks. Then, place your palms flat on the floor, just beyond your feet (see inset). Make sure that both your heels are pressed to the floor and stretch the hamstring muscles at the back of your thighs. The thumb of each hand should

touch the little toe of each foot. Distribute your body weight equally on the toes and heels of both your feet. Breathe evenly, and hold the pose for 1 minute.

SPECIFIC CAUTIONS
Do not practice this variation if you are a beginner or if you are prone to hypertension, headaches, cervical spondylosis, insomnia, migraines, or prolapsed disks.

GETTING INTO THE POSE
Stand with your feet together. Place a block on its broad side on either side of your feet, with the long edges of the blocks parallel to your feet. Follow Steps 1, 2, and 3 of the main asana. Bend from the waist and place your palms on the blocks. Press your chin to your knees. Hold the pose for 1 minute.

PRASARITA PADOTTANASANA
Intense leg stretch

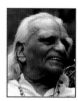

In Sanskrit, *prasarita means* "stretched out" or "spread out," while *pada* means "leg" or "foot." This asana gives an intense stretch to your legs. The torso is inverted in the pose, and the head rests on the floor, or on a block or a bolster. This restful and recuperative asana is usually practiced toward the end of the standing pose cycle, just before Salamba Sirsasana (*see page* 138).

● BENEFITS

Reduces depression, boosts confidence
Soothes the brain and the sympathetic nervous system
Energizes the heart and lungs
Reduces blood pressure
Relieves stress-related headaches, migraines, and fatigue
Tones the abdominal organs
Relieves stomachaches by neutralizing acidity
Relieves lower backaches
Strengthens the knee joint and makes the hip joint supple
Regulates menstrual flow

● CAUTIONS

Do not hold this asana for more than 1 minute, especially if you are a beginner. If you have low blood pressure come out of the pose gradually to avoid dizziness. Do not tilt your head or compress your neck while practicing this pose.

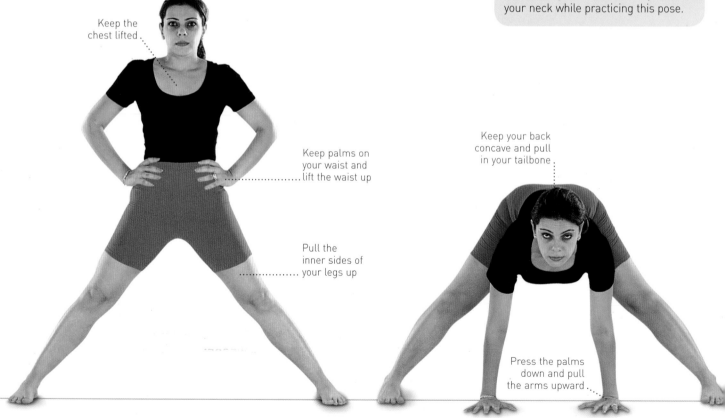

Keep the chest lifted

Keep palms on your waist and lift the waist up

Pull the inner sides of your legs up

Keep your back concave and pull in your tailbone

Press the palms down and pull the arms upward

1 Stand in Tadasana (*see page* 68). Place your hands on your hips, with your thumbs on your back and your fingers on the front of the hips. Inhale, and spread your feet 4ft (1.2m) apart. Your feet should be parallel to each other, the toes pointing forward. Press the outer edges of your feet to the floor. Keep your back erect.

2 Exhale, and lift both kneecaps. Bend forward, extending your spine, and bring your torso down toward the floor. Look up as you bend to ensure that your back is concave. Take both hands off your hips, and lower them to the floor. Place your palms flat on the floor with your fingers spread out.

3 Flex your elbows, keeping your palms flat on the floor. Place the crown of your head on the floor, between your palms. Push your sternum forward and draw the abdomen in. Move the thighbones and groin back to reduce the pressure on your head. Stay in the pose for 1 minute.

Stretch your hamstring muscles

Make sure that your hands and head are in line

Keep your head and neck passive

"Practicing the asana cools the body and brain, and gives you a feeling of tranquillity and repose."

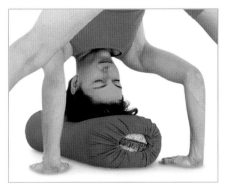

VARIATION 1
HEAD ON BOLSTER

PROPS (SEE PAGE 182)
A BOLSTER helps those with stiff lower backs to achieve the final pose more effectively and without strain.

GETTING INTO THE POSE
Place a bolster on the floor, with its flat end between your feet. Follow Steps 1, 2, and 3 of the main asana. When you bend toward the floor, place your crown on the center of the bolster. Keep your head and neck relaxed. Now, shift your weight onto your heels. Hold the pose for 1 minute.

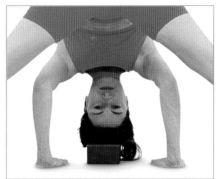

VARIATION 2
HEAD ON BLOCK

PROPS (SEE PAGE 182)
A WOODEN BLOCK will help you if you have a stiff spine and find it difficult to place your head on the floor. Use the block until your spine and the muscles of your back become more flexible. Variations 1 and 2 are progressively advanced steps.

GETTING INTO THE POSE
Place a wooden block on its broad side, on the floor in front of your feet. Follow Steps 1, 2, and 3 of the main asana. Bend forward and place the crown of your head on the block. Hold the pose for 1 minute.

ADHOMUKHA SVANASANA
Downward-facing dog stretch

This inverted stretch brings fresh blood to the heart as well as the lungs, increasing the fitness of the entire body. *Adhomukha* means "facing down" in Sanskrit, while *svan* translates as "dog." This pose and its variations are less strenuous versions of the classic pose (*see page* 88), allowing a better stretch of the limbs, and calming and soothing the mind.

(*see page* 88)

PROPS (SEE PAGE 182)
A WALL AND THREE WOODEN BLOCKS
Two blocks against the wall support the hands, stretch the arms, and reduce strain on the shoulder joints. The third block helps those with stiff backs to achieve the final pose.

SPECIFIC BENEFITS
Helps increase self-confidence. Relieves headaches and hypertension. Helps to rest and rejuvenate the heart. Reduces the "heavy-headed" feeling associated with menopause.

● BENEFITS
Tones and relaxes the nervous system, helping relieve depression and anxiety
Cures breathlessness, palpitations, extreme fatigue, and sunstroke
Stabilizes blood pressure and heart rate
Helps relieve chronic constipation, indigestion, and excess bile formation
Relieves arthritis in the shoulders, wrists, and fingers
Reduces lower backaches
Increases the flexibility of the hip, knee, and ankle joints, and
Strengthens the ligaments and tendons of the legs
Counters the damage to the cartilage of the knee or hamstring muscles, caused by jogging, walking, and other sports
Strengthens the arches of the feet and prevents calcaneal spurs

Push your heels back and pull your inner ankles up ....

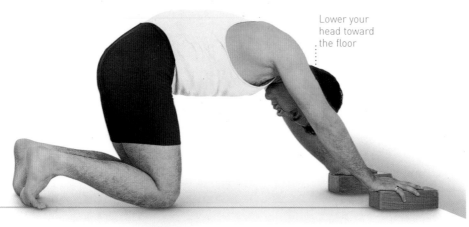

Lower your head toward the floor

Bend the backs of your knees

1 Kneel, facing a wall, about 3.5 ft (1 m) away from it. Place 2 of the blocks on their broad sides, shoulder-width apart, against the wall. Place the third block on its long side, 18 in (45 cm) away from the wall. Separate your feet to a distance of 18 in (45 cm). Place your palms on the two blocks against the wall.

2 Press your palms down on the blocks and walk your feet back, until they are 4 ft (1.2 m) away from your hands. Make sure that your feet are in line with your hands and the same distance apart. Raise both heels, stretch your legs, then lower your heels to the floor. Stretch your arms fully.

Stretch your buttocks
toward the ceiling

3 Consciously stretch each leg from heel to buttock, and from the front of the ankle to the top of the thigh. Raise your buttocks, stretch your chest, and push your sternum toward your hands. Exhale, then rest your head on the third block. Press your hands down on the blocks, extending your arms fully. Stretch your spine and expand your chest. Keep your throat soft and elongated. Relax your eyes and keep your brain passive.

Extend your arms
from the elbows
to the shoulders

Pull your
kneecaps up

Press your feet
down on the floor

VARIATION 1
HANDS AGAINST A WALL

PROPS (SEE PAGE 182)
A WALL AND A WOODEN BLOCK
Placing the fingers against the wall supports the shoulders, reducing strain in the shoulder joints.

SPECIFIC BENEFITS
Helps relieve arthritis of the shoulders, elbows, wrists, and fingers.

GETTING INTO THE POSE
Follow Steps 1 and 2 of the main asana, omitting the blocks for the hands. Place your fingers on the wall, making sure that both palms rest firmly on the floor. Then follow Step 3 of the main asana.

● CAUTIONS
Do not practice this asana if you have diarrhea. Patients of rheumatoid arthritis who have a fever should avoid this asana. If you have a stiff spine or high blood pressure, or are prone to recurrent headaches or varicose veins, always practice all these variations with your head supported by a block. Beginners should not hold the final pose for more than 30 seconds. Gradually increase the duration to 1 minute.

ADHOMUKHA SVANASANA
Variations

"The ethical discipline of the asana comes when you extend your body correctly, evenly, and to the maximum."

VARIATION 2 HEAD ON BOLSTER

PROPS (SEE PAGE 182)
A BOLSTER AND A MAT
The bolster supports the head, helping those with stiff backs to achieve the forward bend easily and without strain. The mat prevents you from slipping when you stretch out.

VARIATION 3 HEELS AGAINST A WALL

PROPS (SEE PAGE 182)
A WALL AND A WOODEN BLOCK
Placing the heels against the wall reduces strain in the knee and hip joints.

SPECIFIC BENEFITS
Strengthens the calf muscles, Achilles' tendons, and the arches of the feet. Reduces cramps in the calf muscles. Stretches the back.

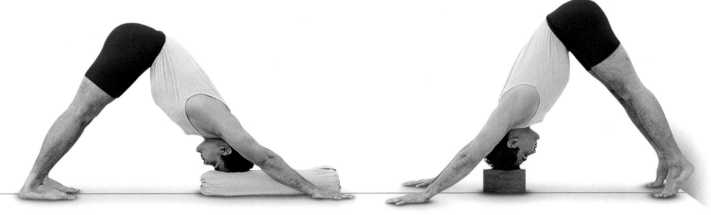

GETTING INTO THE POSE
Place a mat on the floor. Place a bolster on the mat, its long sides parallel to the long sides of the mat. Follow Steps 1, 2, and 3 of the main asana and place your head on the near end of the bolster. In this variation, you should place your palms directly on the floor, omitting the blocks as support for the hands.

GETTING INTO THE POSE
Stand in Tadasana with your back 4 ft (1.2 m) away from the wall. Kneel, then place your hands on the floor. Walk your feet back and place your heels against the wall. Lock your elbows, then follow Step 3 of the main asana.

DANDASANA
Staff pose

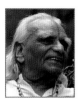

This asana is the starting point of all the seated forward bends and twists. It has many positive effects, the most important being improvement of posture. Dandasana teaches you to sit straight with an absolutely erect spine, and is helpful to those in sedentary professions. Regular practice of this pose massages and stimulates the abdominal and pelvic organs.

● BENEFITS

Improves digestion
Tones the kidneys
Helps prevent sciatic pain
Stretches and activates the muscles of the legs
Prevents fatigue in the feet by stretching the muscles of the feet

● CAUTIONS

If you have asthma, bronchitis, breathlessness, rheumatoid arthritis, ulcers, or bulimia, or are experiencing premenstrual stress, practice the asana with your back supported by a wall. Practice against a wall during menstruation.

PROPS (SEE PAGE 182)

TWO WOODEN BLOCKS AND A FOLDED BLANKET
The folded blanket placed under the buttocks helps the lower spine to extend upward sharply, releasing the hamstrings, while the two blocks under the hands help to extend the torso.

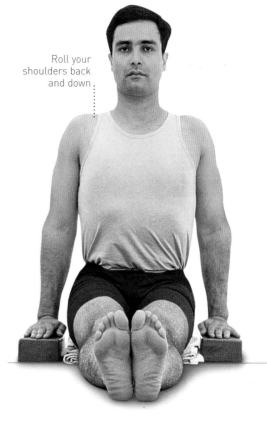

Roll your shoulders back and down

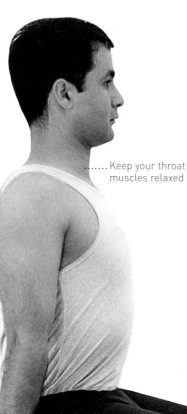

Keep your throat muscles relaxed

1 Sit on a folded blanket, with your spine erect and your knees bent. Position the blocks on their broad sides on either side of your hips. Then place your palms on the blocks. Sit on your buttock bones.

2 Straighten each leg, one at a time, and join the inner sides of your legs and feet. Lengthen the calf muscles, and stretch your knees and toes. Keep your knees straight. Press your palms down on the blocks and stretch your elbows and arms.

3 Lift your abdomen, freeing the diaphragm of tension. Hold the pose for 1 minute. Beginners may find it easier to separate their feet slightly, and should hold the pose for just 30 seconds.

VIRASANA
Hero pose

These versions of the classic asana, Virasana (*see page* 104), using rolled or folded blankets, and a block or bolsters, are designed to make the pose easier for those with stiffness in the hip, knee, or ankle joints. In addition, the extension of the spine enhances the functioning of the heart, and helps improve blood circulation to all parts of the body.

● BENEFITS
Reduces stiffness in the hip joints
Reduces inflammation in the blood vessels of the legs caused by standing for long periods
Alleviates pain or inflammation in the knees and tones knee cartilage
Relieves gout and rheumatic pain
Tones the hamstring muscles
Strengthens the arches of the feet, and relieves pain in the calves, ankles, and heels

● CAUTIONS
If you experience cramps in the legs while practicing this asana, stretch your legs out in Dandasana (*see page* 102). Avoid practicing this asana if you have a headache, migraine, or diarrhea.

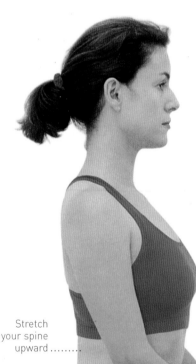

Stretch your spine upward ....

PROPS (SEE PAGE 182)
TWO BOLSTERS AND TWO BLANKETS
The bolsters support the legs and give the torso an upward extension. The blankets—one folded to sit on, the other rolled and placed between the calves and thighs—relieve pressure on the knees and ankles, and distribute body weight evenly.

1 Place 2 bolsters parallel to each other on the floor. Kneel on the bolsters, keeping your knees together. Place the rolled blanket on your shins, and the folded blanket under your buttocks. Sit with your back upright.

2 Keep your chest stretched out. Imagine you are squeezing your kidneys and drawing them into the body. Place your palms on your knees. Look straight ahead. Stay in the pose for 30–60 seconds.

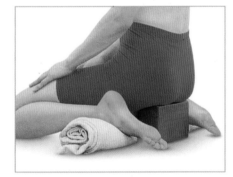

VARIATION 1
SITTING ON A BLOCK

PROPS (SEE PAGE 182)
A BLANKET AND A BLOCK
The blanket eases strain on the knees. The block supports the buttocks.

GETTING INTO THE POSE
Kneel on the floor. Separate your feet and place the block between them. Sit on the block. As you become more supple, replace the block with a folded blanket. Position the rolled blanket in front of the block and place it under both your ankles. Your feet should point back and your toes should rest on the floor. Stretch the soles of your feet. Follow Step 2 of the main asana. Hold the pose for 30–60 seconds.

URDHVAMUKHA JANU SIRSASANA

Upward-facing bent knee pose

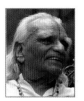

This asana is a creative adaptation of the classic pose (*see page* 114). In this version, the back is erect and the head is tilted back. In Sanskrit, the word *urdhvamukha* means "facing up." In this pose, the action of the eyes facing up, synchronized with the upward movement of the head, stimulates the pineal and pituitary glands. This movement also helps to refresh the mind.

● BENEFITS

Relieves lower and middle backaches
Reduces stiffness in the neck
Tones the kidneys and the abdominal organs
Relieves hemorrhoids
Massages the reproductive and pelvic organs, improving their functioning
Prevents prostate gland enlargement
Regulates menstrual flow and relieves menstrual disorders
Corrects a prolapsed uterus

● CAUTIONS

Avoid this asana if you are tired, have low blood pressure, stress-related headaches, migraines, eye strain, insomnia, or diarrhea. If you have osteoarthritis of the knees, place a block under your bent knee.

Relax the eyes and facial muscles

Do not tilt your head too far back

PROPS (SEE PAGE 182)

A MAT, A BLANKET, AND A YOGA BELT
The blanket supports the buttocks. The belt helps those who are overweight, or have stiff backs and find it hard to reach their feet. It also intensifies the stretch.

1 Spread a mat on the floor and place a folded blanket on it. Then sit in Dandasana (*see page* 102) on the blanket. Bend your right knee, so that the sole of your right foot touches your left thigh. The right heel should rest against the groin. Loop the belt around your left upper heel. Pull strongly on the belt and lift the torso.

2 Straighten and stretch both arms. Press both thighs and the bent knee down on the floor. Tighten your grip on the belt, and stretch your spine up. Tilt your head back, breathing evenly. Hold the pose for 20–30 seconds. Repeat the pose on the other side.

BADDHAKONASANA
Fixed angle pose

In this sitting asana, the knees are bent and the feet are joined to form a fixed angle. *Baddha* means "fixed" or "bound" in Sanskrit, and *kona* translates into "angle." The use of the props makes this version easier and more comfortable than the classic pose (*see page* 108). Regular practice of this asana helps relieve stiffness in the hips, groin, and in the hamstring muscles.

● BENEFITS

Stimulates the heart and improves circulation in the pelvic region
Tones the spine, and the abdominal and pelvic organs
Prevents hernia
Alleviates sciatica and varicose veins
Reduces menstrual pain, irregular periods, and leukorrhea

● CAUTIONS

Practice this asana sitting against a wall if you have asthma, bronchitis, breathlessness, rheumatoid arthritis, cardiac conditions, or premenstrual stress. Make sure that your lower spine does not become concave, as this will strain your waist and hips.

PROPS (SEE PAGE 182)

A BOLSTER AND TWO WOODEN BLOCKS
The bolster below the buttocks lifts the abdomen and relaxes the groin, allowing the knees to descend easily. A block under each knee relieves stiffness in the hips.

1 Sit on a bolster placed at right angles to your body (*see inset below*). Place a block on either side of your hips. Sit in Dandasana (*see page* 102). Bend your knees and join both soles together. Pull your heels closer to the bolster. Beginners may find it easier to use a bolster positioned parallel to the hips (*see inset above*).

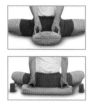

2 Push your knees away from each other and lower them gradually onto the blocks. Take your hands behind your back and press your fingertips to the bolster. Open out your chest and draw in the abdomen. Initially, hold the pose for 1 minute. Gradually increase the duration of the asana to 5 minutes.

Relax your face ....

.... Keep the chest lifted and spread

.... Lift your diaphragm

.. Open the groin

SWASTIKASANA
Cross-legged pose

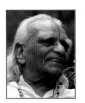

In Sanskrit, *swastika* means "auspicious" and "well-beingness." This asana is one of the basic poses of yoga and symbolizes its meditative spirituality and physical rigor. Regular practice improves blood circulation in the legs. This asana is recommended for those who have to stay on their feet for long periods. The pose also calms and rejuvenates the mind.

● BENEFITS

Rests tired feet and legs
Reduces inflammation of the veins in the legs
Makes the hip joint and groin supple
Strengthens the cartilage of the knees and relieves pain in the knees
Improves circulation and reduces inflammation in the knees

● CAUTIONS

If your legs ache while performing the asana, place a folded blanket under them.

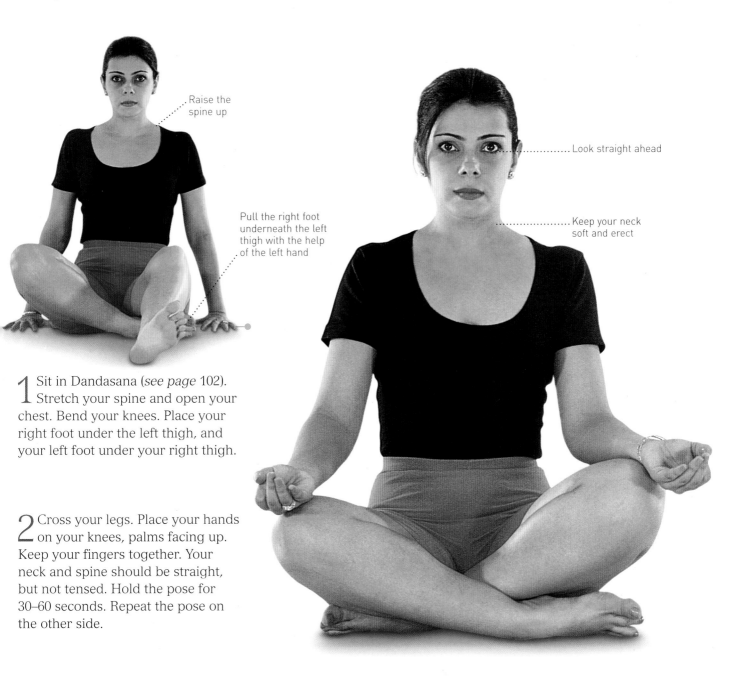

Raise the spine up

Pull the right foot underneath the left thigh with the help of the left hand

Look straight ahead

Keep your neck soft and erect

1 Sit in Dandasana (*see page* 102). Stretch your spine and open your chest. Bend your knees. Place your right foot under the left thigh, and your left foot under your right thigh.

2 Cross your legs. Place your hands on your knees, palms facing up. Keep your fingers together. Your neck and spine should be straight, but not tensed. Hold the pose for 30–60 seconds. Repeat the pose on the other side.

PARIPURNA NAVASANA
Complete boat pose

In this asana, the body takes the shape of a boat. The word *paripurna* means "complete" or "full" in Sanskrit, while *nava* means "boat." The use of props in this asana allows the pose to be held without straining your stomach and back muscles. Regular practice of this asana tones the muscles and abdominal organs.

● BENEFITS

Increases the body's metabolic rate
Improves blood circulation in the abdomen
Tones the abdominal muscles and organs
Relieves indigestion and flatulence
Tones the kidneys
Reduces lower backaches by strengthening the spinal muscles

● CAUTIONS

Do not practice this asana if you have a cardiac condition or low blood pressure. Avoid the pose if you have breathlessness, asthma, bronchitis, a cold and congestion, a migraine, chronic fatigue syndrome, or insomnia, cervical spondylosis, severe backaches, diarrhea, or menstrual disorders.

PROPS (SEE PAGE 182)

A WALL, TWO HALF-HALASANA STOOLS, TWO BLANKETS, A MAT
The stools support the legs and back, freeing the abdomen of tension. The mat is spread on the floor, and the two blankets cushion the back and legs.

SPECIFIC CAUTIONS
The stools are essential until your stomach muscles, arms, legs, and back are strong enough to allow you to hold the pose on your own. Make sure that your neck and head are not strained during practice.

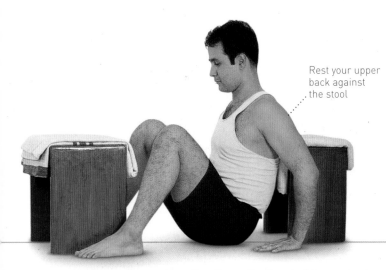

Rest your upper back against the stool

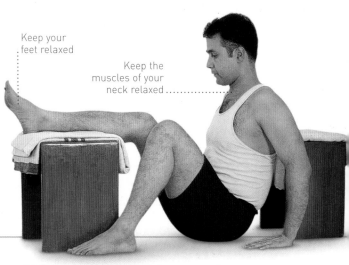

Keep your feet relaxed

Keep the muscles of your neck relaxed

1 Spread a mat on the floor, its short side against a wall. Place a stool against the wall. Place the other stool about 4ft (1.2m) away from the first stool, in line with it. Place a folded blanket on each stool. Sit between both stools, resting your back against the stool touching the wall. Place your palms behind your buttocks, fingers pointing forward. Bend your knees.

2 Sit on your buttock bones and press your palms down on the mat. Raise your right leg and place your calf on the stool in front of you. Your heel should rest on the stool so that it cushions the back and calf. Breathe evenly.

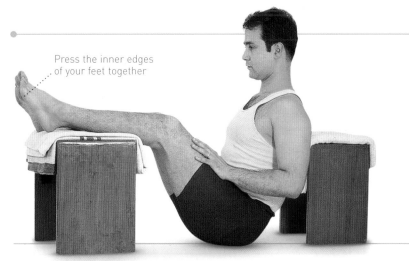

Press the inner edges of your feet together

3 Now raise your left leg, and place the left calf on the stool in front of you. Keep your knees and feet together. Press both heels down on the stool. Place your palms on your thighs.

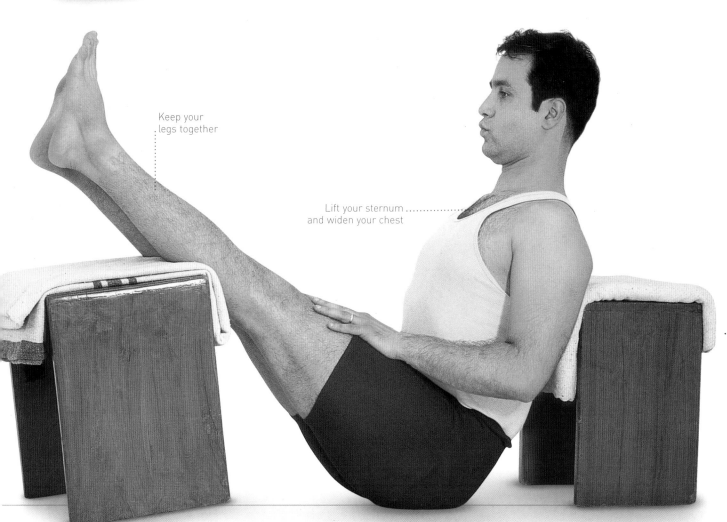

Keep your legs together

Lift your sternum and widen your chest

4 Exhale, and place your palms back on the floor. Press them down and stretch your torso upward. Pull in your shoulder blades. Keeping your legs together, straighten them and lift your calves off the stool. Place your palms back on your thighs. Rotate your thigh muscles inward. Feel the extension of your legs. Keep your abdomen soft. Hold the pose for 1 minute, increasing the duration to 5 minutes with practice.

PARIPURNA NAVASANA
Variation

VARIATION 1
ONE LONG YOGA BELT

PROPS (SEE PAGE 182)
ONE LONG YOGA BELT, OR TWO YOGA BELTS BUCKLED, to support the feet and back.

SPECIFIC CAUTION
Position the belt around your upper back, and not lumbar or middle back since that can cause pain.

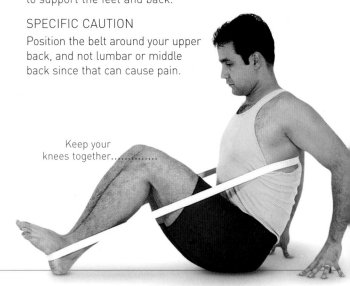

Keep your knees together............

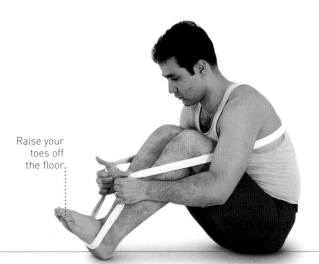

Raise your toes off the floor.

1 Sit on a mat. Bend your knees. Take the belt over your head, and place one end of the belt around the upper back, just below the shoulder blades. Loop the other end around the soles of the feet, just above the heels. Tighten the belt to an appropriate length—it should not feel too slack or too tight.

2 Place your hands behind your hips, approximately 6–8 in (15–20 cm) apart, fingers pointing forward. Press your fingertips to the floor. Move your hands back slightly. Keep both heels on the floor, with the toes pointing forward. Press the knees and feet together. Keep your shoulders and back straight.

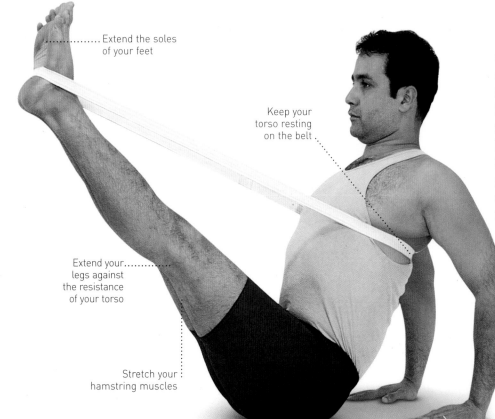

............Extend the soles of your feet

Keep your torso resting on the belt ...:

Extend your...........
legs against
the resistance
of your torso

Stretch your
hamstring muscles

3 Press your palms down firmly on the floor to support your body. Recline your back on the belt. Slowly raise your feet off the floor. Straighten and stretch your legs upward. Keep the spine erect, from the tailbone to the back of your neck. Lift your sternum and open your chest. Relax your facial muscles. Be conscious of the stretch of your legs and torso. Your abdomen should be soft and relaxed. Hold the pose for 1 minute. With practice, increase the duration to 5 minutes. Breathe evenly.

UPAVISTA KONASANA
Seated wide-angle pose

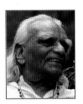

This version of Upavista Konasana is adapted to help beginners and those with stiff backs to stretch the legs out to the sides, omitting the forward bend of the original asana. The pose gets its name from the Sanskrit words *upavista*, which means "seated," and *kona*, which translates into "angle." This asana relaxes stress-related tension in the abdominal muscles.

● BENEFITS

Helps treat arthritis of the hips
Relieves sciatic pain
Helps prevent and relieve hernia
Massages the organs of the reproductive system
Stimulates the ovaries, regulates menstrual flow, and relieves menstrual pain and disorders
Corrects a prolapsed uterus or bladder

● CAUTIONS

If you have asthma, you must practice this asana sitting on a folded blanket close to the wall. Lift and open the chest, allowing for easy breathing.

PROPS (SEE PAGE 182)
A WALL supports the back and eases breathing.

1 Sit against a wall. Then sit in Dandasana (*see page* 102) with your shoulders and back touching the wall. Keep your back erect. Sit on your buttock bones. Place your palms on the floor, beside your hips, fingers pointing forward. Look straight ahead.

2 Press your palms down on the floor to push your torso upward. Exhale, and spread your legs as far apart as possible. Use your hands, one by one, to help you to push your legs even further out to the sides.

Extend your hamstring muscles

3 Move your hands behind your buttocks, and place both palms on the floor. Press your heels and thighs down on the floor. Lift your waist and the sides of your torso. Rotate your thighs to the front so that the kneecaps face the ceiling. Sit on your buttock bones, keeping your pelvic bones parallel to them. Stretch each leg from thigh to heel. Hold the pose for 1 minute (later, increase to 3–5 minutes).

Keep your shoulders rolled toward the wall

Lift the chest up

Push your hamstring muscles down on the floor

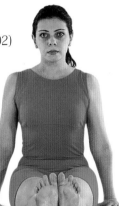

PASCHIMOTTANASANA
Intense back stretch

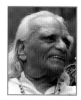

This version of Paschimottanasana uses five combinations of props that make the pose more accessible for those who have stiff backs. These variations, which give a gradually progressive stretch to the back, relieve lower backaches and make the spine supple.

PROPS (SEE PAGE 185)
TWO BOLSTERS support the head and allow people with stiff backs to hold the pose more easily.

SPECIFIC BENEFITS
Those who have sciatica, varicose veins, and arthritis will find relief by doing this variation. When you have a headache or fatigue in the arms and shoulders, adopt this variation in order to relax. Helps treat incontinence.

● BENEFITS

Sharpens memory
Soothes the sympathetic nervous system
Prevents fatigue
Rests the heart, normalizes blood pressure and the pulse rate
Relieves chronic headaches, migraines, and eye strain.
Reduces stress in the facial muscles
Alleviates stress-related compression or a feeling of tightness in the throat and diaphragm
Improves blood circulation in the pelvic area, toning the pelvic organs
Regulates blood supply to the endocrine glands, activating the adrenal glands, and relaxing the thyroid gland
Cools the temperature of the skin
Strengthens the vertebral joints and stretches the ligaments of the spine

● CAUTIONS

Do not practice this asana if you have asthma, bronchitis, or diarrhea. Do not practice this pose if you have cervical spondylosis.

Rest your arms and forehead comfortably on the bolster

1 Sit in Dandasana (*see page* 102). Place 2 bolsters, one on top of the other, across your knees. Make sure that your ankles, heels, and big toes are close together. Stretch your arms over the bolsters and bend forward. Hold your feet just below the toes, keeping both legs straight. Press your thighs and knees together.

2 Bend from the base of your spine and push your waist forward. Elongate your torso toward your feet, stretching it from the groin to the navel. Make sure that your abdominal muscles do not contract. Rest your elbows and forehead on the bolsters. Keep the muscles of your thighs and calves fully stretched.

3 Extend your neck. Push both your shoulders down and back, moving them away from your ears. Rest your forehead evenly on the bolsters, and do not tilt your head to one side. Your arms should be straight, but not tensed. Consciously relax your neck, face, eyes, and ears. Breathe evenly, and stay in this pose for 5 minutes.

"When practiced, this asana cools the brain, calms the mind, and rejuvenates the entire body. It is while practicing yoga asanas that you learn the art of adjustment."

VARIATION 1
THREE BOLSTERS

PROPS [SEE PAGE 185]
THREE BOLSTERS
Sitting on a bolster gives the torso height, making the forward bend easier.

SPECIFIC BENEFITS
Reduces acidity and prevents ulcers. Relieves menstrual pain and premenstrual stress. Helps treat stress-related disorders of the reproductive system. Prevents fibroid formation. Regulates menstrual flow by relaxing the uterine muscles. Relieves vaginal dryness and itching.

SPECIFIC CAUTION
Avoid this variation if you have varicose veins.

VARIATION 2
TWO BOLSTERS AND A BLOCK

PROPS [SEE PAGE 185]
TWO BOLSTERS AND A WOODEN BLOCK
The block under the heels gives the legs an intense stretch.

SPECIFIC BENEFITS
Alleviates osteoarthritis of the knees and ankles. Prevents varicose veins and sciatic pain. Reinvigorates tired feet. Extends the calves and hamstrings, giving relief to the legs.

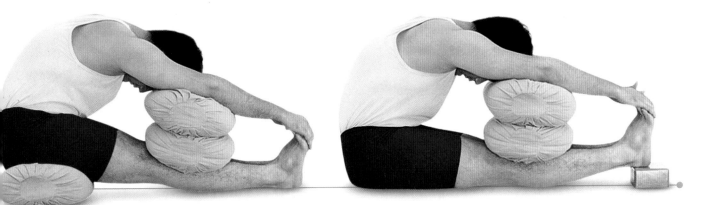

GETTING INTO THE POSE
Place a bolster behind you, so that the center of the long side touches the back of the buttocks. Bend your knees. Press your palms down on the bolster and place your buttocks on it. Now follow Steps 1, 2, and 3 of the main asana.

GETTING INTO THE POSE
Position the block near your feet with its long side facing you. Place your heels, one by one, on the block, supporting the backs of your knees with your hands. Now follow Steps 1, 2, and 3 of the main asana. Make sure that you do not contract your leg muscles. Extend your thigh muscles and keep your knees firmly down on the floor.

PASCHIMOTTANASANA
Variations

"Focus on keeping your spine straight. It is the job of the spine to keep the brain alert."

VARIATION 3
TWO BOLSTERS AND A BELT

PROPS [SEE PAGE 182]
A BELT AND TWO BOLSTERS
The belt helps those who are too stiff to hold their feet.

SPECIFIC BENEFITS
Rests tired feet. Relieves osteoarthritis of the ankles. Prevents sciatica and varicose veins. Helps improve the forward extension of the spine.

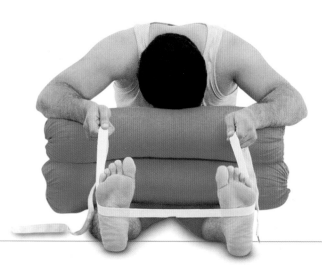

GETTING INTO THE POSE
Follow Step 1 of the main asana, but separate your legs to a distance of 1 ft (30 cm). Point your toes toward the ceiling. Hold one end of the belt in each hand and loop it over your feet. Keep shortening the length of the belt until the pull feels intense. Then follow Steps 2 and 3 of the main asana. Widen your elbows and keep the belt taut.

VARIATION 4
TWO BOLSTERS AND A STOOL

PROPS [SEE PAGE 182]
A LOW, OPEN STOOL AND TWO BOLSTERS
The stool helps you to stretch your arms and spine. It relaxes the back of the head, throat, diaphragm, chest, and back.

SPECIFIC BENEFITS
Helps to relieve depression. Stimulates the liver and kidneys. Reduces ulcers, flatulence, constipation, and indigestion. Prevents varicose veins and sciatic pain. Relieves osteoarthritis of the hips. Prevents fibroids. Relieves vaginal itching. If practiced during menstruation, regulates menstrual flow and reduces menstrual pain. Relieves stress-related headaches and migraines if practiced with a crepe bandage around the eyes. Helps to find muscular alignment since the outer edges of the legs are supported.

GETTING INTO THE POSE
Place the stool on the floor. Sit in Dandasana and stretch your legs through the stool. Separate your legs until they touch the inner sides of the stool. Then follow Steps 1, 2, and 3 of the main asana, but do not hold your toes. Stretch your arms over the bolsters, and hold the farther edge of

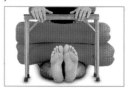

the stool. Rest your forehead on the top bolster and close your eyes. Breathe evenly. This variation, if practiced with the feet together (*see inset*), intensifies the forward extension of the spine.

ADHOMUKHA PASCHIMOTTANASANA
Downward-facing intense back stretch

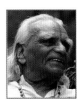

In Sanskrit, *paschim* literally means "west." In yogic terms, this refers to the back of the whole body, from the heels to the head. Although this asana stretches this region intensely, the props enable you to extend the back with ease and hold the pose comfortably, without strain. Regular practice of the asana tones the liver and kidneys. The stretch also alleviates lower backaches.

● BENEFITS

Relieves stress-related appetite loss
Helps in the treatment of acidity, ulcers, anorexia, bulimia, and alcoholism
Tones the liver and kidneys
Relieves lower backaches

● CAUTIONS

Do not practice this asana if you have an episode of diarrhea, or if you are experiencing the symptoms of asthma or bronchitis.

PROPS (SEE PAGE 182)
A LOW STOOL AND TWO BOLSTERS
The stool gives the torso height and helps those with stiff backs to bend forward easily. The bolsters support the torso and help to make the pose restful and relaxing.

1 Sit on the front edge of the stool and place 2 bolsters beside it. Hold the stool and straighten your legs, keeping your legs and feet together. Place a bolster on your legs, parallel to them. Place the second bolster on top of the first, but about 2–3 in (5 cm) closer to your toes. Straighten your back and stretch your torso upward. Take several breaths.

2 Look down and push your torso toward your legs. Stretch your arms out over the bolsters. Make sure that you stretch from the base of the spine. Keep your abdomen soft and breathe normally. Stretch your hands beyond the bolsters and hold the upper soles of your feet.

3 Rest your chest on the bolsters and place your forehead on the top bolster. Now, holding on to your feet, extend your torso down even further. If you cannot reach your toes, rest your hands as far down on the top bolster as possible. Hold the pose for 1 minute. With practice, increase the duration to 5 minutes. Reduce the bolster support as your forward extension improves.

Push your spine forward ....

Stabilize the stool against a wall ....

Keep your legs fully extended

JANU SIRSASANA
Head-on-knee pose

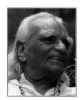

This asana calms the brain and the sympathetic nervous system. The mind detaches itself from the senses and feelings of restlessness and irritability are soothed. This adapted version of the classic pose (*see page* 114) is supported by props. It rests the heart and activates the *anahata* or "heart" chakra (*see page* 57), helping to treat depression and alleviate insomnia.

● BENEFITS

Sharpens the memory
Relieves chronic headaches, migraines, or eye strain
Helps normalize blood pressure
Reduces angina pain
Reduces stress-related appetite loss
Vitalizes the adrenal gland and relaxes the thyroid gland
Improves bladder control
Prevents enlargement of the prostate gland
Reduces menstrual cramps and relieves dryness and itching in the vagina
Prevents fibroids and regulates menstrual flow

● CAUTIONS

Avoid the pose if you have diarrhea because it will aggravate the condition. If your knees are stiff, or if you have osteoarthritis of the knees, practice with a wooden block under the bent knee. If you have a stress-related headache or migraine, practice the asana with a crepe bandage over your eyes.

PROPS (SEE PAGE 182)

A BOLSTER, A BLANKET, AND A LOW, OPEN STOOL
The bolster and blanket support the head and help those with stiff backs to bend forward easily. The low, open stool facilitates the arm extension from the shoulders to the fingers. It also relaxes and stretches the back of the head and neck, creating a tractionlike extension of the spine.

SPECIFIC BENEFITS
If you have a cold, asthma or bronchitis, practice this asana with props because the classical pose will not give relief.

1 Place a low stool on the floor. Sit in Dandasana (*see page* 102) with your feet through it. Sit on your buttock bones. Press your palms to the floor beside your hips and straighten your back. Bend your left leg and bring the heel to your groin. Your toes should touch your right thigh and your legs should be at an obtuse angle. Push the bent knee back. Keep your right leg absolutely straight. Place the bolster across your right calf, and place a folded blanket on top of it for added height.

Keep your back erect

Expand your chest

Press your fingers to the floor

Place the stool in line with your chest

Keep your foot upright

2 Exhale, and bend forward from the base of your spine, not from the shoulder blades. Stretch your arms over the bolster and rest your palms on the stool. Keep your left knee pressed to the floor.

Push your torso forward

Stretch the right leg from thigh to heel

3 Push your torso forward and hold the far edge of the stool. Stretch from the groin to the navel. Do not allow your abdomen to contract as you bend forward. Rest your forehead on the blanket and close your eyes. The height of the bolster or blanket depends upon the flexibility of your back. If you are unable to rest your forehead comfortably, add another blanket. Remove this blanket once you are able to rest your forehead easily. Exhale slowly to release the tension in your neck and head. Stay in this position for approximately 1 minute. Repeat the pose on the other side.

Keep your head and neck relaxed

Extend your spine forward

ADHOMUKHA VIRASANA
Downward-facing hero pose

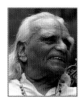

This asana is a variation of the classic pose, Virasana (*see page* 104). *Vira* means "hero" or "warrior" in Sanskrit, *adho* indicates "downward," and *mukha* means "face." This is a very restful asana to practice since it pacifies the frontal brain, reducing stress, soothing the eyes and nerves, and calming the mind. It also helps to rejuvenate you after a tiring day.

● BENEFITS

Relieves breathlessness, dizziness, fatigue, and headaches
Reduces high blood pressure
Stretches and tones the spine, relieving pain in the back and neck
Reduces acidity and flatulence
Alleviates menstrual pain and depression associated with menstruation

● CAUTIONS

Do not practice this asana if you are incontinent. If you have a migraine or a stress-related headache, wrap a crepe bandage around your eyes and forehead.

PROPS (SEE PAGE 185)

A BOLSTER AND TWO BLANKETS
The bolster supports the head and eases stiffness in the back. A blanket supports the chest, while the second blanket under the thighs relieves painful ankles. If you have a migraine, or a stress-related headache, wrap a crepe bandage around your eyes.

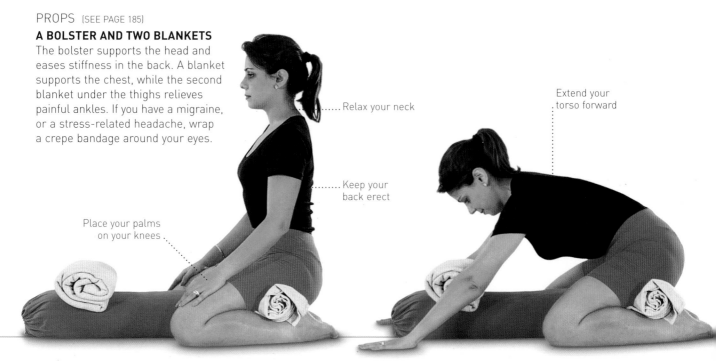

...... Relax your neck

.... Keep your back erect

Place your palms on your knees .

Extend your torso forward

1 Place a bolster on the floor and put a rolled blanket on it. Kneel with the bolster between your knees. Place the second blanket across your calves and heels. Lower your buttocks onto the blanket. Place both palms on your knees, your feet close together. Imagine you are pulling your kidneys into your body. Pause for 30 seconds.

2 Move the bolster toward you. The front end should be in between your knees. Draw the bolster closer to your body so that it is just below your abdomen. Position the rolled blanket on the bolster so that you can rest your face on it. Now exhale, and move your torso forward. Stretch your arms out fully and place your hands on the floor, on either side of the far end of the bolster.

THE GURU'S ADVICE

"The pressure of my hands on the student's sacro-lumbar area is like a fulcrum. In this pose, do not lift the buttocks. Extend the torso and hands forward. Keep the lower back firm, and extend it forward."

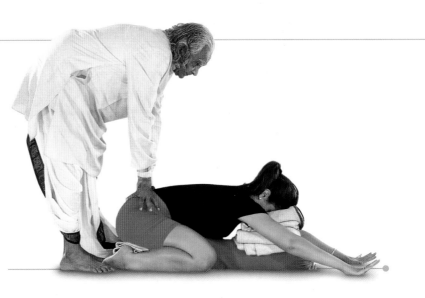

3 Lower your chest to the bolster. Stretch your arms forward, extend the nape of your neck, and rest your forehead and face on the blanket. Push your thighs down, and lower your buttocks toward the floor. Keep your abdomen soft. Open your armpits and extend your sternum. Push your chest forward, broadening your ribs. In order to relax your body, increase the forward stretch of your torso and spine on the bolster. Make sure your buttocks rest on the other blanket. Stay in the pose for 30–60 seconds.

Keep the abdomen elongated and relaxed

Rest on the front of your feet

VARIATION 1 TWO BOLSTERS

PROPS (SEE PAGE 185)
TWO BOLSTERS AND TWO BLANKETS
The bolsters help those with stiff backs to hold the pose easily. The added height makes it easier to lower the chest.

GETTING INTO THE POSE
Place 2 bolsters in front of you and follow Step 1 of the main asana. Now move the bolsters toward you. The front end of the lower bolster should be between your knees. Draw the 2 bolsters closer to your body, so that the end of the top bolster touches your abdomen. Place the rolled blanket on the far edge of the top bolster. Now follow Steps 2 and 3 of the main asana.

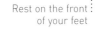

ADHOMUKHA SWASTIKASANA
Downward-facing cross-legged pose

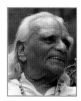

In this asana, you sit cross-legged and rest your head, chest, and shoulders on a bench, bolster, and blanket. This is an extremely relaxing pose and relieves strain in your back, neck, and heart. It also alleviates the symptoms of premenstrual stress. Regular practice of the asana helps people who are prone to anxiety, tension, and frequent mood swings.

● BENEFITS

Soothes the sympathetic nervous system, relieving stress and fatigue
Relieves migraines and stress-related headaches
Relieves palpitations and breathlessness
Helps prevent nausea and vomiting
Relieves pain in the hip joints
Rests tired legs and improves blood circulation in the knees

● CAUTIONS

If you cannot sit in Virasana due to aching feet, you can practice this pose instead. If you have stress-related headaches or a migraine, wrap a crepe bandage around your eyes.

PROPS (SEE PAGE 182)

TWO BOLSTERS, A LONG BENCH, A MAT, AND A BLANKET
The bolster to sit on gives the torso height for the forward stretch. The bench, mat, bolster, and blanket between the chest and the bench, support the head and prevent neck strain.

1 Place a bolster on the floor at right angles to the bench. Place a mat and a bolster along the length of the bench. Place a folded blanket between the front end of the bolster and the front edge of the bench.

2 Sit cross-legged as in Swastikasana (*see page* 209) on a bolster. Make sure that you are sitting on the inner sides of your buttock bones.

3 Exhale, bend forward, and rest your chest on the folded blanket. Place your forehead on the bolster. Bring your arms forward and bend your elbows. Place your right palm on your left forearm, and your left palm on your right forearm. Exhale slowly, and feel the tension in the head and neck dissipate. Keep your neck muscles soft and elongated. Hold the pose for 2 minutes. Breathe evenly.

Relax your upper torso on the blanket

BHARADVAJASANA ON A CHAIR
Torso twist

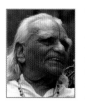

The classic version of this pose (*see page* 128) is the basic seated twist, and can sometimes be difficult for beginners to perform. However, the asana can also be practiced seated on a chair. These adaptations of the classic pose are recommended if you are elderly, overweight, or recovering from a long illness.

PROPS [SSEE PAGE 182]
A CHAIR supports you and allows for effective and safe rotation of the torso.

1 Sit sideways on the chair with the right side of your body against the chair back. Sit erect and exhale. Hold the outer sides of the chair back.

2 Keep the spine lifted and turn the torso toward the right without leaving the spinal axis. Exhale as you rotate, but do not hold your breath. Look over your right shoulder. Hold the pose for 20–30 seconds. Repeat the pose on the other side.

Push the right side of the chair away from your body, while pulling the left side toward you

Keep your legs apart

Do not lift your feet off the floor

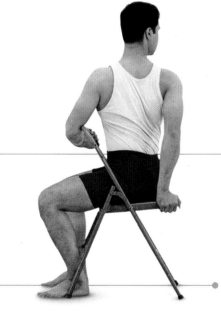

VARIATION 1 LEGS THROUGH THE CHAIR BACK

SPECIFIC BENEFITS
This variation gives a sense of direction, yielding more rotation without disturbing the alignment of the body.

GETTING INTO THE POSE
Step your legs between the chair back and the seat. Hold the seat with your right hand, and the back of the chair with your left hand. Lift and rotate your torso to the right. Hold the pose for 20–30 seconds. Repeat the pose on the other side.

BHARADVAJASANA
Torso stretch

This asana is a variation of the classic seated twist (*see page* 128). It works on the dorsal and lumbar spine, and improves blood circulation in the organs of the abdomen. Regular practice of this pose increases the flexibility of the entire body. It also relieves gout in the knees and helps in the treatment of cervical spondylosis, arthritis, and rheumatism of the heels, knees, hips, and shoulders.

● BENEFITS

Alleviates stiffness and pain in the lower back, neck, and shoulders
Reduces pain in the hip joints, calves, heels, and ankles
Makes the hamstrings supple
Helps treat disorders of the kidneys, liver, spleen, and gall bladder
Relieves indigestion and flatulence
Tones the muscles of the uterus

● CAUTIONS

Do not practice this asana if you have a cardiac condition, migraines, headaches, severe eye strain, a cold or chest congestion, diarrhea, chronic fatigue syndrome, depression, or insomnia.

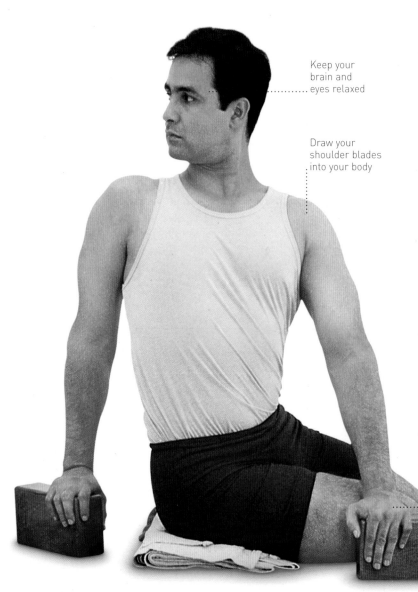

Keep your brain and eyes relaxed

Draw your shoulder blades into your body

Press your hands down on the blocks

PROPS (SEE PAGE 182)

A BLANKET AND TWO WOODEN BLOCKS
The folded blanket supports the buttocks and keeps the body straight. Placing the hands on the blocks gives the pressure needed to keep the spine erect and improve its rotation.

1 Sit in Dandasana (*see page* 102) on a folded blanket. Bend your knees and bring your feet next to your left buttock. Place your left ankle on the arch of your right foot (*see inset*). Press your knees together.

2 Place the blocks on their long sides, one behind the right buttock and the other beside your right knee. Then stretch your spine and inhale.

3 Exhale, and turn to the right. Move your right shoulder back. Place your right hand on the block behind you and your left hand on the block beside you. Press both hands down on the blocks. Raise your spine and chest. Exhale, and look over your right shoulder. Do not hold your breath. Hold the pose for 20–30 seconds. Repeat the pose on the other side.

MARICHYASANA
Torso and leg stretch

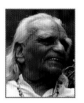

This asana adapts and combines the two classic versions of Marichyasana, one a forward bend, and the other a twist (*see page* 132). The props help to keep the torso centered and erect. They also enhance the rotation of the spine, working the dorsal and lumbar region. Practicing this asana helps reduce stiffness in the back, neck, and shoulders.

● BENEFITS
Alleviates lower backaches and cervical spondylosis
Increases blood circulation to the abdominal organs
Aids digestion and reduces flatulence
Helps in the treatment of hernia
Tones the liver and kidneys

● CAUTIONS
Do not practice if you have a cardiac condition, migraines, headaches, a cold or chest congestion, diarrhea, constipation, chronic fatigue syndrome, insomnia, or depression.

PROPS (SEE PAGE 182)
A BLANKET AND A WOODEN BLOCK
The blanket supports the buttocks and lifts the torso, increasing the spinal twist. It also prevents the bent leg from tilting to the side. The block, placed on its broad side under the hand, improves the spinal twist and keeps the torso erect.

1 Sit in Dandasana (*see page* 102) on a folded blanket. Place a block behind you. Bend your right leg at the knee. Make sure the shin is perpendicular to the floor and your right heel touches your groin. Keep your left leg straight.

2 Bend your right elbow and place your upper right arm against your inner right leg (*see inset*). Place your left hand on the block behind you, keeping your left arm straight. Press your right arm and your right knee against each other, with equal pressure. Press your left hand down on the block.

3 Lift your torso, exhale, and turn to the left. Make sure that your bent leg does not tilt, and that there is no gap between your right arm and knee. Look over your left shoulder. Hold the pose for 20–30 seconds. Repeat the pose on the other side.

Keep your head, eyes, and neck passive

Keep your palm open

Rest your foot on the center of your heel

UTTHITA MARICHYASANA
Intense torso and leg stretch

This variation of the classic pose (*see page* 132) is practiced against the wall with the help of a high stool. This asana works the paraspinal muscles and ligaments, which rarely get exercised in our normal, day-to-day routine. The props allow the twist to be achieved without strain. *Utthita Marichyasana* is recommended for those with lower backaches.

● BENEFITS

Relieves stiffness in the neck and shoulders
Improves the alignment of the spinal column and keeps it supple
Alleviates pain in the lower back, hips, and tailbone
Prevents the shortening of the leg muscles associated with aging
Prevents sciatica
Cures indigestion
Relieves flatulence

● CAUTIONS

Do not practice this asana if you have a serious cardiac condition, blocked arteries, high or low blood pressure, migraines, severe eye strain, a cold, bronchitis, breathlessness, chronic fatigue, depression, insomnia, diarrhea, constipation, or osteoarthritis of the knees. Women should avoid this asana during menstruation.

PROPS (SEE PAGE 182)
A WALL, A HIGH STOOL, AND A ROUNDED BLOCK
The stool makes the twisting action easier for those with stiff backs. The block placed under the left leg allows for a more effective rotation.

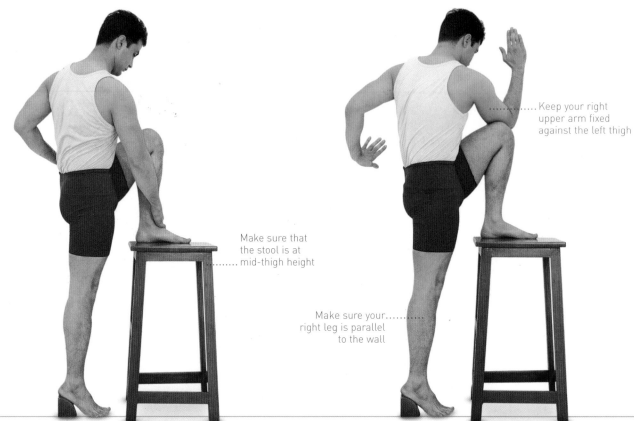

Make sure that the stool is at mid-thigh height

Keep your right upper arm fixed against the left thigh

Make sure your right leg is parallel to the wall

1 Place a stool against a wall. Stand facing the stool, with your left shoulder touching the wall. Put the block under your right heel. Place your left foot on the stool, and your left palm on the wall at waist level. Keep your right leg stretched.

2 Bend your right arm and rest its elbow on the outer side of your left knee. Place your right palm on the wall. Press your left palm against the wall and push your torso away from the wall. Make sure that your body is perpendicular to the floor.

"Total extension brings total relaxation."

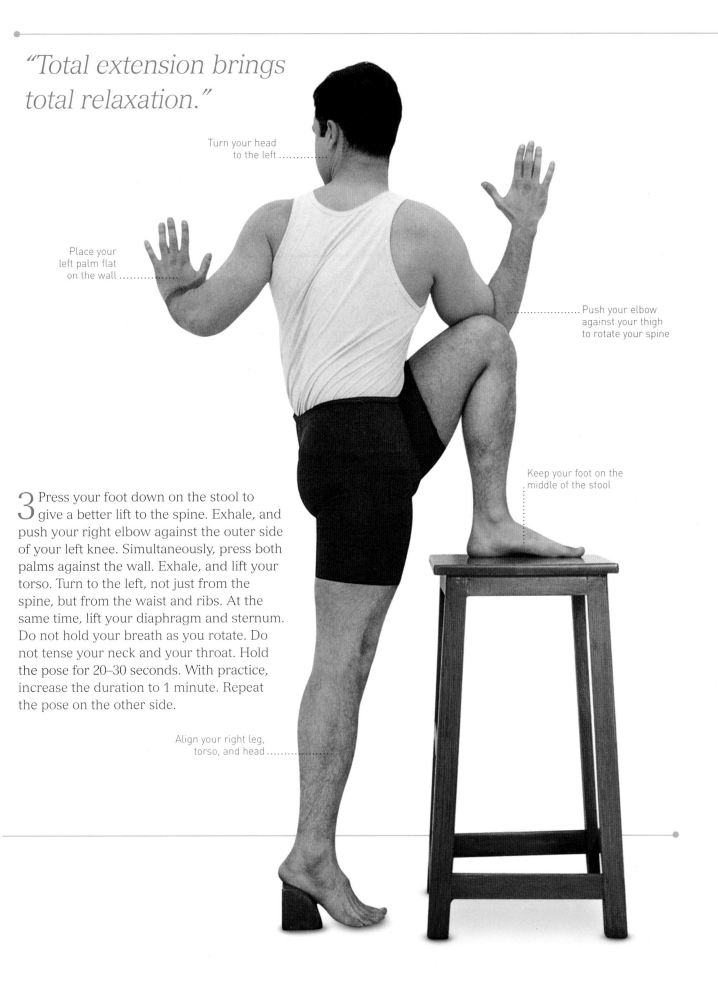

Turn your head to the left ....

Place your left palm flat on the wall ....

Push your elbow against your thigh to rotate your spine

Keep your foot on the middle of the stool

3 Press your foot down on the stool to give a better lift to the spine. Exhale, and push your right elbow against the outer side of your left knee. Simultaneously, press both palms against the wall. Exhale, and lift your torso. Turn to the left, not just from the spine, but from the waist and ribs. At the same time, lift your diaphragm and sternum. Do not hold your breath as you rotate. Do not tense your neck and your throat. Hold the pose for 20–30 seconds. With practice, increase the duration to 1 minute. Repeat the pose on the other side.

Align your right leg, torso, and head ....

PARSVA VIRASANA
Side twist in the hero pose

This asana vigorously stretches the sides of your waist and back, improving blood circulation in the spinal area, and making the shoulders and neck more flexible. *Parsva* means "side" or "flank" in Sanskrit, while *vira* translates as "hero."

● BENEFITS

Improves digestion and cures flatulence by exercising the abdominal muscles
Relieves lower backaches
Alleviates gout, rheumatism, and inflammation of the knees
Lessens stiffness in the hip joints, and makes the hamstrings supple
Reduces pain in the calves, ankles, and heels
Strengthens the arches of the feet and corrects flat feet or calcaneal spurs
Releases a catch or sprain in the shoulders and neck

● CAUTIONS

Avoid this asana if you have migraines, headaches, severe eye strain, bronchitis, a cold and congestion in the chest, or diarrhea. Do not practice if you are prone to depression, extreme fatigue, or insomnia.

PROPS (SEE PAGE 182)

A BLANKET AND A WOODEN BLOCK
Sitting on the blanket reduces pressure on the knees and on the ankle joints. The wooden block, positioned on its long side and placed under your hand, makes it easier for you to rotate your torso and to lift and stretch your spine more effectively.

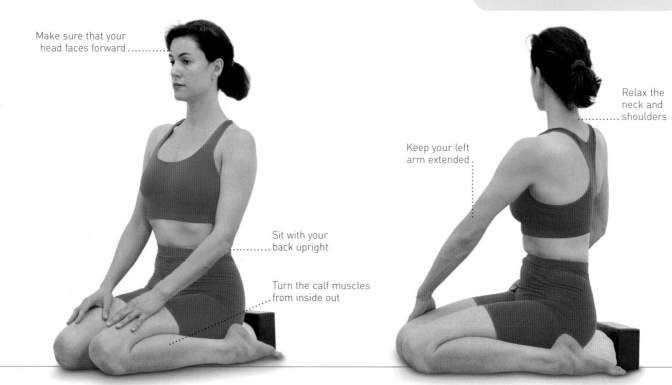

Make sure that your head faces forward

Sit with your back upright

Turn the calf muscles from inside out

Keep your left arm extended

Relax the neck and shoulders

1 Kneel on the mat with your knees close together. Gradually separate your feet. Fold the blanket, and place it between your feet. Lower your buttocks onto the blanket, making sure that you do not sit on your feet. Place the block on the floor, behind your buttocks and parallel to them. Place your palms on your knees. Sit with your head, neck, and back erect. Pause for 30–60 seconds.

2 Exhale, then place your left hand on the outer side of your right thigh and grip it. Rest your right hand on your right hip. The inner sides of your calves should touch the outer sides of your thighs. Push the inner sides of both heels against your hips. Stretch your ankles and then your feet, from the toes to the heels. Feel the energy flow through your feet.

3 Open your chest and focus on your kidneys. Imagine you are pulling them into your body. Keep your spine upright by pulling up the inner portion of your buttocks. Press your knees firmly down to the floor and stretch your torso up further. Exhale, then turn your chest and abdomen to the right. Move your right shoulder blade into your body, and increase the pressure of your left palm against the right thigh.

Move your right shoulder back

Keep your toes on the floor

"This asana rests and rejuvenates tired legs, and is recommended for those who are on their feet for long periods."

4 Turn, lifting your ribs and waist away from your hips, and twisting your torso further to the right. Straighten your left arm and pull your left shoulder blade in toward your spine. Place your right palm on the block and press it down firmly. Make sure that your buttocks rest on the folded blanket. Exhale, and twist your torso even further to the right. If you feel discomfort while rotating your torso, place a rolled towel under each ankle and sit on a wooden block (*see inset*). Hold the pose for 20–30 seconds. With practice, increase the duration to 1 minute. Repeat the pose on the other side.

Tuck your shoulder blades into your body

Turn your neck but keep it relaxed

SALAMBA SARVANGASANA
Shoulderstand

In the classic version of this asana (*see page* 144), your hands and shoulders support your back, making the asana quite strenuous to practice. In this adaptation, a chair allows the pose to be held more easily and without strain.

PROPS [SEE PAGE 182]

A CHAIR, A BOLSTER, AND A BLANKET
The chair supports the body, preventing strain, and helps you to balance better in the pose. Holding the back legs of the chair keeps the chest expanded. The bolster supports the neck and shoulders. It lifts the chest, bringing ease in breathing. The blanket prevents the edge of the chair from cutting into your back.

● BENEFITS
Relieves stress and nervous disorders
Eases migraines and stress-related headaches
Alleviates hypertension and insomnia
Reduces palpitations
Improves the functioning of the thyroid and parathyroid glands
Relieves cervical spondylosis and shoulder pain
Relieves bronchitis, asthma, sinusitis, and congestion
Prevents varicose veins
Alleviates ulcers, colitis, chronic constipation, and hemorrhoids

● CAUTIONS
Do not practice this asana during menstruation. During practice, make sure that your shoulders do not slide off the bolster onto the floor. This will compress the neck and might cause injury.

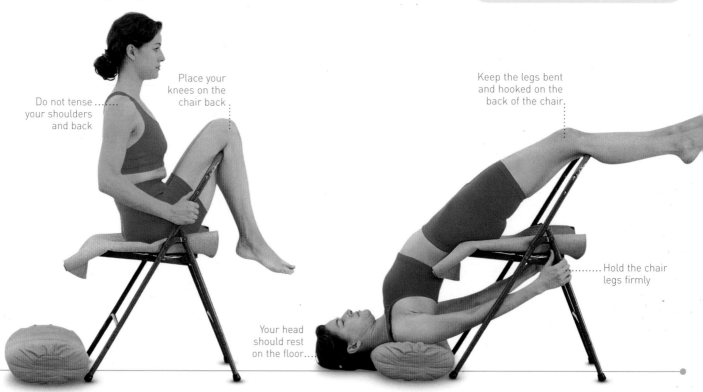

Do not tense your shoulders and back

Place your knees on the chair back

Your head should rest on the floor

Keep the legs bent and hooked on the back of the chair.

Hold the chair legs firmly

1 Place a bolster parallel to the front legs of the chair. Drape a blanket on the chair seat, so that it overlaps its front edge. Sit sideways on the chair with your chest facing the chair back. Hold the chair back, and place your legs on it, one by one. Slide your hands down the chair back and move your buttocks toward the back of the seat.

2 Lower your back onto the chair seat and gradually slide down from the seat of the chair, being careful to keep your buttocks hooked onto the seat. Take your arms under the seat while you are inclining backward. Pass your hands, one by one, through the front legs of the chair and hold the back legs. Straighten your legs and pause for 1 minute.

3 Rest your head comfortably on the floor, and keep your neck and shoulders on the bolster. Hold the back edges of the chair seat. Bend your knees and place your feet on the top edge of the chair back. Make sure that your buttocks rest on the front edge of the chair.

"This asana is recommended during recuperation after a major illness. Regular practice brings benefits to the entire body."

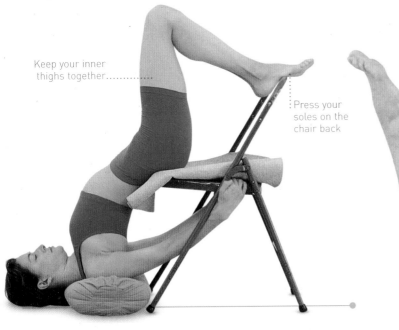

Keep your inner thighs together

Press your soles on the chair back

4 Maintain your grip on the chair seat and straighten your legs, one by one. Your buttocks, lower back, and waist should rest on the front edge of the chair seat. Lift your dorsal spine and shoulder blades. Intensify your grip on the chair seat. Extend your inner legs from the groin to the heels. Rotate your thighs inward. Keep your neck soft. Do not hold your breath. Hold the pose for 5 minutes.

COMING OUT OF THE POSE
Exhale, and place your feet on the chair back. Push the chair away, slightly. Slide your buttocks and back onto the bolster. Rest for a few minutes. Turn on your right, slide off the bolster, and sit up.

Suck in your kneecaps

Rotate your front thighs inward

Press the hips on the seat

Lift the chest upward

Lift the chest upward

HALASANA
Plough pose

This version of Halasana (*see page* 150) uses a chair, a stool, and two bolsters to support the neck, spine, torso, and legs, allowing the pose to be held without strain. Practicing this asana helps alleviate the effects of anxiety and fatigue. The chinlock in this pose soothes the nerves and relaxes the brain. This asana is recommended for those with thyroid disorders.

- BENEFITS

Reduces fatigue, insomnia, and anxiety
Relieves stress-related headaches, migraines, and hypertension
Relieves palpitations and breathlessness
Improves the functioning of the thyroid and parathyroid glands
Alleviates throat ailments, asthma, bronchitis, colds, and congestion
Relieves backaches, lumbago, and arthritis of the back and spine

- CAUTIONS

Do not practice this asana if you have cervical spondylosis. Do not attempt this pose during menstruation. If you suffer from osteoarthritis of the hips, backaches, peptic ulcers, or premenstrual stress; or, if you are overweight, separate your legs in the final pose. If you experience a choking feeling in the throat or heaviness in the head in the final pose, separate your legs.

PROPS (SEE PAGE 182)

A CHAIR, A BLANKET, TWO BOLSTERS, AND A STOOL
The chair helps you to go into and out of the pose with confidence, and allows the spine to be stretched comfortably. The blanket draped over the chair's edge cushions your back. The bolster placed beneath the shoulders prevents strain to the neck and head. The second bolster, placed on the stool, supports the thighs. The stool bears the weight of the body and supports the legs.

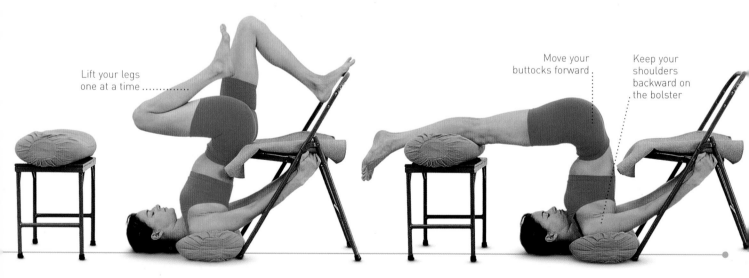

Lift your legs one at a time ....

Move your buttocks forward

Keep your shoulders backward on the bolster

1 Place a folded blanket on the seat of the chair, making sure that it overlaps the chair's front edge. Place a bolster on the floor, its long sides touching the front legs of the chair. Place a stool about 2ft (60cm) away from the bolster, and position the second bolster on top of the stool, in line with the first. Now follow Steps 1, 2, and 3 of Salamba Sarvangasana (*see page* 230). Then, hold the back edge of the chair seat and bring both legs toward the stool. Keep your buttocks against the chair seat.

2 Place your legs, one at a time, on the bolster on the stool. Make sure that your neck is stretched and rests comfortably on the floor. Keep your shoulders on the bolster on the floor. Move your buttocks forward, until your shins rest on the bolster, and your torso is perpendicular to the floor.

3 Bring your arms back through the chair legs. Shift your weight slightly to the back of your shoulders, and bring your arms over your head. Rest them, parallel to each other, on either side of your head, palms facing the floor. Bend your arms, and place your left hand just below your right elbow, and your right hand just below your left elbow. Keep your abdomen and pelvis soft. Stretch both legs from your heels to your thighs. Allow your eyes to recede into their sockets—do not look up. Relax your facial muscles and your throat. It is vital to keep your neck elongated in the pose. You must bring your chest to your chin, and not the other way around. As your brain rests, your breathing will become deeper and longer. Close your eyes. Stay in this pose for 3 minutes.

.... Lift your buttocks

: Extend your legs from
the thighs to the heels

COMING OUT OF THE POSE

After you have held the final pose for the recommended duration, open your eyes slowly. Stretch your arms out on either side of your head. Then follow Steps 1, 2, and 3 carefully (*see below*). Make sure that your movements are not jerky, because this might strain your neck or back. Pause for a few seconds between each step.

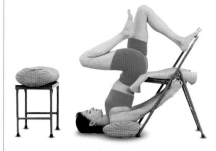

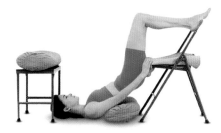

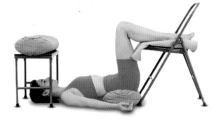

1 Hold the sides of the chair. Move your hips back until your buttocks rest on the front of the chair. Lift your legs, one by one, off the bolster and place your feet on the chair back.

2 Hold the front of the chair. Move your buttocks off the chair. Push your shoulders off the bolster onto the floor. Slide your torso back, until your head moves between the legs of the stool.

3 Rest your arms on the floor, and your buttocks on the bolster. Rest your calves on the seat of the chair. Push the stool back. Bring your legs down. Roll onto your right side and sit up.

VIPARITA KARANI
Inverted pose

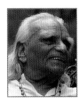

This is a restorative and relaxing asana, but the final pose is quite difficult for beginners and those with stiff backs. The use of props makes the pose easier and more restful. *Viparita* means "upside down" and *karani* means "doing" in Sanskrit, and the blood and hormones circulate better through the body when it is inverted.

● BENEFITS

Regulates blood pressure
Helps treat cardiac disorders
Helps treat ear and eye ailments, stress-related headaches, and migraines
Relieves palpitations, breathlessness, asthma, bronchitis, and throat ailments
Alleviates arthritis and cervical spondylosis
Relieves indigestion, diarrhea, and nausea
Helps treat kidney disorders
Prevents varicose veins

● CAUTIONS

Do not practice during menstruation, although at other times this asana alleviates menstrual disorders. Make sure that you rest your neck and shoulders firmly on the floor. If necessary, use just one bolster.

PROPS (SEE PAGE 182)

A WALL, A WOODEN BLOCK, TWO BOLSTERS, AND A BLANKET
The wall supports the legs. The bolsters support the back and buttocks. A block placed between the wall and the bolsters creates the space to lower the buttocks slightly. The blanket makes the bolsters and block a single unit.

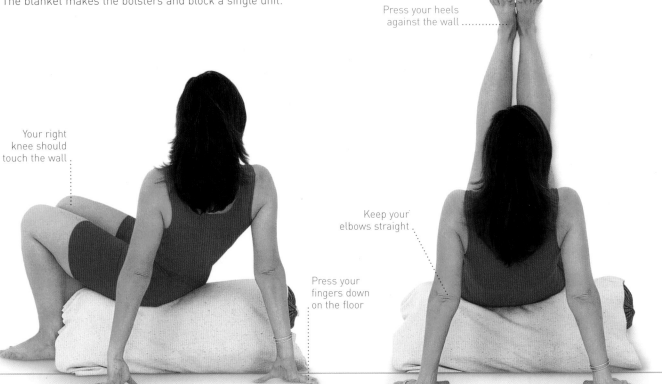

Your right knee should touch the wall

Press your heels against the wall

Keep your elbows straight

Press your fingers down on the floor

1 Place the block on its long side against a wall. Place the bolsters, one on top of the other, parallel to the block. Drape the blanket over the bolsters. Then sit sideways in the middle of the bolsters, and place your fingers flat on the floor behind you.

2 Turn your torso toward the wall, simultaneously lifting your legs, one by one, onto the wall. Keep your knees slightly bent. Support your body on both palms, fingers pointing toward the bolsters. Push both palms down on the floor, and move your buttocks closer to the wall.

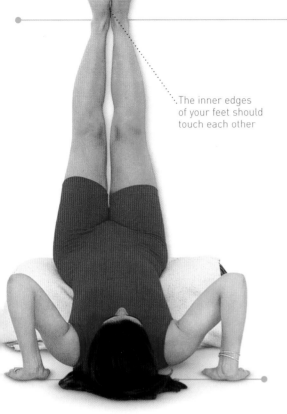

.The inner edges of your feet should touch each other

"This asana alleviates nervous exhaustion, boosts confidence, and reduces depression."

Do not allow your feet to tilt

4 Rest your head and neck on the floor. Lift your chest. Move your shoulders backward toward the bolsters. Spread your arms out to the sides with your palms facing the ceiling. Allow your chest, abdomen, and pelvis to expand and relax. Straighten and stretch your legs. Close your eyes, breathe evenly, and experience the serenity of the pose. Stay in the pose for 3–4 minutes. Gradually increase the duration to 5–8 minutes.

3 Bend your elbows and lower your torso until your shoulders rest on the floor. Straighten your legs fully. If your buttocks have moved away from the wall, bend your knees and place both feet against the wall. Then, press your palms down on the floor, lift your hips, and move the buttocks closer to the wall. Straighten your legs again.

Keep your abdomen soft

Extend your arms away from your torso

Press your shoulders down on the floor

SETUBANDHA SARVANGASANA
Bridge pose

The Sanskrit word *setu* means "bridge," *bandha* translates as "formation," and *sarvanga* means "entire body." In this asana, the body arches to take the shape of a bridge. The chinlock in the asana calms the flow of thoughts and soothes the mind.

PROPS (SEE PAGE 182)
A LONG BENCH, A BOLSTER, TWO BLANKETS, AND A YOGA BELT
The bench stretches the legs and buttocks, and keeps the back arched. A bolster, with a folded blanket on top of it, supports the head and neck. Adjust the height and stability of the bolster by rolling a blanket around it, if required. The belt helps keep the legs together without strain.

SPECIFIC BENEFITS
The reverse movement of the torso in the pose strengthens the back muscles, relieving neck strain and backaches.

● BENEFITS

Helps prevent arterial blockages or cardiac arrest by resting the heart muscles and increasing blood circulation to the arteries
Combats fluctuating blood pressure, hypertension, and depression by soothing the brain and expanding the chest
Relieves eye or ear ailments, migraines, stress-related headaches, nervous exhaustion, and insomnia
Improves digestion and strengthens the abdominal organs
Relieves backaches, strengthens the spine, and relieves neck strain
Helps rest tired legs and prevent varicose veins

● CAUTIONS

Make sure that your lower back touches the edge of the bench in the final pose. Your buttocks should not touch the edge of the bench, but should not be too far from it, otherwise your shoulders will lift, causing neck strain. If you are recovering from a major illness, practice Variation 2.

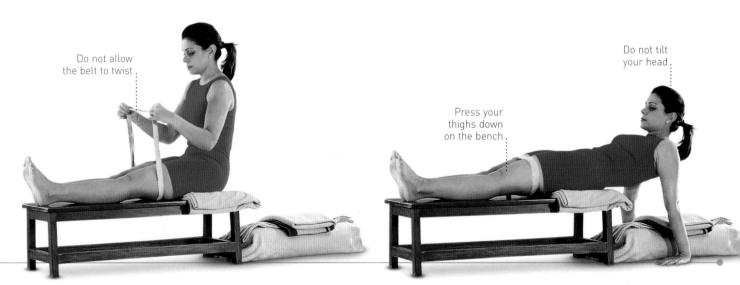

Do not allow the belt to twist

Do not tilt your head

Press your thighs down on the bench

1 Place a folded blanket on one end of the bench. Place a bolster on the floor in line with the bench, and touching one end of it. Place a folded blanket on the bolster. Then sit on the blanket on the bench, with your legs stretched out. Place a yoga belt under your thighs and bind it around the middle of your thighs.

2 Exhale, and lower your back toward the bolster. Press each palm down on the floor on either side of the bolster, your fingers pointing forward. Both arms should support your upper back. Keep your thighs, knees, and feet close together, your heels on the bench, and your toes pointing upward. Lower your arms to the floor.

"The pose sends a fresh supply of blood to the brain, resting and revitalizing the mind and body."

3 Slide further down, until the back of your head and your shoulders rest on the bolster. Straighten your legs, keeping your feet together. Stretch the heels and toes away from the torso to increase the stretch of the legs. Extend your arms to the sides on the floor, with the palms facing the ceiling. Hold the pose for 3 minutes. Gradually increase the time to 5–8 minutes.

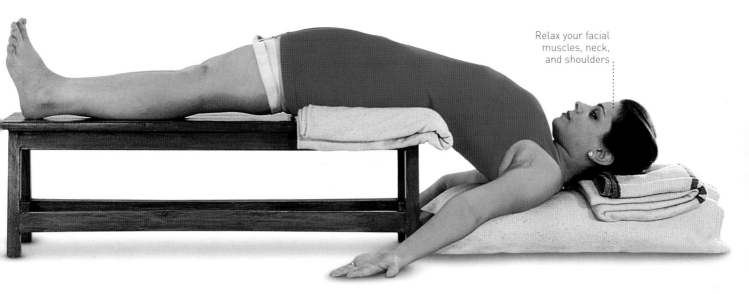

Relax your facial muscles, neck, and shoulders

VARIATION 1 WITH A ROLLED BLANKET

PROPS (SEE PAGE 182)
A LONG BENCH, A MAT, A BLANKET, A YOGA BELT, AND A BOLSTER
The blanket supports the neck.

SPECIFIC BENEFIT
Helps relieve cervical spondylosis.

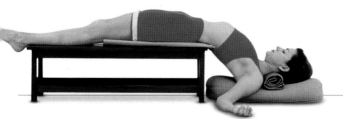

GETTING INTO THE POSE
Roll a blanket and place it on the center of the bolster. Place a mat on the bench. Follow Steps 1, 2, and 3 of the main asana, bending your arms in the final pose. A bolster under the calves (see inset), stretches the legs, prevents varicose veins, and relieves osteoarthritis of the hips and knees.

VARIATION 2 ON 4 BOLSTERS

PROPS (SEE PAGE 182)
FOUR BOLSTERS, A MAT, AND THREE YOGA BELTS
This variation is easier for beginners, and if you are elderly, overweight, or convalescent.

SPECIFIC BENEFITS
The bolsters help to increase chest expansion, relieving breathlessness and chronic bronchitis.

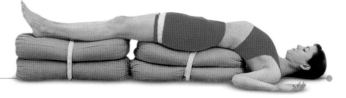

GETTING INTO THE POSE
Place 2 bolsters lengthwise on a mat. Place 2 more bolsters over these. Bind each set and your thighs with yoga belts. Lie on the bolsters. Slide down until your head and shoulders rest on the mat, your palms on either side of your head. Then follow Step 3 of the main asana.

VIPARITA DANDASANA
Inverted staff pose

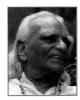

In the classic version of this asana, the feet, hands, and head rest on the earth. The pose is believed to symbolize the yogi's salutation to the divine force. This adaptation with props makes the pose easier to practice, and helps soothe an emotional or restless mind. The word *viparita* means "inverted" in Sanskrit, while *danda* translates as "staff."

PROPS (SEE PAGE 182)
A CHAIR, A BOLSTER, A BLANKET, A MAT, AND A TOWEL
The chair supports your back and increases the flexibility of the neck and shoulders. Holding the chair's legs expands the chest, relieving respiratory and heart ailments. The bolster, with the blanket on top of it, supports the head. This soothes the nerves, and regulates blood pressure. The mat prevents the chair's edge from cutting into your back. The towel supports the lumbar spine.

● **BENEFITS**
Soothes and relaxes the brain
Builds up emotional stability and self-confidence
Stimulates the adrenal, thyroid, pituitary, and pineal glands
Gently massages and strengthens the heart, preventing arterial blockage
Increases lung capacity
Relieves indigestion and flatulence
Increases the flexibility of the spine
Alleviates lower backaches
Corrects a displaced bladder or prolapsed uterus
Relieves menstrual pain and helps treat the symptoms of menopause

● **CAUTIONS**
Do not practice this asana during a migraine. Avoid the pose if you have stress-related headaches, eye strain, constipation, diarrhea, or insomnia. Discontinue the asana if you feel dizzy. If you suffer from backaches, you must practice a few twists before and after this pose.

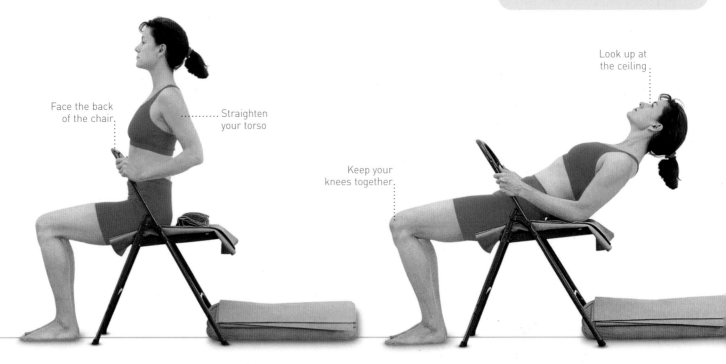

Face the back of the chair.

Straighten your torso

Keep your knees together.

Look up at the ceiling

1 Place the bolster in front of the chair, with one end between the chair's front legs. Place a blanket on the bolster. Drape the mat over the chair's front edge and place the folded towel on the mat. Step your feet through the back of the chair, and sit down. If needed, tie a yoga belt round your legs to keep them together (*see inset*).

2 Hold the sides of the chair back and slide your hips toward the back of the chair until your buttocks rest on the back edge of the chair. Exhale, and lift your chest, arching your entire back. Lower your torso, making sure that the folded towel supports your lumbar spine.

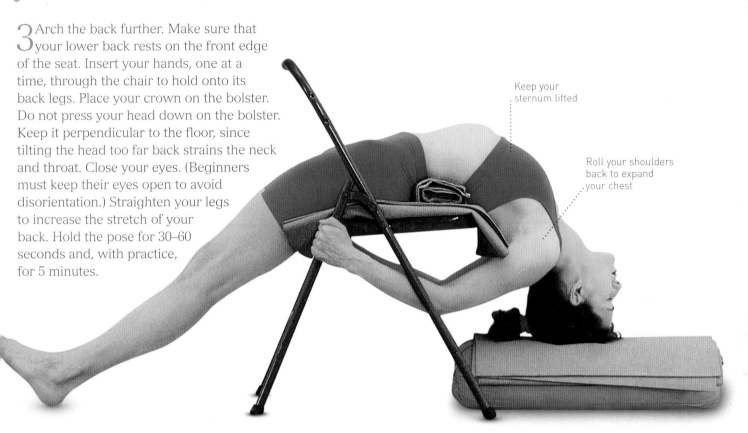

3 Arch the back further. Make sure that your lower back rests on the front edge of the seat. Insert your hands, one at a time, through the chair to hold onto its back legs. Place your crown on the bolster. Do not press your head down on the bolster. Keep it perpendicular to the floor, since tilting the head too far back strains the neck and throat. Close your eyes. (Beginners must keep their eyes open to avoid disorientation.) Straighten your legs to increase the stretch of your back. Hold the pose for 30–60 seconds and, with practice, for 5 minutes.

Keep your sternum lifted

Roll your shoulders back to expand your chest

VARIATION 1 FEET ON A STOOL

PROPS (SEE PAGE 182)
A CHAIR, A LOW OPEN STOOL, A ROLLED TOWEL, A FOLDED BLANKET, A MAT, A BOLSTER, AND A YOGA BELT
The stool supports the feet. The belt keeps the legs together.

SPECIFIC BENEFITS
Relieves diarrhea, abdominal cramps, and indigestion. Alleviates cervical spondylosis. Reduces pain in the back, shoulders, and neck.

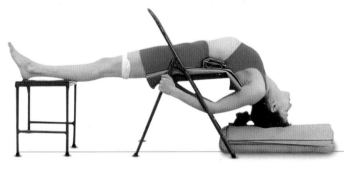

GETTING INTO THE POSE
Place a stool 2 ft (60 cm) from the chair. Follow Step 1 of the main asana. Place your legs on the stool, and follow Steps 2–3.

VARIATION 2 FEET AGAINST A WALL

PROPS (SEE PAGE 182)
A WALL, A CHAIR, A ROLLED TOWEL, A FOLDED BLANKET, AND A MAT
The wall supports the feet and intensifies the final stretch

SPECIFIC BENEFITS
Gives intensive extension to the abdomen and chest, increasing the arch of the spine.

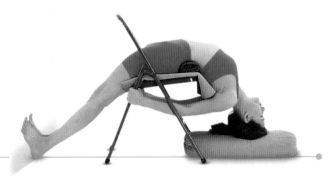

GETTING INTO THE POSE
Place the chair about 2 ft (60 cm) from the wall. Follow Steps 1, 2, and 3 of the main asana, but press your soles against the wall. Stretch your legs, pushing the chair a little away from the wall, if necessary.

USTRASANA
Camel pose

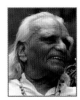

This version of the classic pose (*see page 156*), uses props to support the back, making the asana less strenuous to practice. The expansion of the chest in the pose alleviates stress by calming turbulent emotions. If you are feeling depressed, or are prone to mood swings or anxiety, this will help to boost your self-confidence. The pose is especially beneficial to adolescents.

● BENEFITS

Enhances resistance to infections
Stimulates the adrenal, pituitary, pineal, and thyroid glands
Increases lung capacity, and helps maintain the elasticity of lung tissue
Tones the liver, kidneys, and spleen
Tones the spine, relieving lower backaches and arthritic pain in the back
Helps prevent varicose veins by toning the legs, hamstrings, and ankles
Helps correct a prolapsed uterus, by stretching the pelvic area
Improves blood circulation to the ovaries and tones them
Relieves menstrual pain and the symptoms of menopause

● CAUTIONS

Avoid this asana if you have migraines, stress-related headaches, eye strain, rheumatoid arthritis, osteoarthritis of the knees, diarrhea, constipation, or if you are prone to insomnia. Do not practice the pose during menstruation.

PROPS (SEE PAGE 182)

A LOW, OPEN STOOL, A HALF-HALASANA STOOL, TWO BOLSTERS, AND TWO FOLDED BLANKETS
The stools support the back, gently massaging the heart and increasing coronary blood flow. This helps to prevent arterial blockages and to relieve anginal pain. The pose lifts the torso and diaphragm, expands the lungs, and rests the brain. The bolsters, one placed on each stool, support the back and head, so that the back is symmetrically curved in the pose. The blankets support the head and neck.

Straighten your shoulders

Bend your elbows

Both stools must be the same height

Distribute your weight on both knees

Lift your sternum

Lower your head gradually

1 Place the stool with the open sides on the floor, with a bolster across it. Place the second stool behind it. Position a bolster on this stool and put the blankets on it. Kneel in front of the stool with the open sides, and rest your palms on the bolster placed on it. Move your calves, one by one, between the legs of the stool. Your buttocks should touch the bolster on the stool.

2 Gradually arch your back, and lower your torso toward the bolster on the low, open stool. Broaden your chest as you move your elbows down on the first bolster. Then press your elbows down on the bolster, and place your palms on your hips. Move your head back, toward the folded blankets on the second stool.

THE GURU'S ADVICE

"Once your head is placed on the folded blankets, you must ensure that you open the ribs, and move the shoulder blades into the body. Look at how I am pressing my student's shoulders back with my thumbs. Roll the armpits and chest forward and up. Lift your sternum. As your chest moves up, make sure that your head extends back on the blankets."

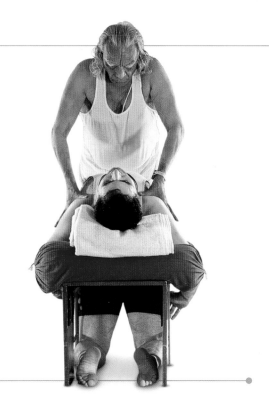

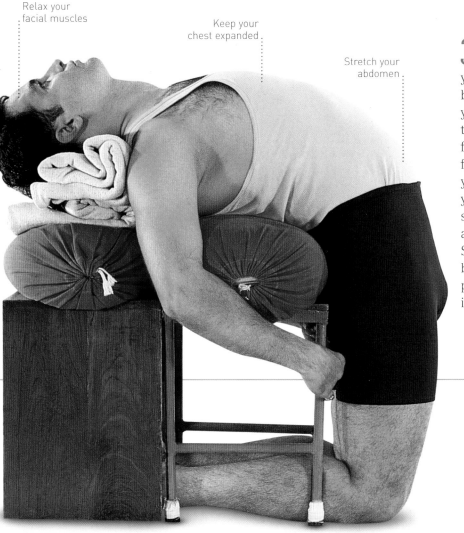

Relax your facial muscles

Keep your chest expanded

Stretch your abdomen

3 Lower your torso onto the bolster on the open stool, until your head rests on the folded blankets on the second stool. Arch your neck, but do not strain your throat. Press your shins to the floor, and push the thighbones forward, away from the stool. Roll your shoulders back and move your shoulder blades toward your spine. Pull your spine, tailbone, and back muscles into your body. Stretch your thighs, hips, and buttocks. Breathe evenly. Hold the pose for 1 minute. With practice, increase the duration to 3 minutes.

SUPTA PADANGUSTHASANA
Reclining leg, foot, and toe stretch

In Sanskrit, *supta* means "lying down," *pada* means "foot," and *angustha* is the big toe. Since the fingers do not reach the toe easily, a yoga belt is used. It is placed around the sole of one foot, and the resultant stretch to the legs increases flexibility in the pelvic area and improves blood circulation in the legs.

PROPS (SEE PAGE 182)
A MAT, A WALL, AND A YOGA BELT
The wall steadies the outstretched foot, preventing it from tilting. It also ensures that the body is correctly aligned. The yoga belt, looped around the sole of the raised foot, makes the asana easier for those who are stiff in the hips and pelvic area.

1 Place a mat against a wall. Sit Dandasana (*see page* 102) facing the wall. Keep a yoga belt beside you. The soles of your feet should touch the wall comfortably, with your toes pointing upward. Press both your palms down on the mat.

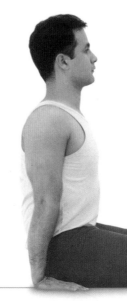

Straighten your legs

2 Lower your back onto the mat, supporting your torso on your palms until your head rests on the mat. Bend your right knee, and bring it to your chest. Keep your left sole pressed against the wall. Loop the belt around the sole of your right foot. Hold one end of the belt in each hand. Make sure that you hold the yoga belt as close to your foot as possible. This opens your chest, and keeps your breathing regular and even. Keep your extended leg pressed down on the mat.

Keep the lumbar pressed to the floor

Press the back of the left leg down on the mat

Do not allow your head to tilt

"Supta Padangusthasana makes the muscles of the legs stronger."

Stretch the sole of your right foot

Relax your facial muscles and neck

3 Inhale, and raise your right leg until it is perpendicular to the floor. Hold both ends of the belt with the right hand. Place your left arm beside your left hip. Press the left foot against the wall, and the left thigh on the mat. Stretch your right leg up further, simultaneously pulling your toes toward you with the belt. Feel the stretch in your right calf. Keep your left leg firmly pressed to the floor. Do not bend either knee or allow the left leg to tilt out. Initially, stay in this position for 20-30 seconds. With practice, increase the time to 1 minute. Repeat the pose on the other side.

Press the thigh into its socket. Press the right hip and waist down

Extend the hamstring muscles of both legs

VARIATION 1 FOOT ON BLOCK

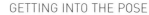

PROPS [SEE PAGE 182]
A MAT, A WALL, A YOGA BELT, AND A WOODEN BLOCK
The block under the foot makes the pose easier for those who are stiff in the pelvic area.

SPECIFIC CAUTION
You must keep your leg straight as you lower it onto the block. Allowing it to bend during this action might lead to injury.

GETTING INTO THE POSE
Place the wooden block on your right. Follow Steps 1, 2, and 3 of the main asana. After you raise your right leg, exhale, then lower your leg to the right, keeping it absolutely straight. Place your right foot on the block. Pull on the belt and stretch your leg. Hold the pose for 20–30 seconds. Repeat the pose on the other side.

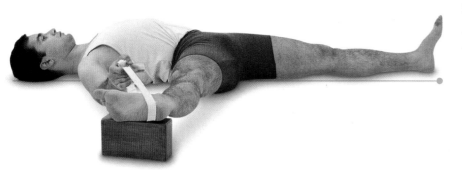

SUPTA BADDHAKONASANA
Reclining fixed angle pose

The Sanskrit word *supta* means "reclining," *baddha* means "fixed," while *kona* translates as "angle." This is a very restful asana that can be practiced even by those who have had bypass surgery. It gently massages the heart and helps open blocked arteries. The pose also improves blood circulation in the abdomen, massaging and toning the abdominal organs.

PROPS (SEE PAGE 182)
A BOLSTER, A BLANKET, A YOGA BELT, AND TWO WOODEN BLOCKS
The bolster supports the back and lifts the chest. The blanket supports the head, alleviating stress and heaviness in the head and neck. The belt helps maintain the angle of the legs easily and holds the feet together. The wooden blocks support the thighs, reducing strain in the groin.

● BENEFITS

Regulates blood pressure
Prevents hernia as the hips and groin become more supple
Relieves lower backaches
Relieves varicose veins and sciatica
Reduces the pain caused by hemorrhoids
Relieves indigestion and flatulence
Tones the kidneys and improves poor bladder control
Improves blood circulation in the ovarian region, and is particularly beneficial during puberty and menopause
Alleviates menstrual pain and leukorrhea
Corrects a prolapsed uterus

● CAUTIONS

If you feel any strain while getting into the pose, use two bolsters instead of one. If you feel strain in the region of the groin, place a folded towel or blanket on both blocks placed below the knees.

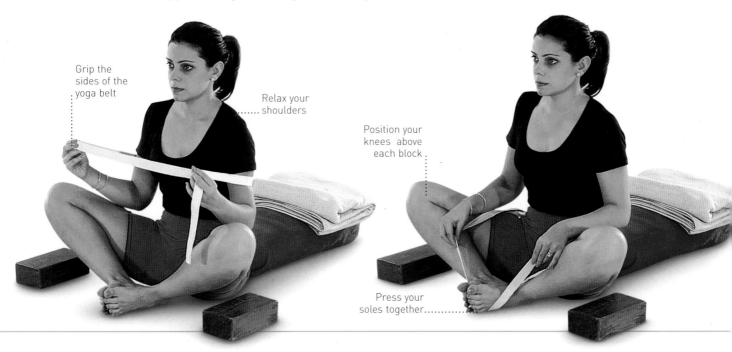

Grip the sides of the yoga belt

Relax your shoulders

Position your knees above each block

Press your soles together

1 Sit in Dandasana (*see page* 102). Place a bolster behind you, its short end against your buttocks, and place a folded blanket on its far end. Place 2 wooden blocks on their broad sides on either side of your hips. Bend your knees, and join the soles of your feet together. Draw your heels toward your groin. Buckle the belt and loop it over your shoulders.

2 Bring the belt down to below your waist. Pass it under both feet to stretch it over your ankles and the insides of the thighs. Move your feet closer to your groin. The belt should feel neither too tight nor too slack, so adjust the buckle accordingly. Make sure that the end of the bolster touches your buttocks. Position a block under each thigh.

THE GURU'S ADVICE

"To bring your knees down to the floor, you must first widen the inside of your thighs to stretch the ligaments of the inner knees. Push the inner sides of your legs toward your knees and widen the groin. Then your knees will descend easily. The belt's position is also important. Here, I am adjusting the student's belt to flatten the thighs as much as possible."

3 Place your elbows on the floor, and lower your head and back onto the bolster. Make sure that the bolster comfortably supports the length of your back and your head. Your spine should be on the center of the bolster. Stretch your arms out to the sides, with the palms facing the ceiling. Relax, and extend your groin out to the sides. Feel the expansion of the pelvis, and the release of tension in your ankles and knees. Initially, stay in the pose for 1 minute. With practice, increase the duration to 5–10 minutes.

Open and lift your chest

Keep your eyes passive

Stretch your thighs out to the sides

SUPTA VIRASANA
Reclining hero pose

This asana is a less strenuous version of the classic pose (*see page* 166). Practice the asana at the beginning of your yoga session, since it calms a restless and agitated mind, and induces the right mood for your practice.

PROPS (SEE PAGE 182)
A BOLSTER AND A ROLLED BLANKET
The bolster helps people with stiff backs to practice easily. It helps prevent the knees from lifting off the floor. It also helps to maintain the lift of the chest and the stretch of the torso. The folded blanket under the head prevents eye strain, and ensures that the head and neck do not tilt to one side.

● BENEFITS

Helps prevent arterial blockages by gently massaging and strengthening the heart and increasing coronary blood flow
Increases the elasticity of lung tissue
Enhances resistance to infections
Relieves indigestion, acidity, and flatulence
Corrects a prolapsed uterus, and tones the pelvic organs
Relieves lower backaches
Reduces inflammation in the knees, and relieves gout and rheumatic pain
Relieves pain in the legs and feet and rests them, alleviating the effects of long hours of standing
Helps correct flat feet

● CAUTIONS

If you have angina or partially blocked arteries, or are recovering from bypass surgery, only practice the pose under expert supervision.

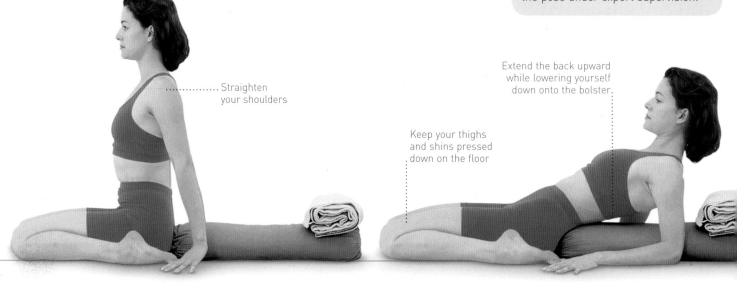

.... Straighten your shoulders

Extend the back upward while lowering yourself down onto the bolster

Keep your thighs and shins pressed down on the floor

1 Kneel in Virasana (*see page* 104) and place a bolster behind you, the short end touching your buttocks. Place a rolled blanket on the far end. Make sure that the inner sides of your feet touch your hips. Keep your back straight. Place your fingers on the floor beside your toes.

2 Press your palms on the floor, bend both elbows, and lean back toward the bolster. Place your elbows and forearms, one at a time, on the floor. Gradually lower your back onto the bolster. To avoid strain in the pelvic area or the thighs, make sure that your knees remain firmly on the floor.

Feel the stretch .... in your knees

"The chest expansion in the asana is particularly beneficial for the heart. The pose reduces fatigue and stimulates the entire body."

Do not raise your shoulders

Keep your thighs close together

3 Once you lower your back onto the bolster, rest the back of your head on the rolled blanket. Keep your chest fully expanded. Press your shoulder blades down on the bolster to lift your chest. Extend your toes and ankles toward the bolster. Push your feet closer to your hips with your hands. Extend the pelvis, and press your thighs close together.

4 Move your arms out to the sides, with the palms facing upward. Extend your neck, but keep your throat relaxed. Drop your eyelids down gently. Experience the relaxation of the thighs and the abdomen, and the lift of the chest. Feel the continuous stretch from the cervical spine to the tailbone. Initially, stay in the pose for 1 minute. With practice, increase the duration to 5–10 minutes.

Open your chest, and lift your ribs

Relax your facial muscles

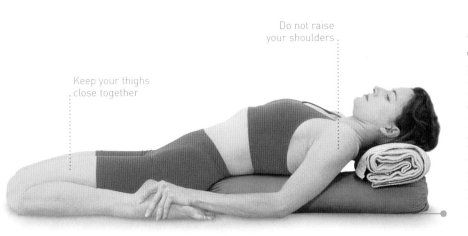

SAVASANA
Corpse pose

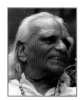

In this version of the classic asana (*see page* 170), subtle adjustments in the final pose are made easier with the help of props. The steady, smooth breathing in the pose allows energy to flow into the body, invigorating it, and reducing the stress of everyday life.

PROPS (SEE PAGE 182)

A FOLDED BLANKET, A BOLSTER, A CREPE BANDAGE, AND A MAT
The bolster supports the back, raises the chest, and releases the diaphragm. The folded blanket lifts the head and neck, soothing and clearing the mind. If you have a cold, cough, or asthma, keeping your head and chest raised in this pose, helps you to breathe comfortably. The bandage shields the eyes from light. It also soothes the eyes, ears, and brain by softening and relaxing the facial skin, muscles, and ligaments. (You can practice Ujjayi Pranayama and Viloma Pranayama with this arrangement of props too.)

● BENEFITS
Removes physical and mental fatigue
Relaxes and soothes the sympathetic nervous system
Helps treat high blood pressure, and relieves migraines and stress-related headaches
Alleviates the symptoms of respiratory diseases and eases breathing
Speeds recuperation after an illness
Helps toward refreshing, dreamless sleep, especially for those with sleep disorders

● CAUTIONS
This asana is usually practiced at the end of a yoga session. Do not practice it more than once in a single session. Beginners should practice Savasana without props for 5 weeks before attempting this version, and should hold the pose for 5 minutes. For the first 10 weeks of practice with props, wrap the bandage around your forehead, but not your eyes. If at any time you experience feelings of isolation, anxiety, fear, or depression when your eyes are covered, practice without the bandage.

Extend your spine ....

Stretch out your legs .

1 Spread the mat on the floor. Place a bolster on the mat, with its long sides parallel to the long sides of the mat. Sit in Dandasana (*see page* 102) with the short end of the bolster against your buttocks, and place the folded blanket on the far end. If you have

osteoarthritis of the knees or if your legs are feeling tired, place a bolster under your knees (*see inset*).

2 Wrap the bandage around your forehead, following the instructions for Ujjayi Pranayama (*see page* 252). Now place your elbows and forearms on the mat. Lower your back, vertebra by vertebra, onto the bolster until your head rests comfortably on the folded blanket. Position your buttocks evenly on the center of the mat. Spread out your arms to the sides, palms facing up, and rest them on the floor.

"The stillness in the pose is not meditation, but reflects a mastery of the inner self and a surrender to a higher, sublime consciousness."

COMING OUT OF THE POSE

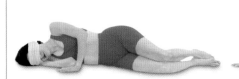

1 When you come out of the pose, do not tense your neck and throat. Bring your arms to your sides and bring your legs together. Gently roll off the bolster onto your right side, and place your right palm under your head. Keep your left palm down near the chest and your knees slightly bent. Pause and rest for a few moments. Allow your body and mind to determine when you should sit up.

2 When you feel ready, push yourself into a sitting position with your left hand. Sit cross-legged and unwrap the bandage gently. Do not take it off when you are lying down, since this can strain the facial and cranial nerves. Open your eyes slowly. If you open them too abruptly, your vision may blur. Straighten your legs and sit in Dandasana.

Rest your head evenly on the blanket

Keep your thigh muscles relaxed

Let your feet drop out to the sides naturally

3 Straighten your legs and stretch them evenly away from each other, without disturbing the extension of your waist. Exhale, focusing on your breathing, then lift and stretch your diaphragm, keeping it free of tension. Keep your arms at a comfortable distance from your body. If they are placed too near or too far away, your shoulders will lift off the bolster. Stretch your shoulders away from your neck. The center of your back should be on the center of the bolster. Keep your abdomen soft and relaxed. Expand your chest and relax your throat, until you feel a soothing sensation in the neck. Make sure that your head does not tilt back. Relax your facial muscles and your jaw. Do not clench your teeth.

4 Keep your breathing smooth and free of tension, but do not breathe deeply. Let your eyeballs relax into their sockets, and allow external surroundings to recede. Feel the energy flow from your brain to your body as the physical, physiological, mental, intellectual, and spiritual planes come together. Stay in the pose for 5–10 minutes.

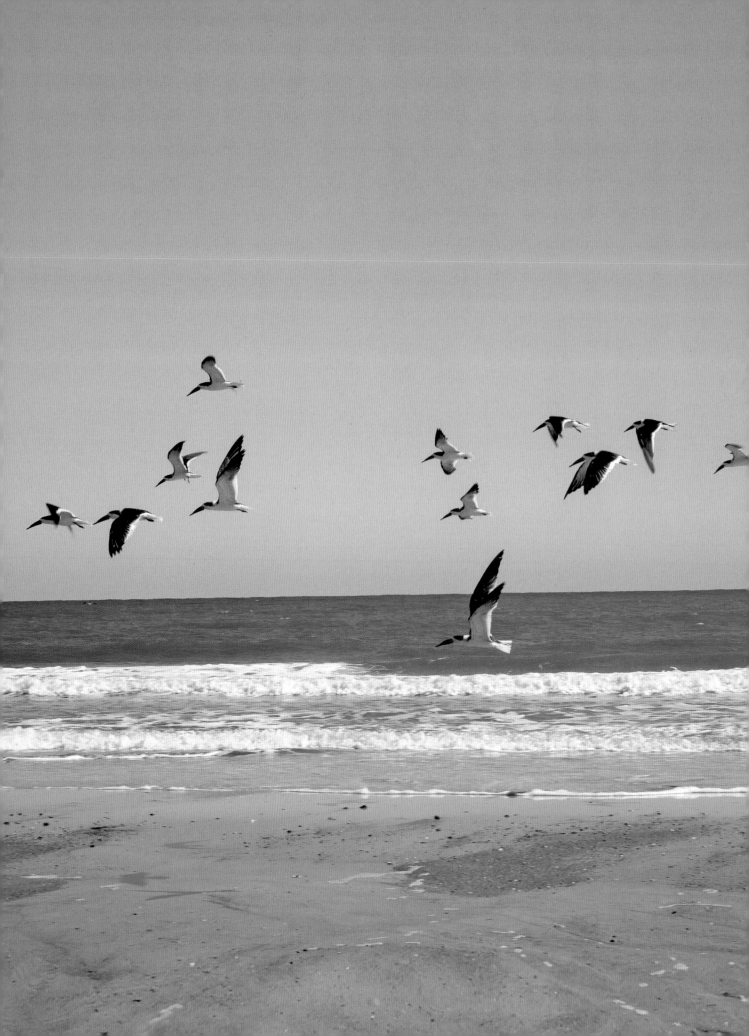

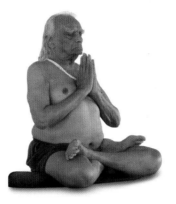

CHAPTER 6

PRANAYAMA WITH PROPS

*"The **rhythm** of the body, the melody of the **mind**, and the **harmony** of the **soul** create the symphony of **life**."*

Breath is the essence of life and *prana* is the life force, or energy. The art of pranayama seeks to harness this life force. By focusing the mind totally on the breath, blockages in the body's channels are unlocked, allowing energy to flow freely and connect with the life force. The sage Patanjali said that concentration and clarity of thought were developed through pranayama, opening the path to deeper relaxation and eventually meditation. The use of props in pranayama stills the body, freeing the mind to unite completely with the breath and fully absorb the life force, or *prana*.

The Importance of Pranayama

by Yogacharya B.K.S. Iyengar

In pranayama, breathing is elevated to a controlled, extended process of exhalation and inhalation. This generates the cosmic energy of *prana*, the life force that provides the strength, power, and vitality required for any activity.

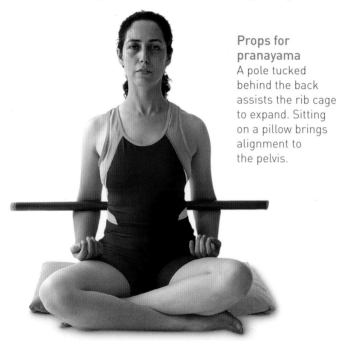

Props for pranayama
A pole tucked behind the back assists the rib cage to expand. Sitting on a pillow brings alignment to the pelvis.

Although *prana* is usually translated as breath, it is actually the energizing force that is in the breath. The essence that we breathe in and out contains *prana*, which manifests itself as our life force. The moment breathing stops, the life force departs.

The practice of pranayama

Prana means breath and *ayama* means regulation of breath. Pranayama is the science of breath. It is the process of the elongation, extension, expansion, length, and breadth of each breath. Pranayama also involves the retention of breath, which is a deliberate and rhythmic controlling of the breath. This control of the breath together with the extended inhalation and exhalation is the art of pranayama.

Just as some view God as the creator, sustainer, and destroyer, *prana* and pranayama act as a generating life force, the exhalation of breath throwing out the toxins that can destroy life, while the inhalation and retention distributes energy throughout the body.

The mind and breath

It is said that the mind and breath are one's constant companions. Where there is breath, there the mind is focused and where there is an active mind, so is the breath focused. The practice of pranayama seeks to quiet the mind, bringing it under control through the deep and rhythmic flow of inhalations and exhalations.

The sound of the breath

The pranayamic breath has a sound of its own: *Soham*. The sound of the inhalation is "sa" and that of the exhalation is "ham." "Soham" has been interpreted as "He, I am and I am He." During pranayama, concentration is drawn solely to the action of the breath, and it is this attentive awareness of the breath that leads to the art of *dhyana*, or meditation.

The art of inhaling not only focuses the mind on the breath, but also brings one into contact with their essence, or soul. With the retention of the breath during the inhalation, the soul

*"In **pranayama**, your **intellect** should be as **firm** as a **burning candle** in a **windless place**."*

becomes wedded to the body. This is the divine union of the soul with our nature, or body. During the process of exhalation, the soul re-enters into an unfathomable space. The mind dissolves and the divine marriage of *Prakriti,* the body, and *Purusha,* the soul, occurs.

The path to meditation

Pura means dwelling place, or city, and the person who dwells in that place is *Purusha.* The body, therefore, is the dwelling place and the dweller is the *Purusha,* or the soul. The benefits of pranayama can be seen in the devotional and spiritual path, leading from self-realization to a more spiritual realization. Pranayama plays the role of *Brahma,* the Creator, *Vishnu,* the Protector, and *Maheshwara,* the Destroyer.

The stages of the breath

Just as *Brahma* is seen as the creator, the inhalation becomes the creator of life. The retention of the breath after an inhalation is the protector of life, known as *Vishnu.* The release of the breath during the exhalation is the process of throwing out the destructive life force, known as *Maheshwara,* who destroys

vicious things within the body and enhances the life span. Finally, the retention of the breath after exhalation allows one to surrender totally both the breath and the mind to the self, or soul, that resides within.

In this way, pranayama can be compared to God who plays the three roles of creation, protection, and destruction. Inhalation creates the life force, retention protects it, and exhalation prolongs life.

Just as the practice of the asanas, or poses, is seen as the yoga of action, developing the individual's knowledge of the body, mind, and consciousness, the practice of pranayama is said to lead one toward the path of love minus lust, which is known as *Bhakti Marga.* Among the eight aspects, or limbs, of yoga (*see pages 52–53*), pranayama is therefore seen as the heart of the practice.

Without the energy of *prana,* nothing can be attempted or achieved. *Prana* is the foundation of everything that exists in the world, while the art of pranayama is the process of generating that energy, making constructive use of it to live in the path of holistic health. The benefits of pranayama can be felt from the skin to the soul, and from the soul to the skin wholly and completely.

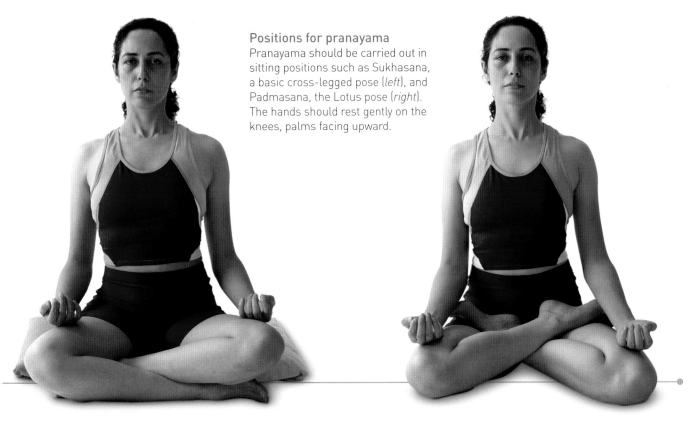

Positions for pranayama
Pranayama should be carried out in sitting positions such as Sukhasana, a basic cross-legged pose (*left*), and Padmasana, the Lotus pose (*right*). The hands should rest gently on the knees, palms facing upward.

UJJAYI PRANAYAMA
Conquest of energy

This is the basic form of pranayama (*see page* 54). *Ut* means "expand" in Sanskrit, *jaya* means "conquest," *prana* means "life force," and *ayama* is the "distribution" of that force or energy. Pranayama is not just cycles of inhalation and exhalation, nor is it merely deep breathing. The practice of pranayama goes beyond these to link our physiological and spiritual dimensions.

● BENEFITS

Relieves depression and boosts confidence
Alleviates cardiac disorders
Normalizes blood pressure
Relieves asthma
Invigorates the nervous system

● CAUTIONS

This is not recommended for beginners. Intermediate students must practice with props. Never swallow your saliva during or between inhalation and exhalation. Swallow after a complete exhalation. Do not practice if you have a severe backache or constipation. Do not practice this pranayama if you are feeling tired, because exertion can be harmful for the lungs and the heart. Do not practice strenuous yoga asanas after pranayama. Before pranayama, practice a few reclining asanas to expand the abdominal cavity and the diaphragm.

PROPS (SEE PAGE 182)

TWO FOAM BLOCKS, TWO WOODEN BLOCKS, A ROLLED BLANKET, A CREPE BANDAGE, AND A MAT

The blanket and the two wooden blocks raise the head above the level of the chest, freeing and expanding the diaphragm. They also support the middle back and ribs and help stretch the intercostal muscles. The foam blocks lift the chest and keep the abdominal muscles soft. The rolled blanket helps relax the head and brain, stopping the flow of thought. The crepe bandage helps focus the mind and turn it inward.

PREPARATION

Hold one end of the bandage just above your ear, and wrap it around your forehead 3 times, winding it over your eyes and ears. Make sure you tuck in the end of the bandage at your temple, as Geeta Iyengar (see left), demonstrates on the student. If you tuck it in at the back of the head, you will not be able to rest your head evenly on the blanket. Make sure that the bandage is neither too tight nor too loose. It should cover your forehead and eyes, but should not press down on your nose.

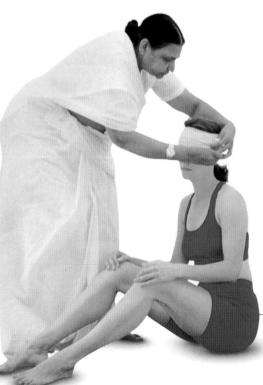

Allow your feet to tilt outward

THE GURU'S ADVICE

"Follow the instructions carefully. Remember that faulty practice can strain the lungs and diaphragm. Set aside 40–60 minutes at a fixed time of day for the pranayama. Never practice just after a meal, or immediately after an energetic session of asanas."

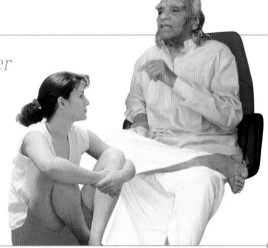

1 Spread a mat on the floor. Place 2 foam blocks about 1 ft (30 cm) from the mat's edge, the top one protruding over the right end of the lower one (*see inset*). Place the wooden blocks on their long sides, one parallel to the foam blocks, and the other at right angles to the first.

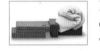 Place a rolled blanket on the second wooden block.

2 Sit in Dandasana (*see page* 102) and put on the bandage. Place your elbows and forearms on the mat and lower your back onto the foam blocks. There should be a slight gap between your buttocks and the blocks, as Geeta Iyengar demonstrates to the student (*see below*). Place your shoulders on the first wooden block, and push your lower shoulder blades into your chest, away from your spine and not toward your ears. This helps to broaden your thoracic cavity, allowing you to inhale deeply. Rest the back of your head comfortably on the rolled blanket, but do not allow it to tilt back. Relax your jaws, and rest your tongue on your lower jaw, as this helps prevent the accumulation of saliva.

3 Relax your throat. Stretch your legs out slowly, one at a time. Relax every part of your body, consciously, including your skin. Imagine that you are pushing the skin of your scalp toward your brow. This calms the frontal brain and at the same time, keeps it alert. This is the key to complete physical, psychological, and neuro-physiological relaxation. Focus on an imaginary point inside your chest to exclude all external disturbances. Drop your eyelids completely, but gently. Do not close your eyes tightly. If your pupils move upward, your mind will fill with thoughts and tension. Look inward and feel your senses withdraw.

Make sure the bandage is not too tight

Relax your neck muscles

Move your shoulders away from your neck

UJJAYI PRANAYAMA

"There are four stages to this pranayama. Attempt each stage sequentially, one at a time."

STAGES

Attempt the four stages in sequence. Each cycle of breath begins with an inhalation and ends with an exhalation, both of equal duration. Do not worry about the duration or retention of your breath; with practice, it will become steady, resonant, and rhythmic. Beginners should not attempt more than the advised cycles of the pranayama. Always stop before reaching the limit of your endurance. Practice each stage for 5–8 minutes.

Keep your facial muscles passive

Lift your sternum

Relax your legs

1 This is a preparatory stage and consists of normal inhalation and exhalation. Breathe naturally, but consciously. When you breathe in, expand your chest fully but do not tense your diaphragm. Be conscious of your breathing, but do not breathe deeply. Practice 10 cycles.

2 This stage involves normal inhalation and deep exhalation. Inhale, then exhale slowly, deeply, and steadily, releasing all the air in your lungs. Keep your sternum lifted. Synchronize the movements of your diaphragm and abdomen, keeping the flow of breath smooth and uniform. Practice 15 cycles.

3 This stage involves deep inhalation and normal exhalation. Exhale without strain, then inhale slowly and deeply. Feel your breath move up from the pelvis to the pit of the throat, and then spread to each side of your torso. Practice 15–20 cycles.

4 The final stage consists of deep inhalation and deep exhalation. Exhale, emptying your lungs without strain. Then, inhale slowly, deeply, and smoothly. Exhale silently, until the lungs feel completely empty. Practice 15–20 cycles. End the pranayama with an exhalation.

COMING OUT OF THE POSE

Roll gently off the foam blocks onto your right side. Sit up slowly and move the blocks away. Now lie down in Savasana (*see page 248*), with a blanket under your head and neck. Remain in the pose for 5 minutes, breathing normally. Then turn onto your right side again. Place your left hand on the right hand. Pause, then supporting yourself on your left hand, sit up slowly, and sit cross-legged. Unwrap the bandage and open your eyes gently. Rest for a few moments.

VILOMA 2 PRANAYAMA
Interrupted breathing cycle

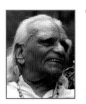

This pranayama is practiced in three stages and each stage can take 3–4 weeks to perfect. Each stage is more subtle than the preceding one, and requires a greater level of awareness. *Viloma* means "against the natural course" in Sanskrit, because in this pranayama you have to hold your breath for two seconds during each breathing cycle.

● BENEFITS
Brings lightness to the body and serenity to the mind
Regulates blood pressure
Reduces eye strain and headaches
Relieves symptoms of colds, coughs, and tonsillitis
Helps treat menorrhagia and metrorrhagia
Reduces mood swings and PMS-related headaches
Helps treat the symptoms of menopause

● CAUTIONS
Do not practice if you have a severe backache, constipation, or diarrhea. If you feel out of breath or fatigued, finish the cycle you are on, take a few normal breaths, then resume your practice. Swallow your saliva only after a complete exhalation. Practice a few cycles of Stage 1, followed by Stage 2, before attempting all 3 stages sequentially. Never start your practice with Stage 3. Always stop before you reach your limit. Beginners should not practice more than 6 cycles.

PROPS (SEE PAGE 182)
TWO FOAM BLOCKS, TWO WOODEN BLOCKS, A CREPE BANDAGE, AND A MAT

The foam blocks support the back, lift the chest, and keep the abdominal muscles relaxed. The two wooden blocks lift the head above the chest, expanding the diaphragm, middle back, and ribs, helping to stretch stiff intercostal muscles. The bandage helps turn the mind inward.

GETTING INTO THE POSE
Place the foam and wooden blocks as in Ujjayi Pranayama (*see page* 254). Follow the steps for Savasana (*see page* 248). Then practice a few cycles of Ujjayi Pranayama. This will open your chest and stimulate your intercostal muscles.

Keep your abdomen soft and relaxed ....

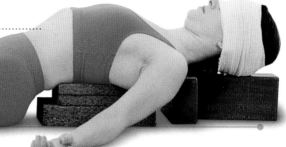

1 Keep your sternum lifted and your diaphragm firm. Inhale and exhale without strain, slowly and deeply. Your exhalation should last for 2–3 seconds. Then, pause for 2 seconds before inhaling. This constitutes a single cycle. Repeat this 3–5 times.

2 Your breathing should now fade away effortlessly at each pause and resume equally easily. Follow the instructions for Stage I, with your exhalations longer than your pauses. Practice 15–20 cycles over 7–10 minutes. Rest in Savasana.

3 Do a few cycles of Steps 1 and 2. Focus on the silence of the pauses. Experience a feeling of serenity.

COMING OUT OF THE POSE
Practice a cycle of Ujjayi Pranayama (*see page* 256). Then follow the coming out of the pose sequence for Savasana (*see page* 248).

CHAPTER 7

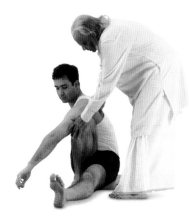

YOGA FOR AILMENTS

*"Yoga is the golden **key** which unlocks the door to **peace, tranquillity**, and **joy**."*

Yoga can heal parts of our bodies that have been injured, traumatized, or simply ignored and neglected. Medical treatment can accelerate the healing process but, all too often, cannot tackle the source of the problem. The ancient yogis realized that the cure for diseases lay within ourselves. They formulated a therapy which worked on our very natures, to enable the systems of the body to function as effectively and efficiently as possible, both preventing and curing disease. Yoga asanas involve movements that stimulate injured parts of the body by increasing the blood supply to them. The practice of asanas also increases our ability to bear pain.

Yoga Therapy

Yoga's system of healing is based on the premise that the body should be allowed to function as naturally as possible. Practicing the recommended asanas will first rejuvenate your body, and then tackle the causes of the ailment.

The four pillars of yoga therapy are the physician, the medication, the attendant, and the patient. In the yogic worldview, the sage Patanjali is the physician, asanas are the medication, the yoga instructor is the attendant, and the student is the patient. Asanas are recommended to "patients" according to their ailment and their physical and emotional condition. This has to be done with care. If a doctor's diagnosis is wrong or the dosage is inappropriate, the treatment can actually harm the patient. Similarly, asanas that are not suited to an individual's requirements can adversely affect his or her health. Follow the recommended sequence of asanas carefully.

The human body is a very complex piece of machinery, a finely connected network of muscles, joints, nerves, veins, arteries, and capillaries. It is a hard task to keep all these elements coordinated and in good working order under the best of circumstances. More often than not, ailments, whether minor or major, affect the body. The science of yoga, as well as that of Ayurveda (a traditional Indian system of healing based on herbal remedies), classify ailments that afflict the body and the mind under three basic categories. These are, firstly, self-inflicted ailments, caused by neglect or abuse of the body; secondly, congenital ailments, present from birth; and thirdly, ailments caused by the imbalance of any of the five elements of ether, air, fire, water, and earth, in our system. Yoga can treat all three, but the pace and effectiveness of the cure depends on the type of ailment, its progression, the patient's constitution, and his or her commitment to the treatment.

How the therapy works

The process of yoga therapy is based on selecting and sequencing asanas which stretch specified parts of the body, and block others. You must remember, however, that in the case of serious or congenital disabilities, yoga asanas may not effect a full recovery, but in many cases can alleviate some of the suffering associated with the condition. For instance, the asana sequence prescribed

Yoga therapy rejuvenates the body
Yogacharya Iyengar in Paripurna Matsyendrasana

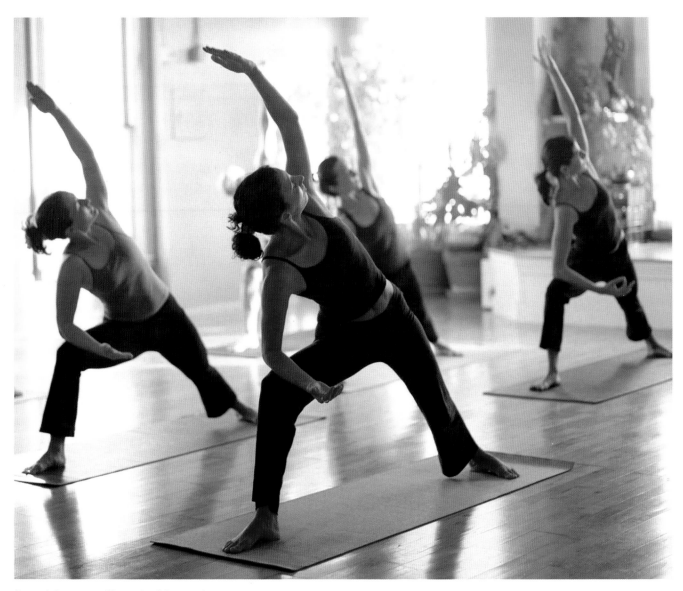

Practicing steadily and with persistence
Yoga therapy involves stretching certain parts of the body and relaxing others

for AIDS (*see page* 309), may relieve some of the symptoms, and the relief can boost morale and self-confidence.

Another benefit of yoga therapy is that it has been known to raise the threshold of pain and endurance. This only happens, however, if the recommended asanas are practiced with patience and dedication. Yoga calms the brain and soothes the nerves, reducing the apprehension of pain, which is, in many cases, as damaging as pain itself.

Medication accelerates the healing process, but is not a cure in itself. Nature alone is the ultimate cure. The belief underlying yoga therapy is to enable the human system to function as efficiently, effectively, and naturally as it can. This natural process, however, operates at its own rhythm and pace, and the pace may sometimes be slow.

Yoga therapy begins with understanding the entire human body and the way it functions. The origins and development of the ailment in question are carefully studied, particularly the parts of the body most affected. The aim is not simply to cure the specific symptom, but to target the cause.

*"**Health** is **not** a **commodity** to be bargained for. It has to be **earned through sweat**."*

Asanas and health

Asanas make your body supple, bringing alertness to your mind, while soothing your nerves and glands, relaxing your brain, and maintaining a physical, physiological, and emotional balance. Regular practice of asanas improves your self-confidence and will power. The practice of asanas lubricates joints, and increases mobility, bringing about an awareness of each muscle, joint, and organ. Different combinations of asanas improve the range of movement for each muscle and joint, helping to align the left and the right sides of the body.

How asanas heal you

Asanas are based on the simple principles of stretching, bending, rotating, and relaxing. These movements have diverse effects on the body's systems, and will either heal, stimulate, or seal off specific parts of the body. At the same time, the approach is holistic, aimed at purifying and strengthening each organ, bone, and cell of the

body. Yoga is a combination of physical therapy, psychotherapy, and spiritual therapy, a healing science which does not distinguish between the physical and physiological bodies. Asanas are bio-physio-psychological poses, through which we build up many "dams" inside our body. Blood and energy are brought to these "dams," which then open very gradually, allowing the organs to absorb fresh healing blood and energy. When a part of the body is affected by disease, it loses its sensitivity. During the practice of specifically therapeutic asanas, energy from these "dams" flows uninterruptedly to the affected area, allowing the healing process to begin.

It is important to work gradually from the periphery to the affected area. First, the peripheral parts of the body should be toned, strengthened, and put into good working order. Only then can the ailment be tackled. Sometimes, however, in the case of a fresh problem, the affected part should be worked upon directly, before it degenerates further.

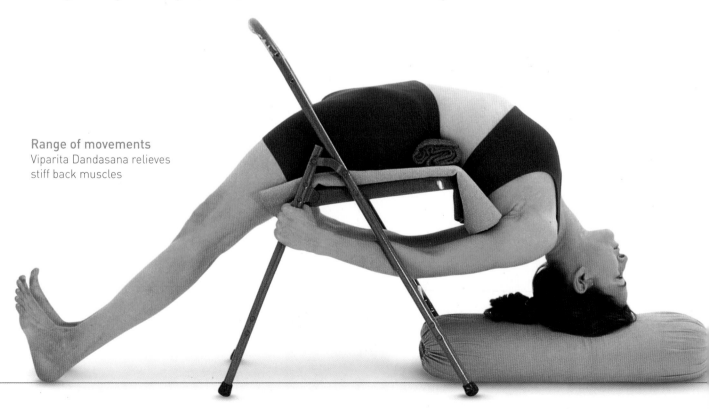

Range of movements
Viparita Dandasana relieves
stiff back muscles

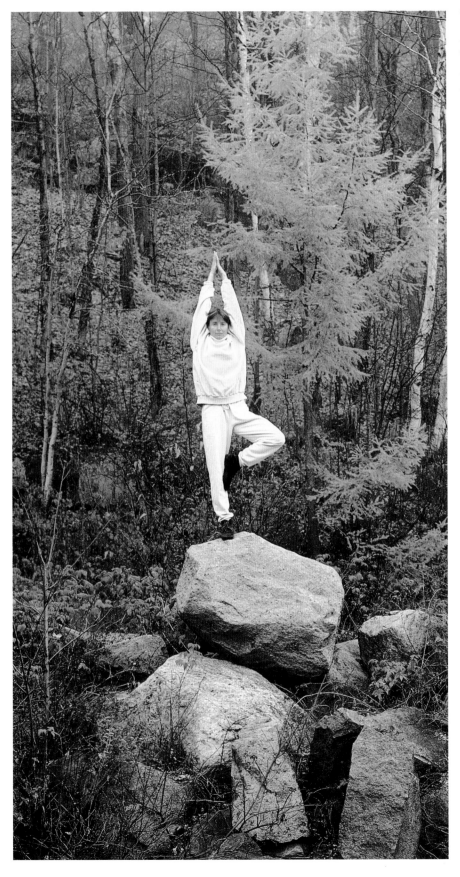

The brain and the body

A very important aspect of yoga therapy is that it teaches us to control the effect of the brain upon the body. The term "brain" is used here in the broadest sense, covering the mind and intellect, and including thought, experience, and imagination. Energy from the brain is diffused to various parts of the body in the form of vital, healing energy. Practicing yoga teaches the brain to be calm and passive, to accept and subdue pain, not fight it. The energy that is otherwise dissipated in coping with stress and pain, is diverted to healing.

Ultimately, the aim of yoga therapy is to teach the brain and body to work in harmony. Specific asanas work on the various systems of the body, whether respiratory, circulatory, digestive, hormonal, immune, or reproductive. Therefore, the combination and sequencing of the asanas must be followed for the healing process to be effective. Follow the sequence prescribed for your particular ailment, setting up a schedule for practicing the recommended asanas (*see page* 408). Do not get discouraged if the healing of your ailment takes time. Remember, perseverance is the essence of yoga.

Holistic therapy
Yoga addresses every organ, bone, muscle, and cell of the body

HEART AND CIRCULATION

The heart is the organ that pumps blood to all parts of the body. It is located in the thoracic cavity, nestled between the lungs. The circulatory system, composed of arteries, veins, and capillaries, carries blood to and from the heart to the entire body, supplying oxygen and nutrients, and carrying away waste products. The following sequences of asanas address some common disorders of this system.

COLD EXTREMITIES

This is caused by a slowdown in circulation, when blood collects in the torso and fails to correctly reach the extremities. It gives rise to ailments of the chest and of the intestinal and abdominal organs. It is often the result of a sluggish thyroid, stress, or nervousness.

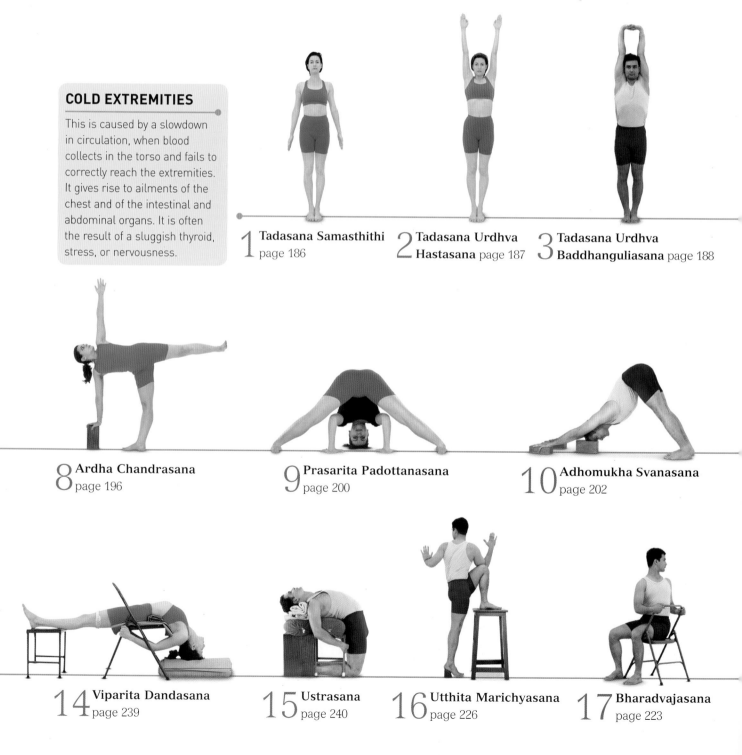

1 **Tadasana Samasthithi** page 186

2 **Tadasana Urdhva Hastasana** page 187

3 **Tadasana Urdhva Baddhanguliasana** page 188

8 **Ardha Chandrasana** page 196

9 **Prasarita Padottanasana** page 200

10 **Adhomukha Svanasana** page 202

14 **Viparita Dandasana** page 239

15 **Ustrasana** page 240

16 **Utthita Marichyasana** page 226

17 **Bharadvajasana** page 223

*"Never perform asanas mechanically.
If you do, your body stagnates."*

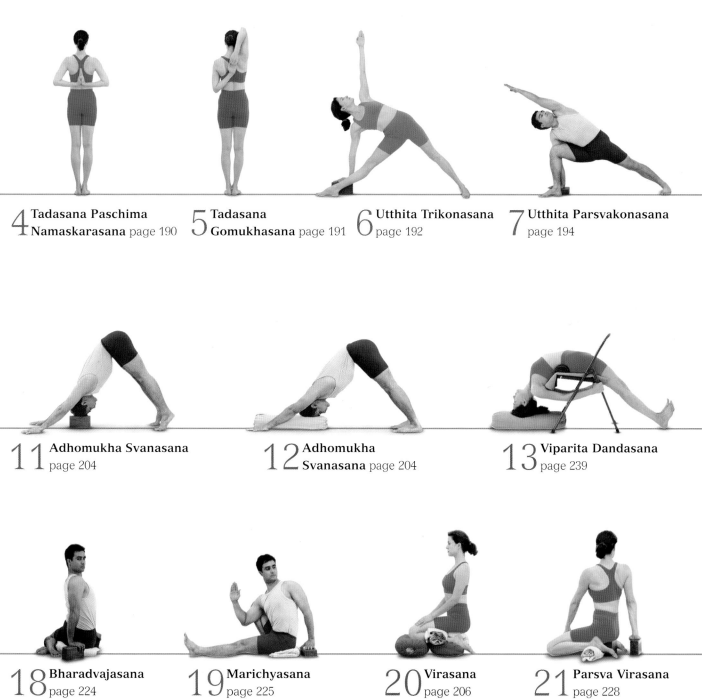

4 **Tadasana Paschima Namaskarasana** page 190

5 **Tadasana Gomukhasana** page 191

6 **Utthita Trikonasana** page 192

7 **Utthita Parsvakonasana** page 194

11 **Adhomukha Svanasana** page 204

12 **Adhomukha Svanasana** page 204

13 **Viparita Dandasana** page 239

18 **Bharadvajasana** page 224

19 **Marichyasana** page 225

20 **Virasana** page 206

21 **Parsva Virasana** page 228

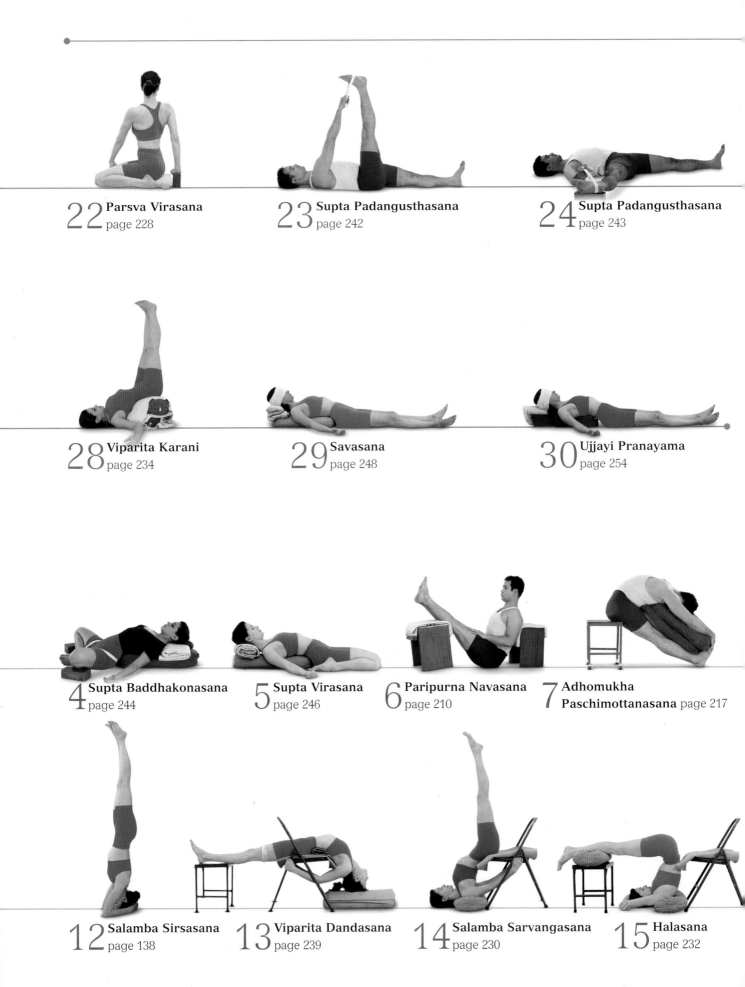

22 **Parsva Virasana**
page 228

23 **Supta Padangusthasana**
page 242

24 **Supta Padangusthasana**
page 243

28 **Viparita Karani**
page 234

29 **Savasana**
page 248

30 **Ujjayi Pranayama**
page 254

4 **Supta Baddhakonasana**
page 244

5 **Supta Virasana**
page 246

6 **Paripurna Navasana**
page 210

7 **Adhomukha Paschimottanasana** page 217

12 **Salamba Sirsasana**
page 138

13 **Viparita Dandasana**
page 239

14 **Salamba Sarvangasana**
page 230

15 **Halasana**
page 232

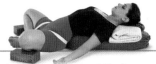
25 Supta Baddhakonasana
page 244

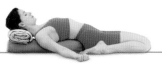
26 Supta Virasana
page 246

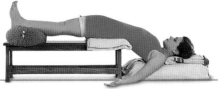
27 Setubandha Sarvangasana
page 237

VARICOSE VEINS

In this condition, veins just beneath the skin of the legs are elongated and dilated, leading to aching legs, fatigue, and muscle cramps. The condition often occurs during pregnancy and menstruation, and also affects those who have to stay on their feet for long periods.

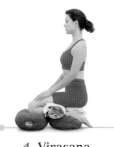
1 Virasana
page 206

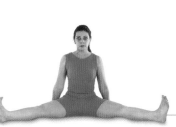
2 Upavista Konasana
page 213

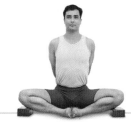
3 Baddhakonasana
page 208

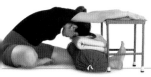
8 Janu Sirsasana
page 218

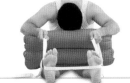
9 Paschimottanasana
page 216

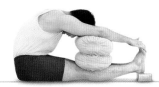
10 Paschimottanasana
page 215

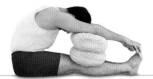
11 Paschimottanasana
page 214

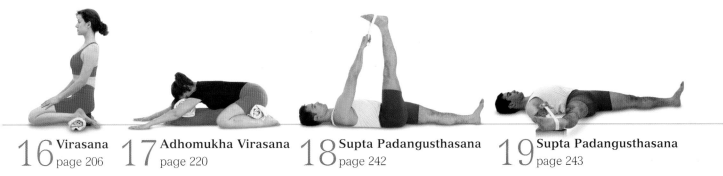
16 Virasana
page 206

17 Adhomukha Virasana
page 220

18 Supta Padangusthasana
page 242

19 Supta Padangusthasana
page 243

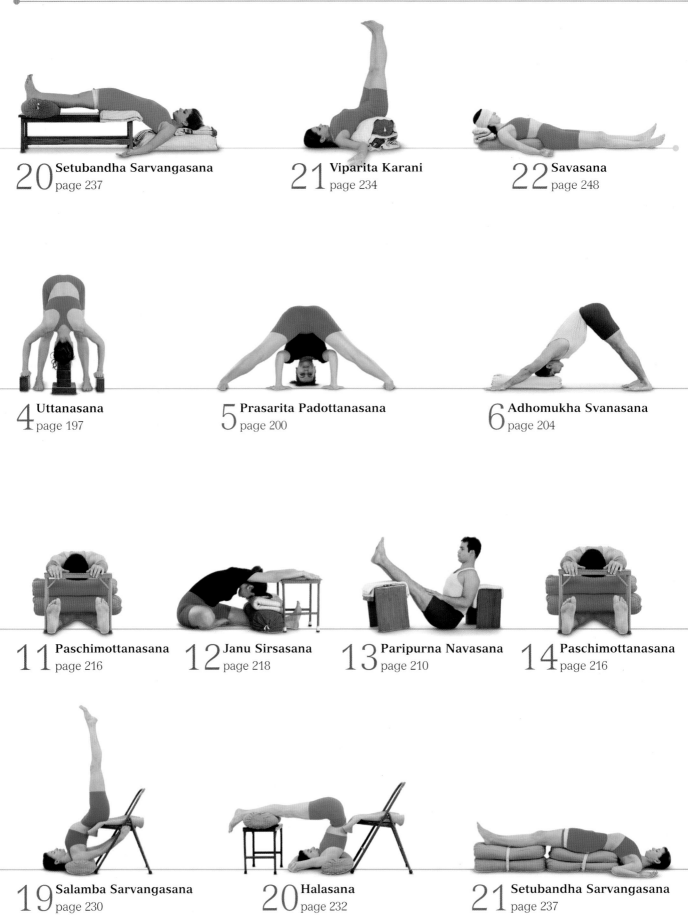

20 **Setubandha Sarvangasana**
page 237

21 **Viparita Karani**
page 234

22 **Savasana**
page 248

4 **Uttanasana**
page 197

5 **Prasarita Padottanasana**
page 200

6 **Adhomukha Svanasana**
page 204

11 **Paschimottanasana**
page 216

12 **Janu Sirsasana**
page 218

13 **Paripurna Navasana**
page 210

14 **Paschimottanasana**
page 216

19 **Salamba Sarvangasana**
page 230

20 **Halasana**
page 232

21 **Setubandha Sarvangasana**
page 237

HIGH BLOOD PRESSURE

This condition is defined as sustained, elevated blood pressure, and is also known as hypertension. It has many causes, which include psychological, physiological, and environmental factors.

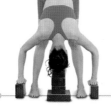

1 **Uttanasana** page 197

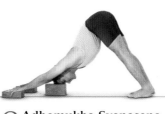

2 **Adhomukha Svanasana** page 202

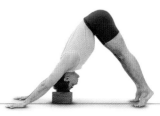

3 **Adhomukha Svanasana** page 204

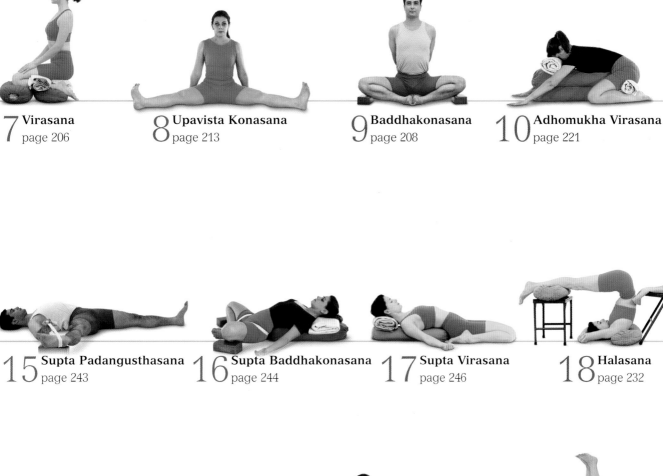

7 **Virasana** page 206

8 **Upavista Konasana** page 213

9 **Baddhakonasana** page 208

10 **Adhomukha Virasana** page 221

15 **Supta Padangusthasana** page 243

16 **Supta Baddhakonasana** page 244

17 **Supta Virasana** page 246

18 **Halasana** page 232

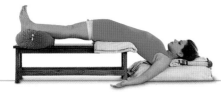

22 **Setubandha Sarvangasana** page 237

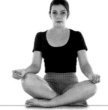

23 **Swastikasana** page 209

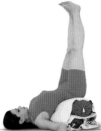

24 **Viparita Karani** page 234

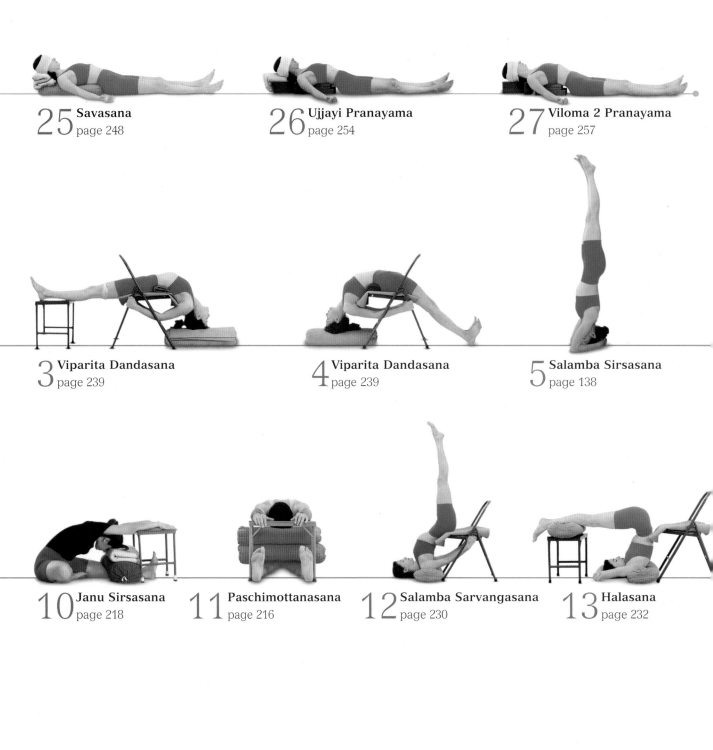

25 **Savasana**
page 248

26 **Ujjayi Pranayama**
page 254

27 **Viloma 2 Pranayama**
page 257

3 **Viparita Dandasana**
page 239

4 **Viparita Dandasana**
page 239

5 **Salamba Sirsasana**
page 138

10 **Janu Sirsasana**
page 218

11 **Paschimottanasana**
page 216

12 **Salamba Sarvangasana**
page 230

13 **Halasana**
page 232

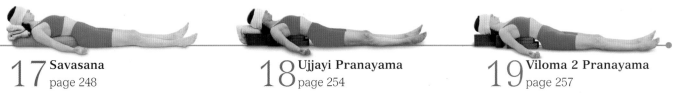

17 **Savasana**
page 248

18 **Ujjayi Pranayama**
page 254

19 **Viloma 2 Pranayama**
page 257

LOW BLOOD PRESSURE

This condition, also called hypotension, occurs when blood pressure is less than normally required to transport blood to all parts of the body. This can reduce blood supply to the brain, resulting in fatigue, fainting spells, light-headedness, blurred vision, or nausea.

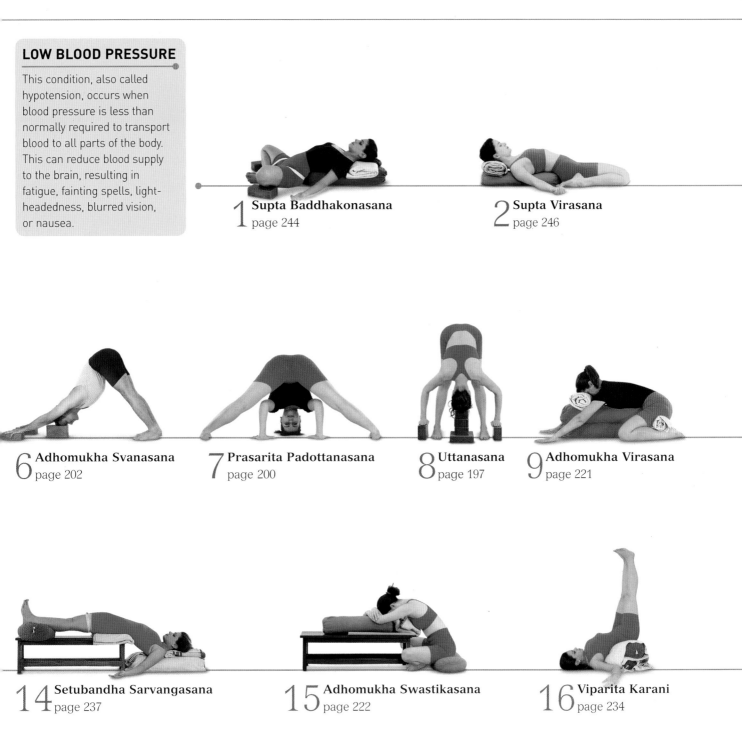

1 **Supta Baddhakonasana**
page 244

2 **Supta Virasana**
page 246

6 **Adhomukha Svanasana**
page 202

7 **Prasarita Padottanasana**
page 200

8 **Uttanasana**
page 197

9 **Adhomukha Virasana**
page 221

14 **Setubandha Sarvangasana**
page 237

15 **Adhomukha Swastikasana**
page 222

16 **Viparita Karani**
page 234

BLOCKED ARTERIES

This occurs when the coronary vessels are blocked, reducing blood flow to the cardiac muscles. This process eventually damages these muscles, and is a major cause of heart attacks. A common symptom is angina or chest pain (*see page* 272).

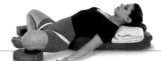

1 **Supta Baddhakonasana**
page 244

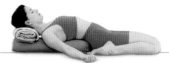

2 **Supta Virasana**
page 246

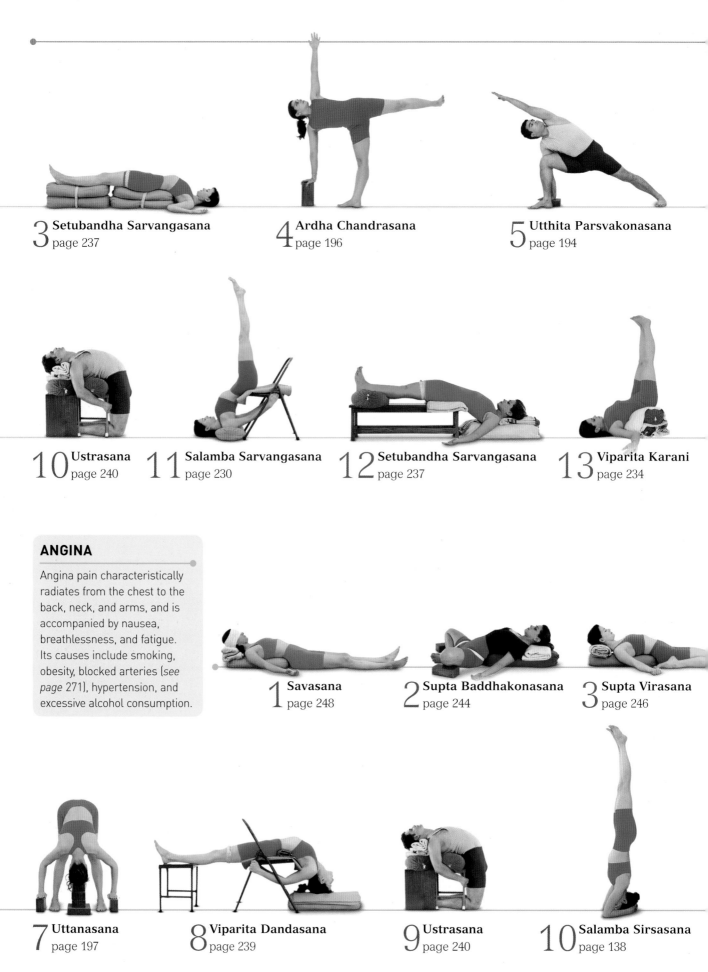

3 **Setubandha Sarvangasana**
page 237

4 **Ardha Chandrasana**
page 196

5 **Utthita Parsvakonasana**
page 194

10 **Ustrasana**
page 240

11 **Salamba Sarvangasana**
page 230

12 **Setubandha Sarvangasana**
page 237

13 **Viparita Karani**
page 234

ANGINA

Angina pain characteristically radiates from the chest to the back, neck, and arms, and is accompanied by nausea, breathlessness, and fatigue. Its causes include smoking, obesity, blocked arteries (*see page* 271), hypertension, and excessive alcohol consumption.

1 **Savasana**
page 248

2 **Supta Baddhakonasana**
page 244

3 **Supta Virasana**
page 246

7 **Uttanasana**
page 197

8 **Viparita Dandasana**
page 239

9 **Ustrasana**
page 240

10 **Salamba Sirsasana**
page 138

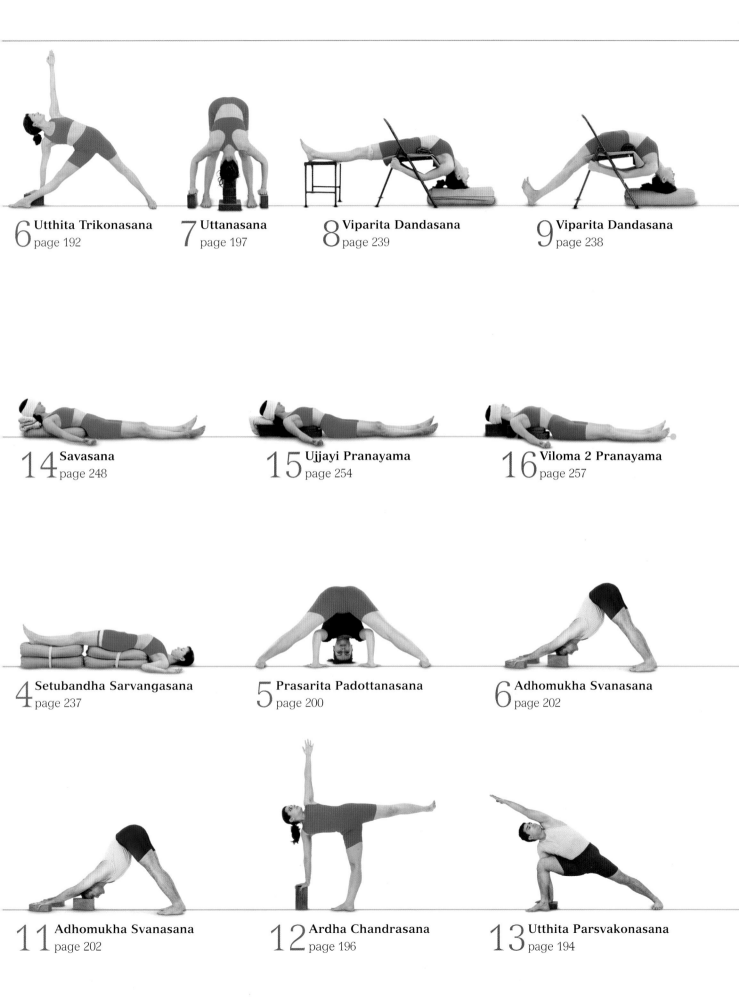

6 **Utthita Trikonasana** page 192

7 **Uttanasana** page 197

8 **Viparita Dandasana** page 239

9 **Viparita Dandasana** page 238

14 **Savasana** page 248

15 **Ujjayi Pranayama** page 254

16 **Viloma 2 Pranayama** page 257

4 **Setubandha Sarvangasana** page 237

5 **Prasarita Padottanasana** page 200

6 **Adhomukha Svanasana** page 202

11 **Adhomukha Svanasana** page 202

12 **Ardha Chandrasana** page 196

13 **Utthita Parsvakonasana** page 194

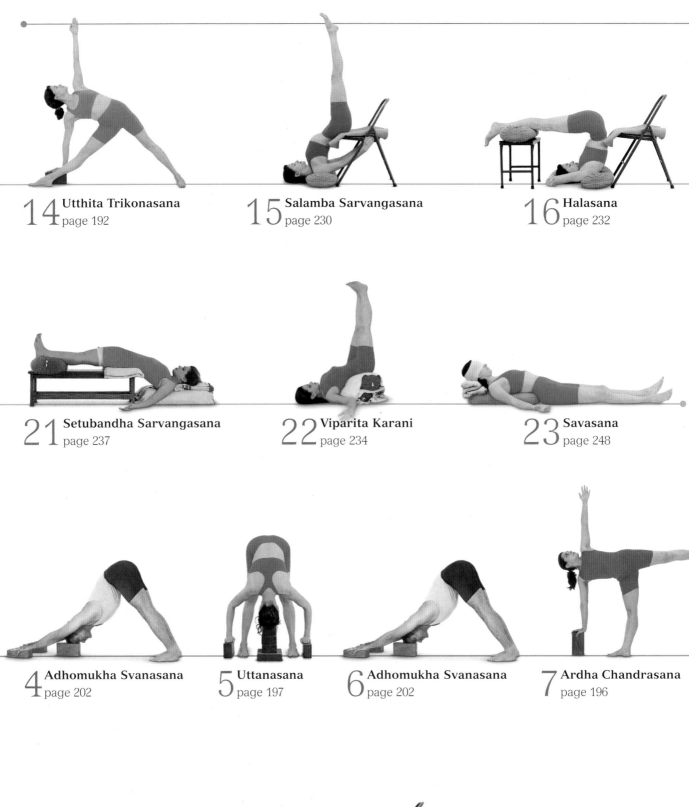

14 **Utthita Trikonasana** page 192

15 **Salamba Sarvangasana** page 230

16 **Halasana** page 232

21 **Setubandha Sarvangasana** page 237

22 **Viparita Karani** page 234

23 **Savasana** page 248

4 **Adhomukha Svanasana** page 202

5 **Uttanasana** page 197

6 **Adhomukha Svanasana** page 202

7 **Ardha Chandrasana** page 196

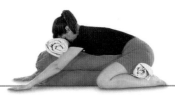

12 **Adhomukha Virasana** page 221

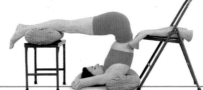

13 **Halasana** page 232

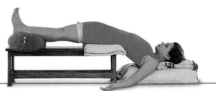

14 **Setubandha Sarvangasana** page 237

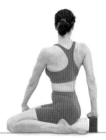

17 Parsva Virasana
page 228

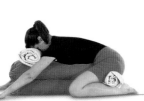

18 Adhomukha
Virasana page 221

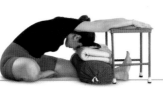

19 Janu Sirsasana
page 218

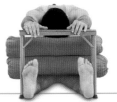

20 Paschimottanasana
page 216

HEART ATTACK

Inadequate blood supply to the heart muscles results in myocardial infarction or a heart attack. It is often due to the gradual blocking of the coronary arteries (*see page* 272).

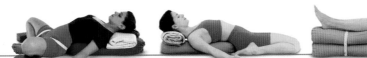

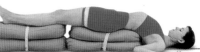

1 Supta Baddhakonasana
page 244

2 Supta Virasana
page 246

3 Setubandha
Sarvangasana page 237

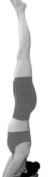

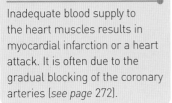

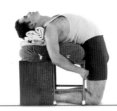

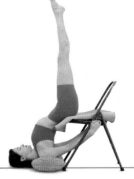

8 Salamba Sirsasana
page 138

9 Viparita Dandasana
page 239

10 Ustrasana
page 240

11 Salamba Sarvangasana
page 230

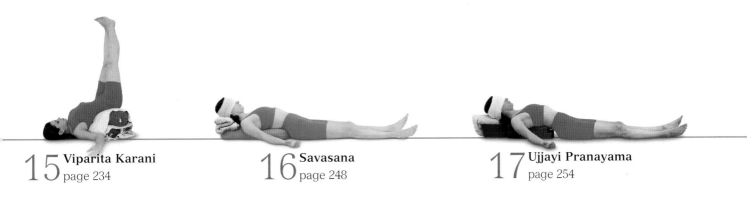

15 Viparita Karani
page 234

16 Savasana
page 248

17 Ujjayi Pranayama
page 254

RESPIRATORY SYSTEM

Respiration starts from the upper respiratory tract in the nose and the pharynx (the throat). Then inhaled air passes through to the trachea (the windpipe), and the two major bronchi. These airways conduct air into the lungs. Carbon dioxide from the body's cells is exhaled through the lungs. Yoga asanas are particularly beneficial for all respiratory disorders if the recommended sequences are practiced regularly.

COLDS

These are minor viral infections of the mucous membranes that line the upper respiratory tract, including the nose and throat. The most common symptoms are nasal obstruction and discharge, sinusitis, sore throat, sneezing, coughing, and headaches.

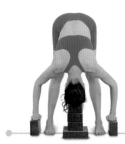

1 **Uttanasana**
page 197

2 **Prasarita Padottanasana**
page 200

3 **Adhomukha Svanasana** page 202

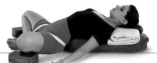

8 **Supta Baddhakonasana**
page 244

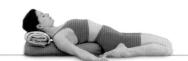

9 **Supta Virasana**
page 246

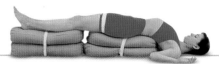

10 **Setubandha Sarvangasana**
page 237

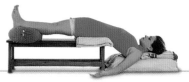

14 **Setubandha Sarvangasana**
page 237

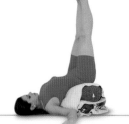

15 **Viparita Karani**
page 234

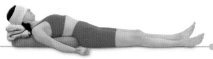

16 **Viloma 2 / Savasana**
pages 257, 248

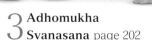

"Hence, control the breath to restrain the wandering mind."

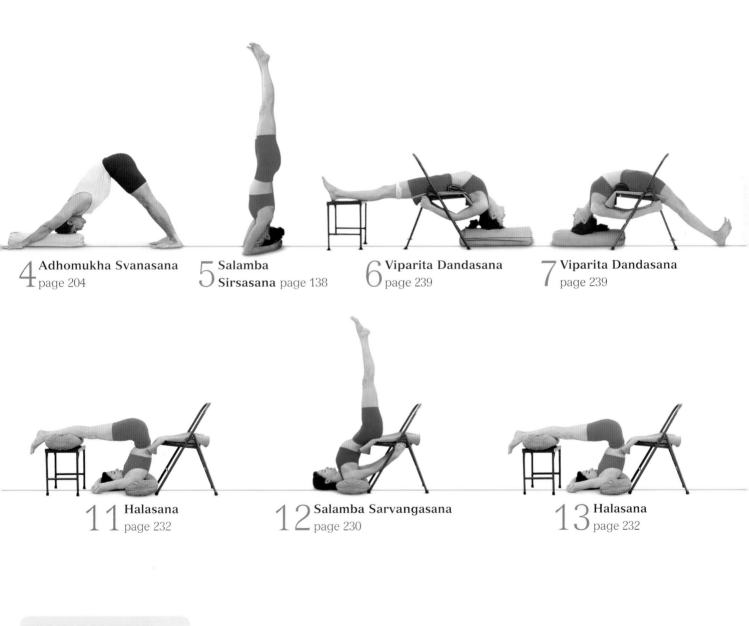

4 **Adhomukha Svanasana**
page 204

5 **Salamba Sirsasana** page 138

6 **Viparita Dandasana**
page 239

7 **Viparita Dandasana**
page 239

11 **Halasana**
page 232

12 **Salamba Sarvangasana**
page 230

13 **Halasana**
page 232

BREATHLESSNESS

This condition, also called dyspnea, is caused by deficiencies in the elastic recoil of the lungs. Air is retained in the lungs, which then become distended. The diaphragm is squeezed and the effort to breathe strains the chest.

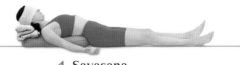

1 **Savasana**
page 248

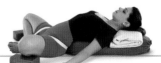

2 **Supta Baddhakonasana**
page 244

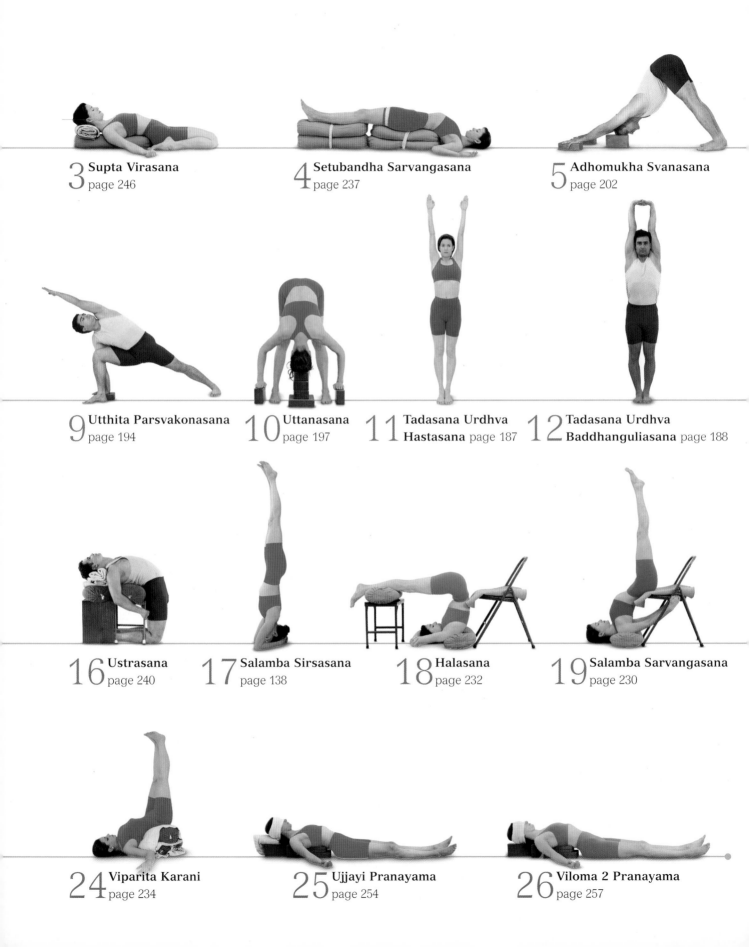

3 **Supta Virasana**
page 246

4 **Setubandha Sarvangasana**
page 237

5 **Adhomukha Svanasana**
page 202

9 **Utthita Parsvakonasana**
page 194

10 **Uttanasana**
page 197

11 **Tadasana Urdhva Hastasana** page 187

12 **Tadasana Urdhva Baddhanguliasana** page 188

16 **Ustrasana**
page 240

17 **Salamba Sirsasana**
page 138

18 **Halasana**
page 232

19 **Salamba Sarvangasana**
page 230

24 **Viparita Karani**
page 234

25 **Ujjayi Pranayama**
page 254

26 **Viloma 2 Pranayama**
page 257

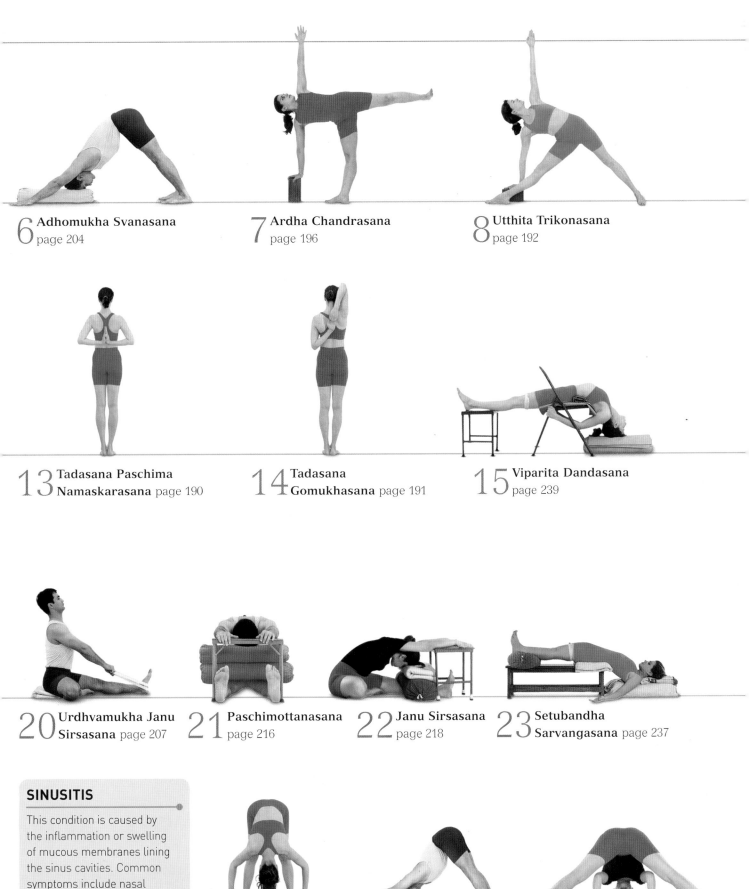

6 **Adhomukha Svanasana**
page 204

7 **Ardha Chandrasana**
page 196

8 **Utthita Trikonasana**
page 192

13 **Tadasana Paschima Namaskarasana** page 190

14 **Tadasana Gomukhasana** page 191

15 **Viparita Dandasana**
page 239

20 **Urdhvamukha Janu Sirsasana** page 207

21 **Paschimottanasana**
page 216

22 **Janu Sirsasana**
page 218

23 **Setubandha Sarvangasana** page 237

SINUSITIS

This condition is caused by the inflammation or swelling of mucous membranes lining the sinus cavities. Common symptoms include nasal congestion and discharge, headaches, and pain in the region of the upper jaw, eyes, cheeks, or ears.

1 **Uttanasana**
page 197

2 **Adhomukha Svanasana** page 202

3 **Prasarita Padottanasana** page 200

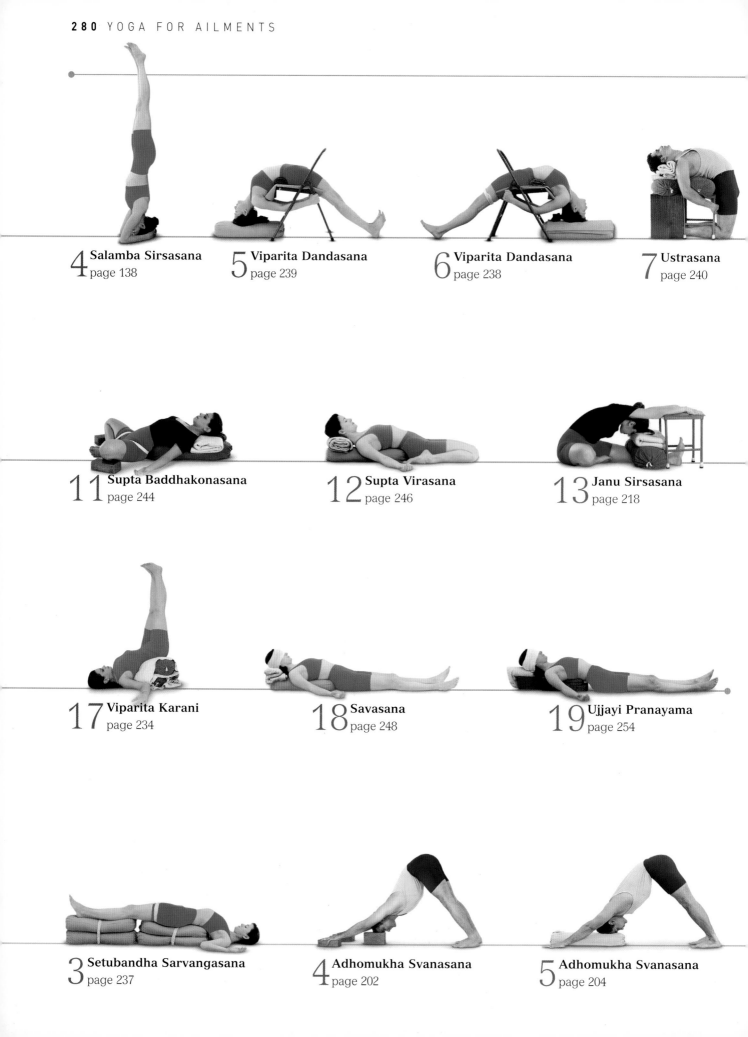

4 **Salamba Sirsasana**
page 138

5 **Viparita Dandasana**
page 239

6 **Viparita Dandasana**
page 238

7 **Ustrasana**
page 240

11 **Supta Baddhakonasana**
page 244

12 **Supta Virasana**
page 246

13 **Janu Sirsasana**
page 218

17 **Viparita Karani**
page 234

18 **Savasana**
page 248

19 **Ujjayi Pranayama**
page 254

3 **Setubandha Sarvangasana**
page 237

4 **Adhomukha Svanasana**
page 202

5 **Adhomukha Svanasana**
page 204

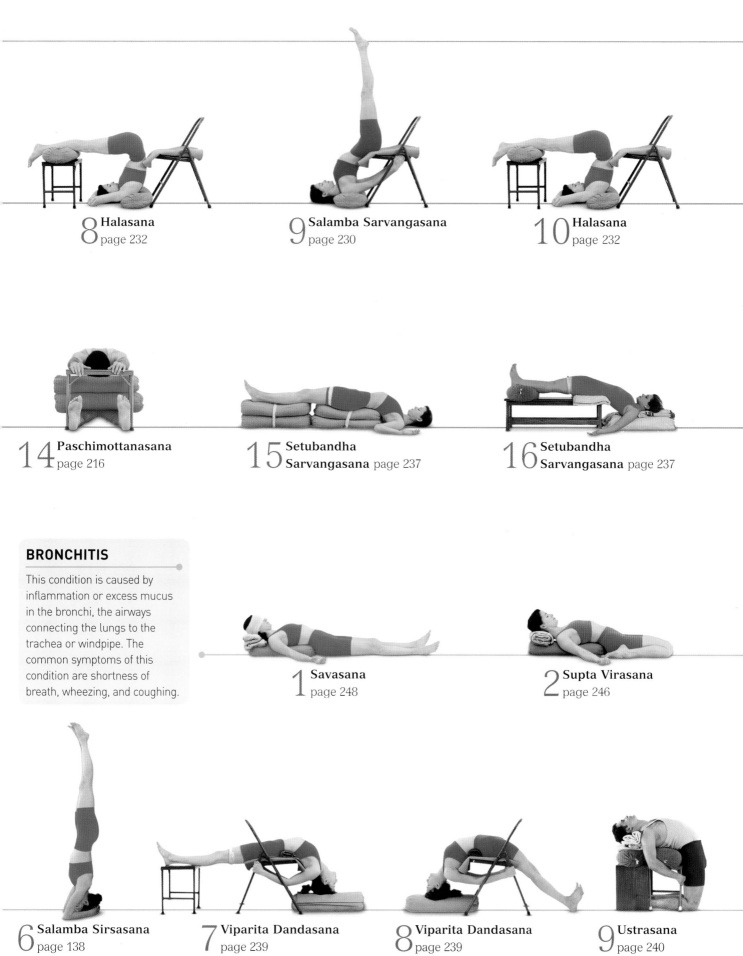

8 **Halasana**
page 232

9 **Salamba Sarvangasana**
page 230

10 **Halasana**
page 232

14 **Paschimottanasana**
page 216

15 **Setubandha Sarvangasana** page 237

16 **Setubandha Sarvangasana** page 237

BRONCHITIS

This condition is caused by inflammation or excess mucus in the bronchi, the airways connecting the lungs to the trachea or windpipe. The common symptoms of this condition are shortness of breath, wheezing, and coughing.

1 **Savasana**
page 248

2 **Supta Virasana**
page 246

6 **Salamba Sirsasana**
page 138

7 **Viparita Dandasana**
page 239

8 **Viparita Dandasana**
page 239

9 **Ustrasana**
page 240

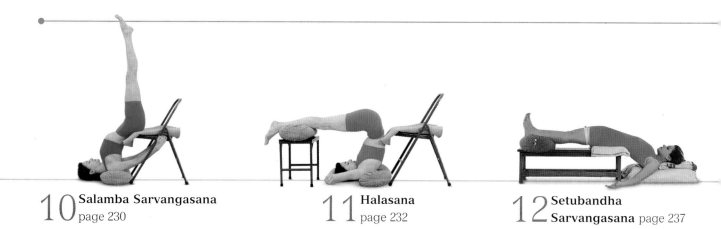

10 **Salamba Sarvangasana** page 230

11 **Halasana** page 232

12 **Setubandha Sarvangasana** page 237

ASTHMA

In this condition, the airways of the lungs are constricted, causing tightness in the chest, bouts of coughing, wheezing, and breathing difficulties. The inflammation of the air passages can become chronic. Asthma is usually caused by allergies or stress.

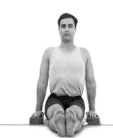

1 **Dandasana** page 205

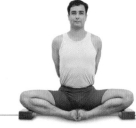

2 **Baddhakonasana** page 208

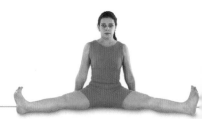

3 **Upavista Konasana** page 213

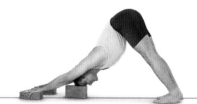

7 **Setubandha Sarvangasana** page 237

8 **Adhomukha Svanasana** page 202

9 **Uttanasana** page 197

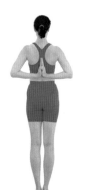

13 **Tadasana Paschima Namaskarasana** page 190

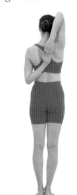

14 **Tadasana Gomukhasana** page 191

15 **Ardha Chandrasana** page 196

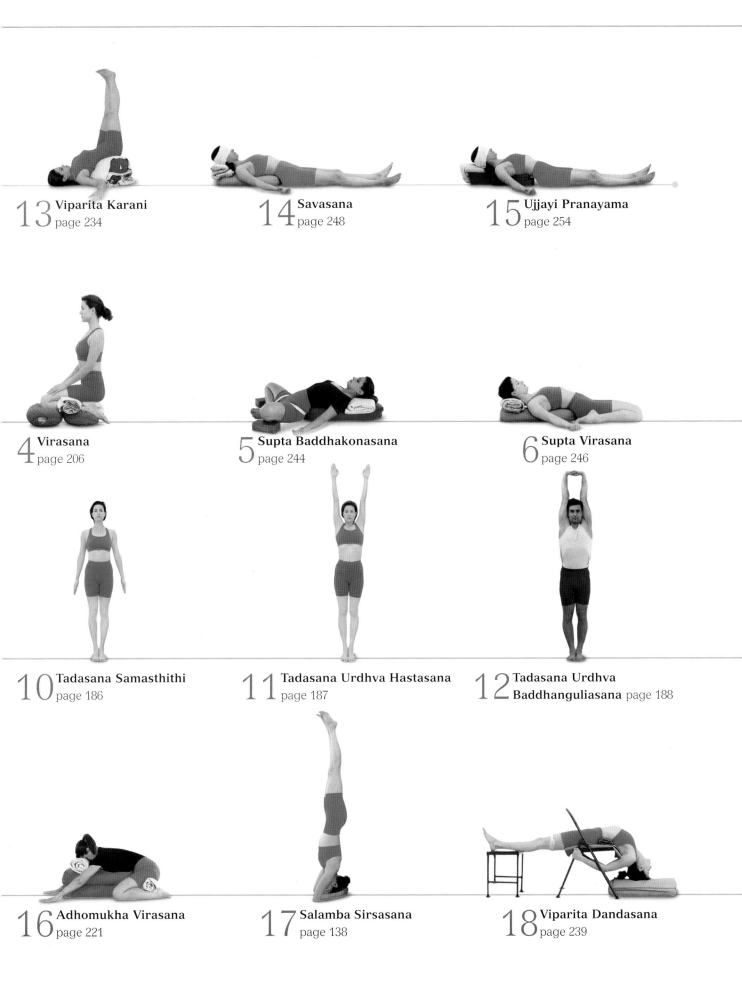

13 **Viparita Karani**
page 234

14 **Savasana**
page 248

15 **Ujjayi Pranayama**
page 254

4 **Virasana**
page 206

5 **Supta Baddhakonasana**
page 244

6 **Supta Virasana**
page 246

10 **Tadasana Samasthithi**
page 186

11 **Tadasana Urdhva Hastasana**
page 187

12 **Tadasana Urdhva Baddhanguliasana** page 188

16 **Adhomukha Virasana**
page 221

17 **Salamba Sirsasana**
page 138

18 **Viparita Dandasana**
page 239

"Fear and fatigue block the mind. Confront both squarely, and then courage and confidence will flow into you."

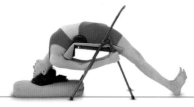

19 **Viparita Dandasana** page 239

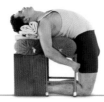

20 **Ustrasana** page 240

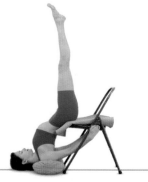

21 **Salamba Sarvangasana** page 230

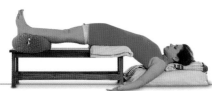

22 **Setubandha Sarvangasana** page 237

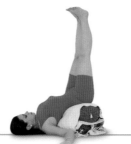

23 **Viparita Karani** page 234

24 **Savasana** page 248

DIGESTIVE SYSTEM

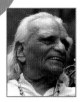

All the food we eat has to travel an average distance of almost 35 ft (11 m) through the body. It passes through the mouth, esophagus, small intestine, and large intestine. Food interacts with the saliva and with the secretions of the pancreas, gall bladder, and liver, and is broken down by digestive enzymes and acids. During this process, nourishment is absorbed by the body. Regular practice of these recommended asanas effectively alleviates digestive disorders.

INDIGESTION

This condition is associated with upper abdominal pain, discomfort, or distension which is either intermittent or chronic. Other indications are nausea, vomiting, belching, acidity, flatulence, and a constant feeling of being full.

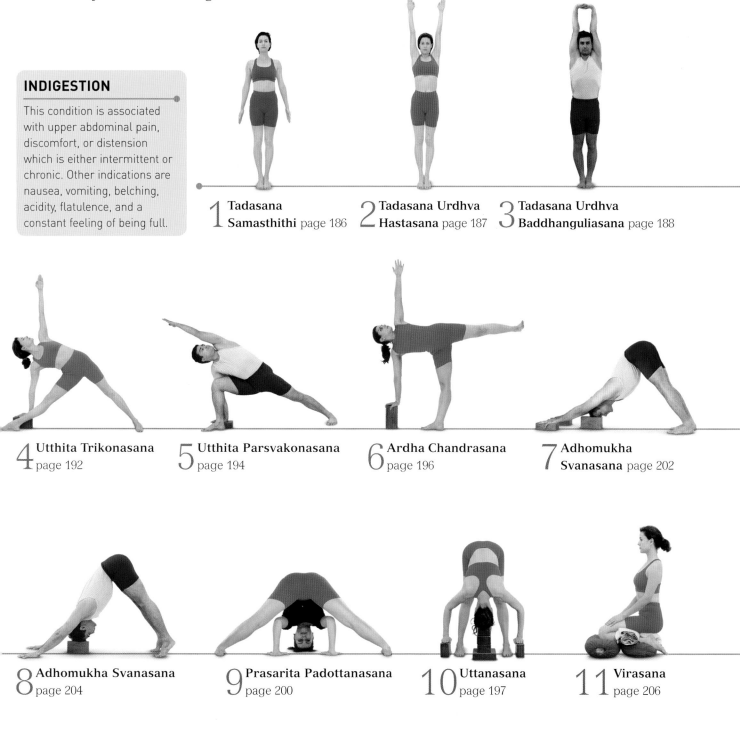

1 **Tadasana Samasthithi** page 186

2 **Tadasana Urdhva Hastasana** page 187

3 **Tadasana Urdhva Baddhanguliasana** page 188

4 **Utthita Trikonasana** page 192

5 **Utthita Parsvakonasana** page 194

6 **Ardha Chandrasana** page 196

7 **Adhomukha Svanasana** page 202

8 **Adhomukha Svanasana** page 204

9 **Prasarita Padottanasana** page 200

10 **Uttanasana** page 197

11 **Virasana** page 206

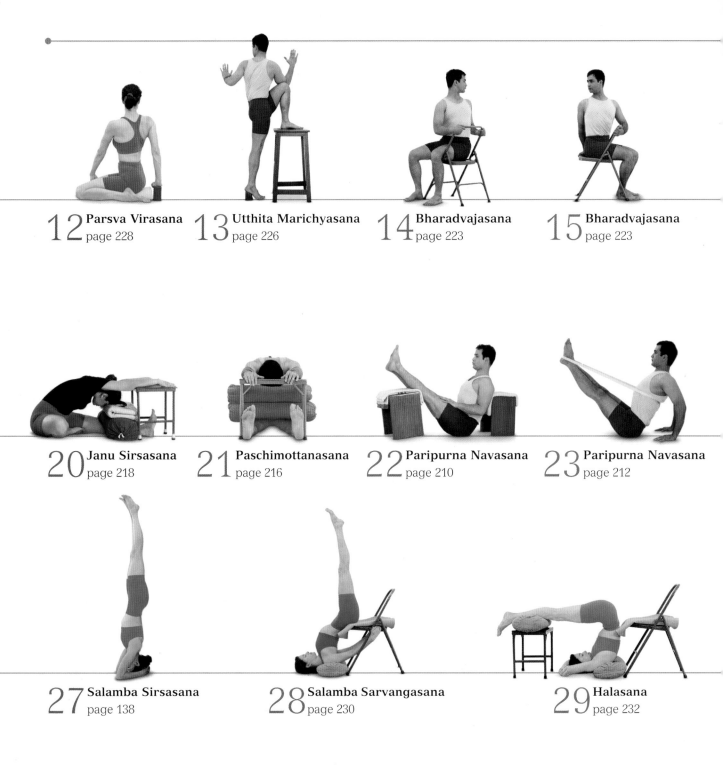

12 **Parsva Virasana**
page 228

13 **Utthita Marichyasana**
page 226

14 **Bharadvajasana**
page 223

15 **Bharadvajasana**
page 223

20 **Janu Sirsasana**
page 218

21 **Paschimottanasana**
page 216

22 **Paripurna Navasana**
page 210

23 **Paripurna Navasana**
page 212

27 **Salamba Sirsasana**
page 138

28 **Salamba Sarvangasana**
page 230

29 **Halasana**
page 232

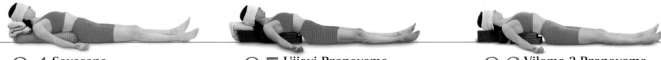

34 **Savasana**
page 248

35 **Ujjayi Pranayama**
page 254

36 **Viloma 2 Pranayama**
page 257

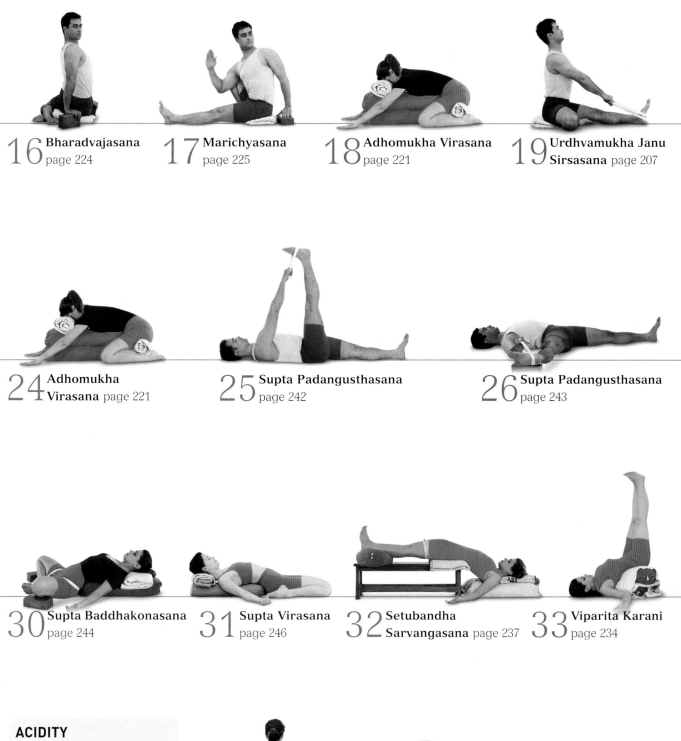

16 **Bharadvajasana** page 224

17 **Marichyasana** page 225

18 **Adhomukha Virasana** page 221

19 **Urdhvamukha Janu Sirsasana** page 207

24 **Adhomukha Virasana** page 221

25 **Supta Padangusthasana** page 242

26 **Supta Padangusthasana** page 243

30 **Supta Baddhakonasana** page 244

31 **Supta Virasana** page 246

32 **Setubandha Sarvangasana** page 237

33 **Viparita Karani** page 234

ACIDITY

This is commonly indicated by a sharp, burning sensation in the lower chest, just below the sternum. It can be caused by overeating, the intake of highly spiced or rich food, excessive alcohol, or drugs, such as aspirin or cortisone.

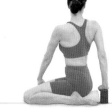

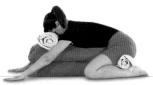

1 **Parsva Virasana** page 228

2 **Adhomukha Paschimottanasana** page 217

3 **Adhomukha Virasana** page 221

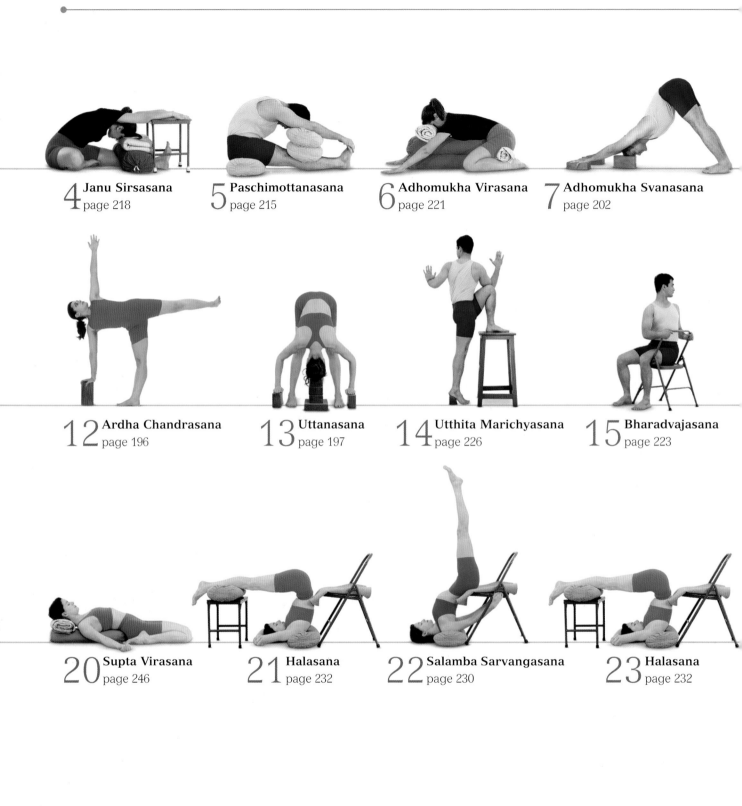

4 **Janu Sirsasana**
page 218

5 **Paschimottanasana**
page 215

6 **Adhomukha Virasana**
page 221

7 **Adhomukha Svanasana**
page 202

12 **Ardha Chandrasana**
page 196

13 **Uttanasana**
page 197

14 **Utthita Marichyasana**
page 226

15 **Bharadvajasana**
page 223

20 **Supta Virasana**
page 246

21 **Halasana**
page 232

22 **Salamba Sarvangasana**
page 230

23 **Halasana**
page 232

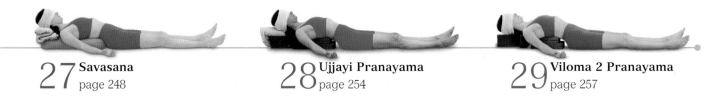

27 **Savasana**
page 248

28 **Ujjayi Pranayama**
page 254

29 **Viloma 2 Pranayama**
page 257

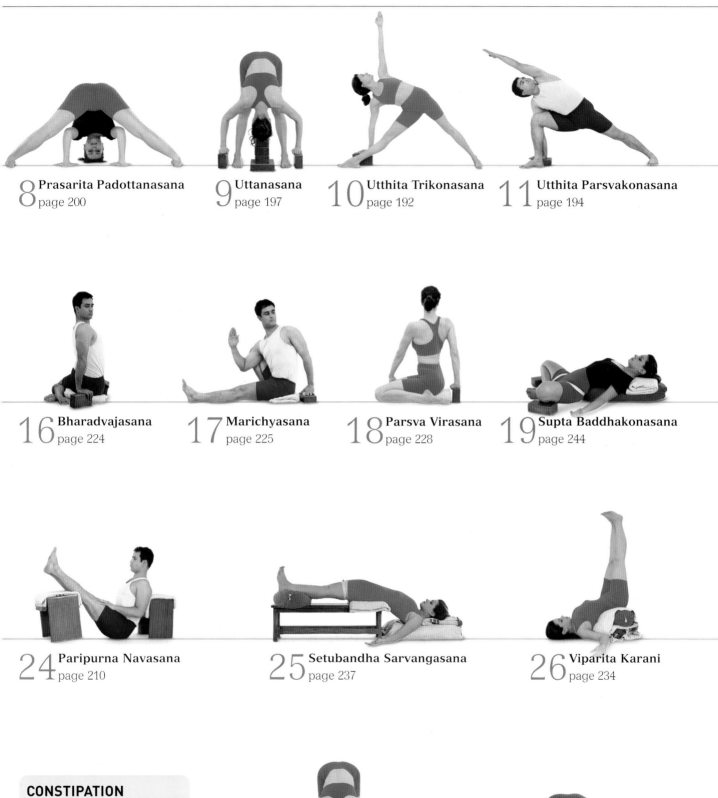

8 **Prasarita Padottanasana**
page 200

9 **Uttanasana**
page 197

10 **Utthita Trikonasana**
page 192

11 **Utthita Parsvakonasana**
page 194

16 **Bharadvajasana**
page 224

17 **Marichyasana**
page 225

18 **Parsva Virasana**
page 228

19 **Supta Baddhakonasana**
page 244

24 **Paripurna Navasana**
page 210

25 **Setubandha Sarvangasana**
page 237

26 **Viparita Karani**
page 234

CONSTIPATION

For some people, the elimination of waste from the body is difficult, infrequent, and sometimes painful. This is often accompanied by a feeling that the bowels have not been completely emptied.

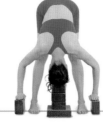

1 **Uttanasana**
page 197

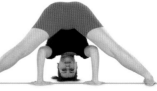

2 **Prasarita Padottanasana**
page 200

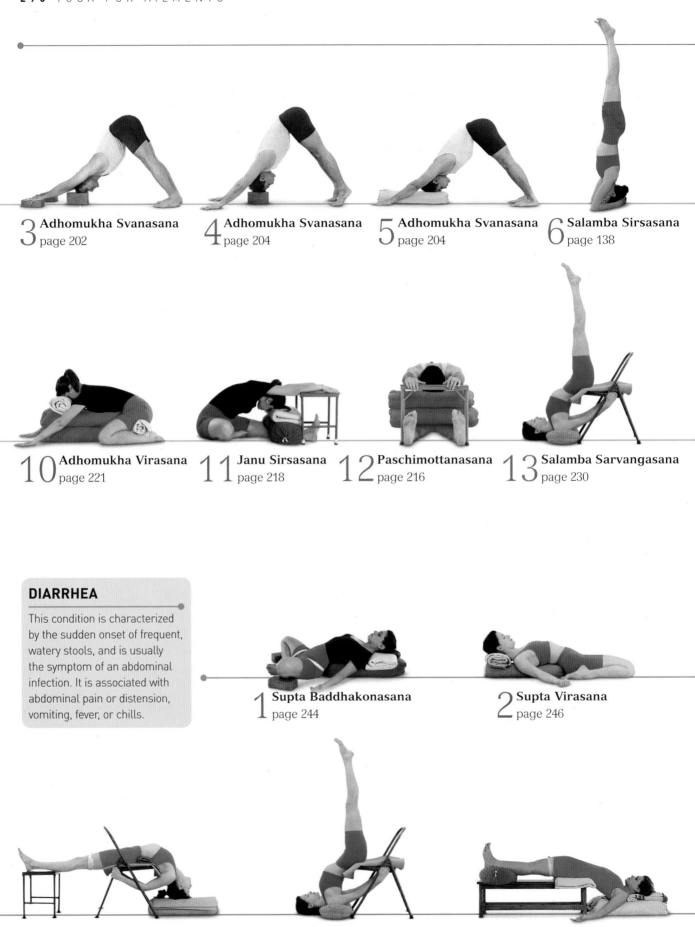

3 **Adhomukha Svanasana** page 202

4 **Adhomukha Svanasana** page 204

5 **Adhomukha Svanasana** page 204

6 **Salamba Sirsasana** page 138

10 **Adhomukha Virasana** page 221

11 **Janu Sirsasana** page 218

12 **Paschimottanasana** page 216

13 **Salamba Sarvangasana** page 230

DIARRHEA

This condition is characterized by the sudden onset of frequent, watery stools, and is usually the symptom of an abdominal infection. It is associated with abdominal pain or distension, vomiting, fever, or chills.

1 **Supta Baddhakonasana** page 244

2 **Supta Virasana** page 246

6 **Viparita Dandasana** page 239

7 **Salamba Sarvangasana** page 230

8 **Setubandha Sarvangasana** page 237

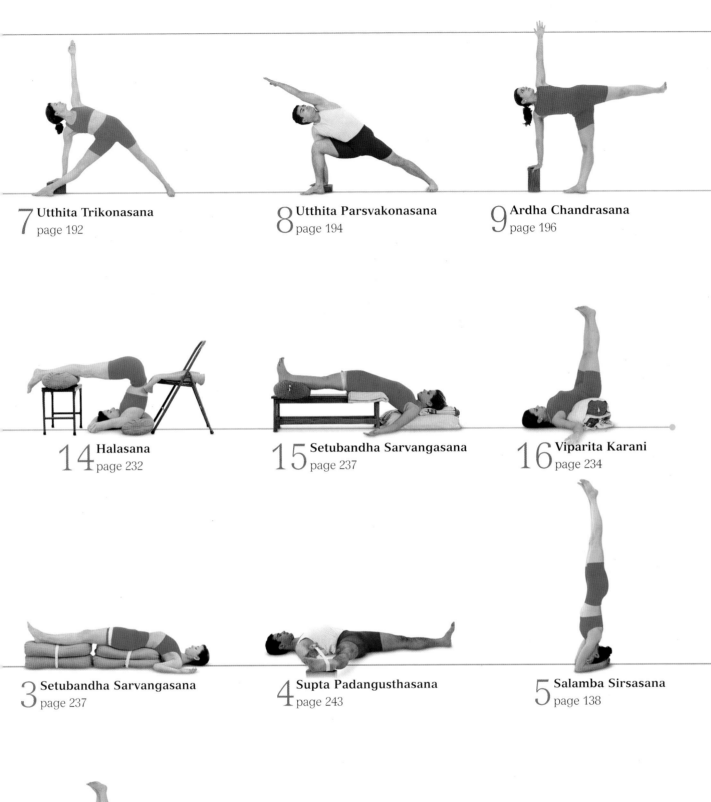

7 **Utthita Trikonasana**
page 192

8 **Utthita Parsvakonasana**
page 194

9 **Ardha Chandrasana**
page 196

14 **Halasana**
page 232

15 **Setubandha Sarvangasana**
page 237

16 **Viparita Karani**
page 234

3 **Setubandha Sarvangasana**
page 237

4 **Supta Padangusthasana**
page 243

5 **Salamba Sirsasana**
page 138

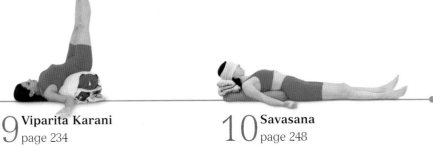

9 **Viparita Karani**
page 234

10 **Savasana**
page 248

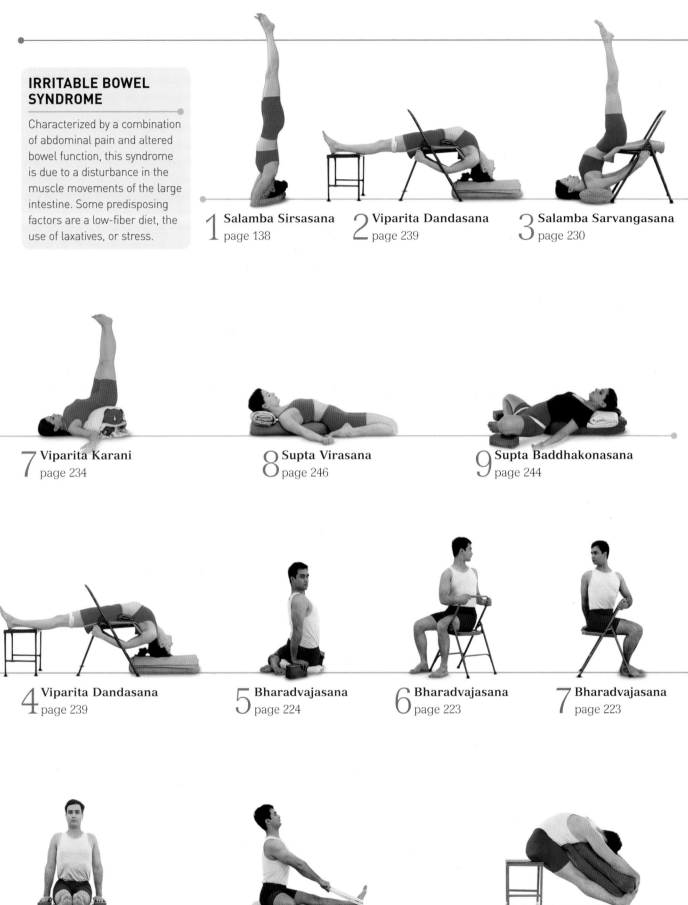

IRRITABLE BOWEL SYNDROME

Characterized by a combination of abdominal pain and altered bowel function, this syndrome is due to a disturbance in the muscle movements of the large intestine. Some predisposing factors are a low-fiber diet, the use of laxatives, or stress.

1 **Salamba Sirsasana** page 138

2 **Viparita Dandasana** page 239

3 **Salamba Sarvangasana** page 230

7 **Viparita Karani** page 234

8 **Supta Virasana** page 246

9 **Supta Baddhakonasana** page 244

4 **Viparita Dandasana** page 239

5 **Bharadvajasana** page 224

6 **Bharadvajasana** page 223

7 **Bharadvajasana** page 223

12 **Dandasana** page 205

13 **Urdhvamukha Janu Sirsasana** page 207

14 **Adhomukha Paschimottanasana** page 217

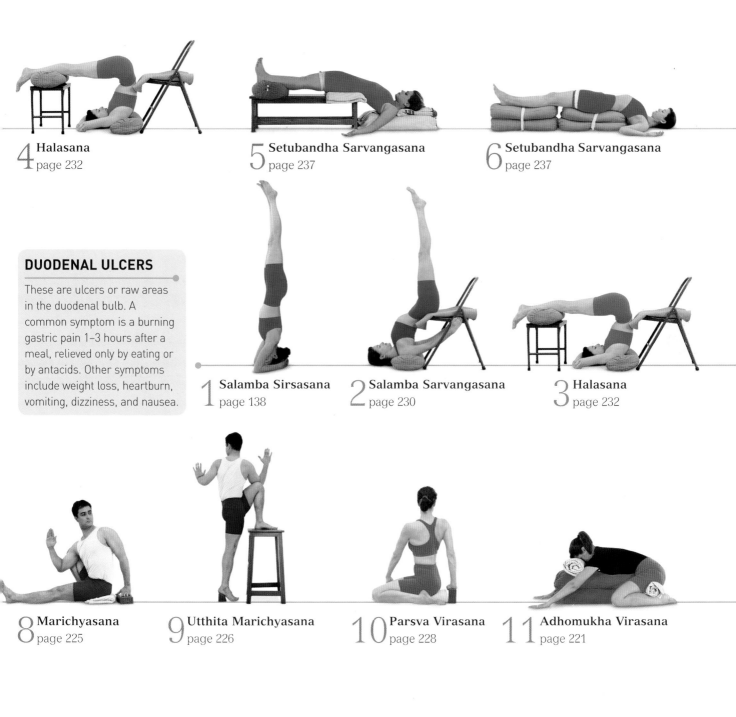

4 **Halasana**
page 232

5 **Setubandha Sarvangasana**
page 237

6 **Setubandha Sarvangasana**
page 237

DUODENAL ULCERS

These are ulcers or raw areas in the duodenal bulb. A common symptom is a burning gastric pain 1–3 hours after a meal, relieved only by eating or by antacids. Other symptoms include weight loss, heartburn, vomiting, dizziness, and nausea.

1 **Salamba Sirsasana**
page 138

2 **Salamba Sarvangasana**
page 230

3 **Halasana**
page 232

8 **Marichyasana**
page 225

9 **Utthita Marichyasana**
page 226

10 **Parsva Virasana**
page 228

11 **Adhomukha Virasana**
page 221

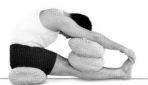

15 **Paschimottanasana**
page 215

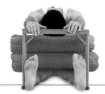

16 **Paschimottanasana**
page 216

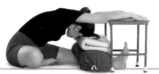

17 **Janu Sirsasana**
page 218

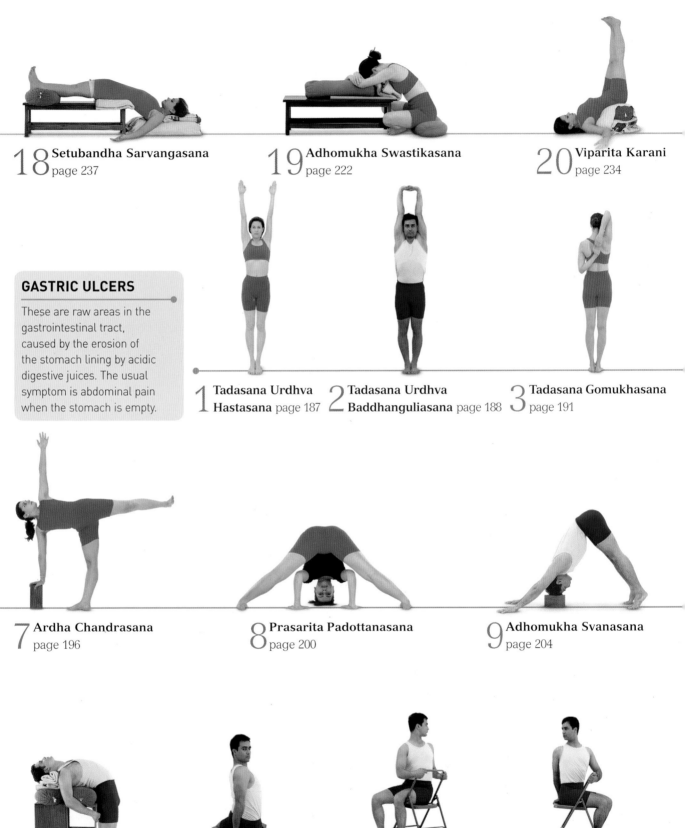

18 **Setubandha Sarvangasana** page 237

19 **Adhomukha Swastikasana** page 222

20 **Viparita Karani** page 234

GASTRIC ULCERS

These are raw areas in the gastrointestinal tract, caused by the erosion of the stomach lining by acidic digestive juices. The usual symptom is abdominal pain when the stomach is empty.

1 **Tadasana Urdhva Hastasana** page 187

2 **Tadasana Urdhva Baddhanguliasana** page 188

3 **Tadasana Gomukhasana** page 191

7 **Ardha Chandrasana** page 196

8 **Prasarita Padottanasana** page 200

9 **Adhomukha Svanasana** page 204

13 **Ustrasana** page 240

14 **Bharadvajasana** page 224

15 **Bharadvajasana** page 223

16 **Bharadvajasana** page 223

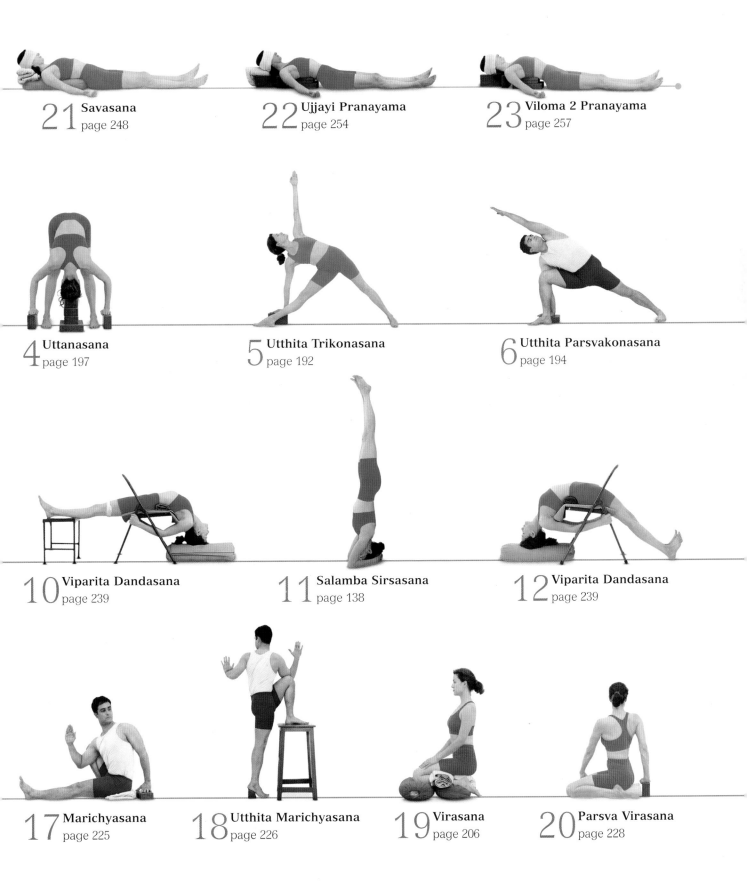

21 **Savasana** page 248

22 **Ujjayi Pranayama** page 254

23 **Viloma 2 Pranayama** page 257

4 **Uttanasana** page 197

5 **Utthita Trikonasana** page 192

6 **Utthita Parsvakonasana** page 194

10 **Viparita Dandasana** page 239

11 **Salamba Sirsasana** page 138

12 **Viparita Dandasana** page 239

17 **Marichyasana** page 225

18 **Utthita Marichyasana** page 226

19 **Virasana** page 206

20 **Parsva Virasana** page 228

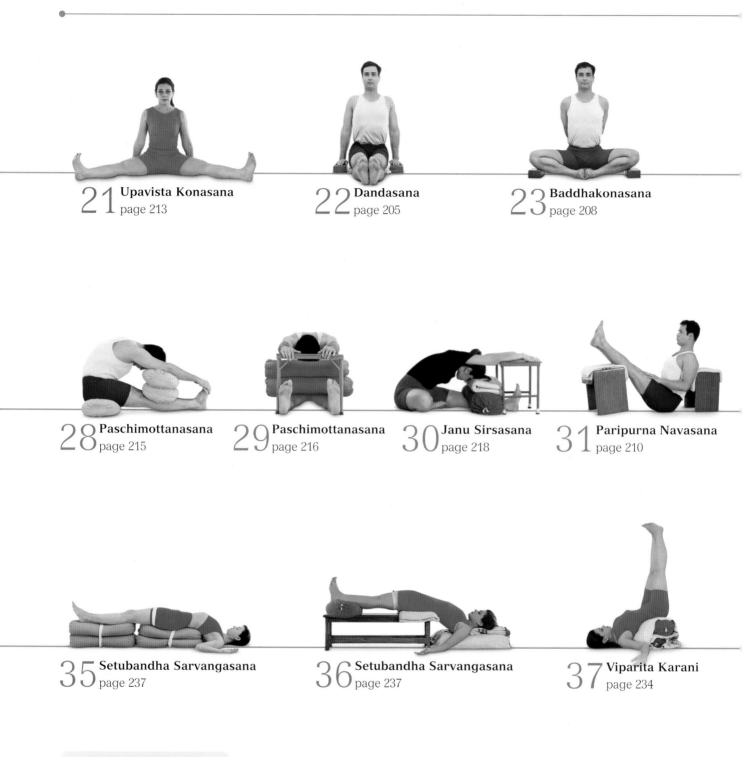

21 **Upavista Konasana**
page 213

22 **Dandasana**
page 205

23 **Baddhakonasana**
page 208

28 **Paschimottanasana**
page 215

29 **Paschimottanasana**
page 216

30 **Janu Sirsasana**
page 218

31 **Paripurna Navasana**
page 210

35 **Setubandha Sarvangasana**
page 237

36 **Setubandha Sarvangasana**
page 237

37 **Viparita Karani**
page 234

ULCERATIVE COLITIS

This condition is caused by the inflammation of the colon and rectum. The common symptoms include diarrhea with blood in the stools, abdominal pain or cramps, and rectal bleeding. Attacks can be frequent or can occur after long intervals.

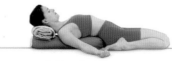

1 **Supta Virasana**
page 246

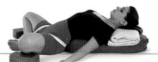

2 **Supta Baddhakonasana**
page 244

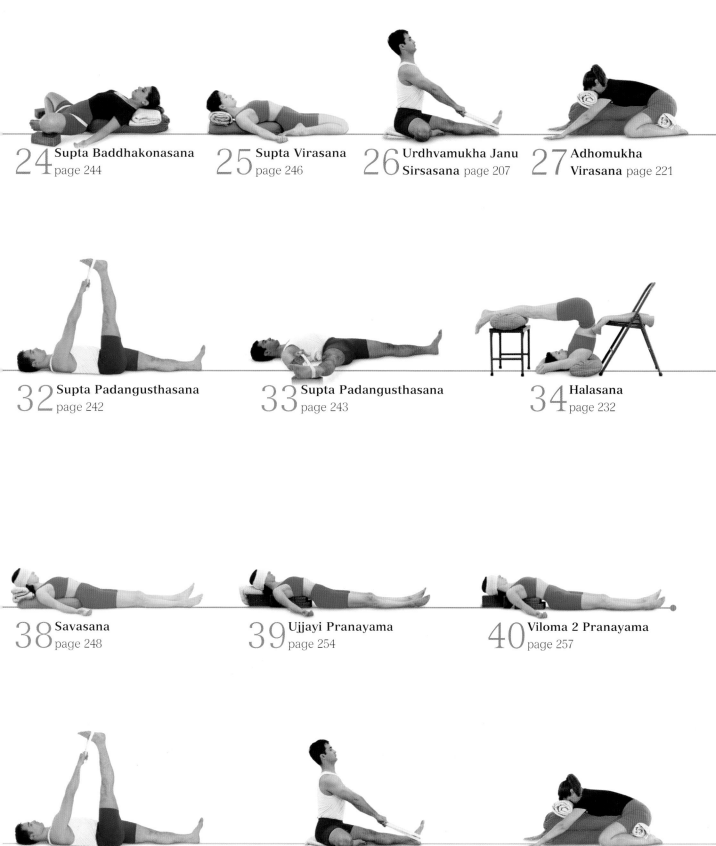

24 **Supta Baddhakonasana** page 244

25 **Supta Virasana** page 246

26 **Urdhvamukha Janu Sirsasana** page 207

27 **Adhomukha Virasana** page 221

32 **Supta Padangusthasana** page 242

33 **Supta Padangusthasana** page 243

34 **Halasana** page 232

38 **Savasana** page 248

39 **Ujjayi Pranayama** page 254

40 **Viloma 2 Pranayama** page 257

3 **Supta Padangusthasana** page 242

4 **Urdhvamukha Janu Sirsasana** page 207

5 **Adhomukha Virasana** page 221

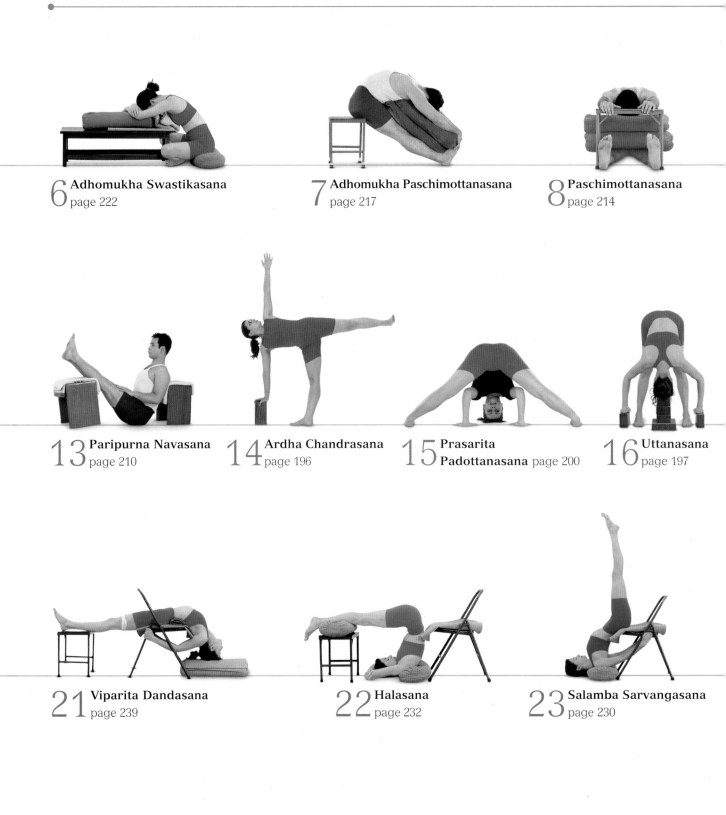

6 **Adhomukha Swastikasana** page 222

7 **Adhomukha Paschimottanasana** page 217

8 **Paschimottanasana** page 214

13 **Paripurna Navasana** page 210

14 **Ardha Chandrasana** page 196

15 **Prasarita Padottanasana** page 200

16 **Uttanasana** page 197

21 **Viparita Dandasana** page 239

22 **Halasana** page 232

23 **Salamba Sarvangasana** page 230

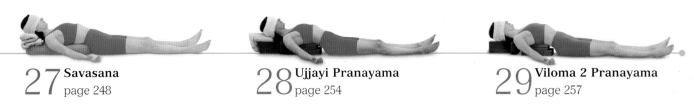

27 **Savasana** page 248

28 **Ujjayi Pranayama** page 254

29 **Viloma 2 Pranayama** page 257

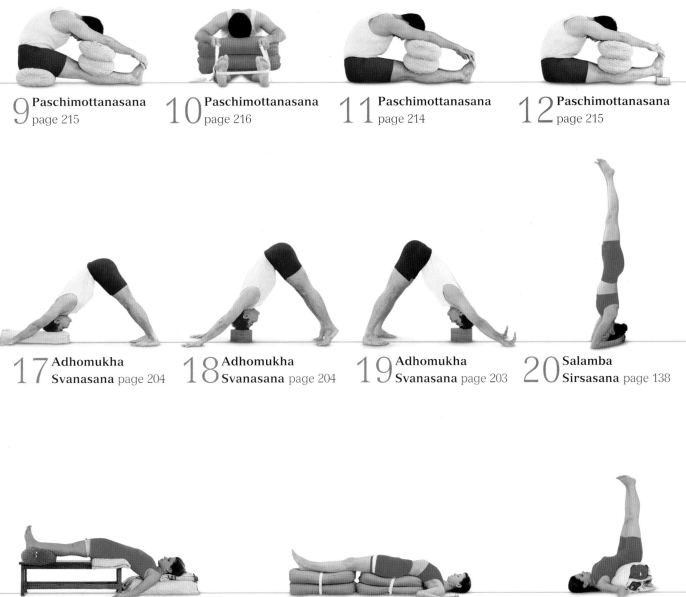

9 **Paschimottanasana** page 215

10 **Paschimottanasana** page 216

11 **Paschimottanasana** page 214

12 **Paschimottanasana** page 215

17 **Adhomukha Svanasana** page 204

18 **Adhomukha Svanasana** page 204

19 **Adhomukha Svanasana** page 203

20 **Salamba Sirsasana** page 138

24 **Setubandha Sarvangasana** page 237

25 **Setubandha Sarvangasana** page 237

26 **Viparita Karani** page 234

"When stability becomes a habit, maturity and clarity follow."

URINARY SYSTEM

This system comprises the kidneys, ureters, bladder, and the urethra. The kidneys manufacture urine, which consists of water and the waste products of metabolism, such as protein. Urine is excreted from the body, enabling the kidneys to maintain the body's electrolyte and acid base balance. The ureters transport urine to the bladder, while the urethra is the canal for the passage of urine to the exterior. Yoga asanas help treat many common urinary disorders.

INCONTINENCE

This is the involuntary loss of urine from the bladder. The condition becomes more common with age. The causes include weakening of the pelvic floor muscles, strokes, bladder irritation, and loss of control in the central nervous system.

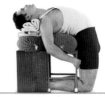

1 Uttanasana
page 197

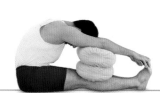

2 Prasarita Padottanasana
page 200

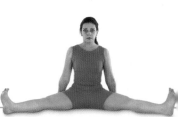

3 Adhomukha Svanasana
page 204

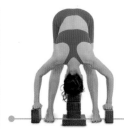

8 Viparita Dandasana
page 239

9 Ustrasana
page 240

10 Paschimottanasana
page 214

11 Upavista Konasana
page 213

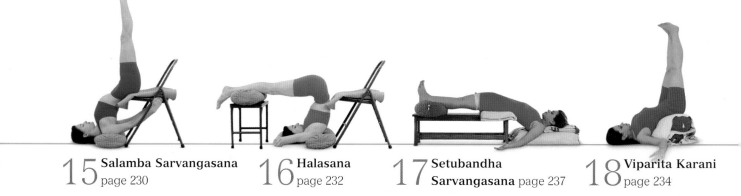

15 Salamba Sarvangasana
page 230

16 Halasana
page 232

17 Setubandha Sarvangasana page 237

18 Viparita Karani
page 234

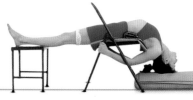

"Intensified action in yoga brings intensified intelligence."

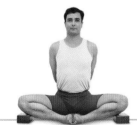

4 **Urdhvamukha Janu Sirsasana** page 207

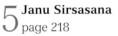
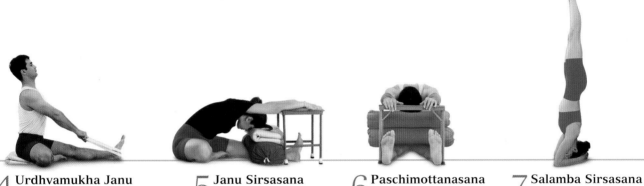

5 **Janu Sirsasana** page 218

6 **Paschimottanasana** page 216

7 **Salamba Sirsasana** page 138

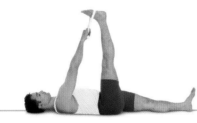

12 **Baddhakonasana** page 208

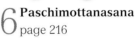

13 **Supta Padangusthasana** page 242

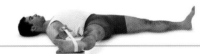

14 **Supta Padangusthasana** page 243

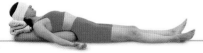

19 **Savasana** page 248

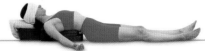

20 **Ujjayi Pranayama** page 254

21 **Viloma 2 Pranayama** page 257

HORMONAL SYSTEM

Hormones are natural chemical substances which control certain major functions of the body. Hormones are secreted by glands, which include the thyroid, parathyroid, pituitary, pineal, and adrenal glands, the testes and the ovaries, as well as the islets of Langerhans in the pancreas. Regular practice of the recommended asanas helps to ensure an effective secretion of hormones into the bloodstream.

OBESITY

This is a condition of excess body fat that is 20 percent greater than the individual's desired weight. Obesity is often caused by Cushing's syndrome, hypothalamic disorders, genetic factors, taking corticosteroid drugs, excess calorie intake, or lack of exercise.

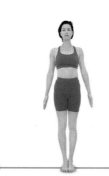

1 **Tadasana Samasthithi** page 186

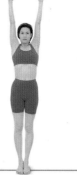

2 **Tadasana Urdhva Hastasana** page 187

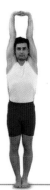

3 **Tadasana Urdhva Baddhanguliasana** page 188

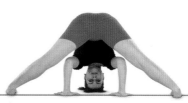

8 **Ardha Chandrasana** page 196

9 **Prasarita Padottanasana** page 200

10 **Adhomukha Svanasana** page 202

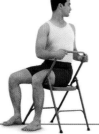

15 **Bharadvajasana** page 223

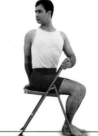

16 **Bharadvajasana** page 223

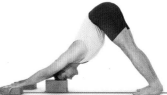

17 **Virasana** page 206

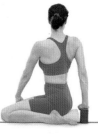

18 **Parsva Virasana** page 228

"Yoga is a mirror, to look at ourselves from within."

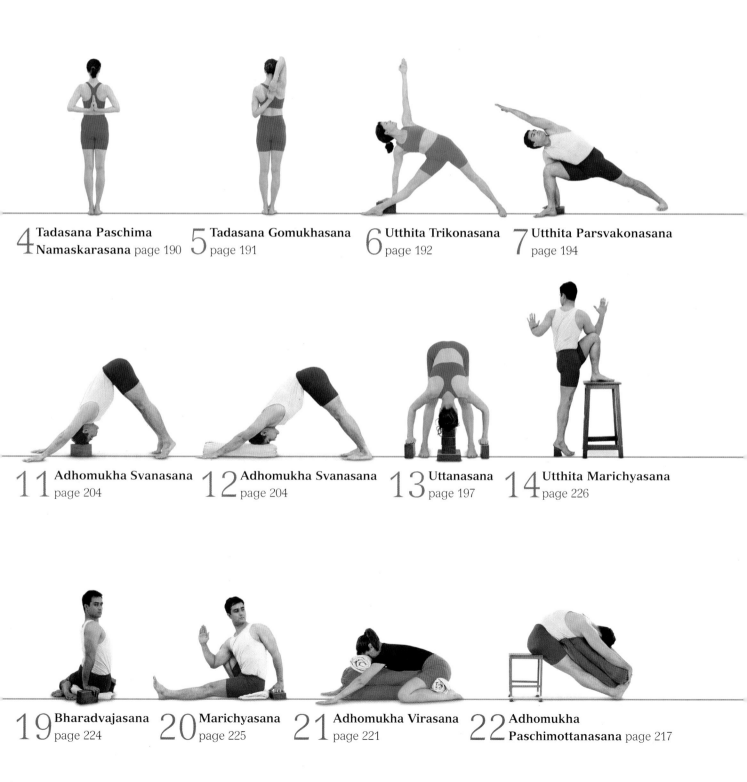

4 **Tadasana Paschima Namaskarasana** page 190

5 **Tadasana Gomukhasana** page 191

6 **Utthita Trikonasana** page 192

7 **Utthita Parsvakonasana** page 194

11 **Adhomukha Svanasana** page 204

12 **Adhomukha Svanasana** page 204

13 **Uttanasana** page 197

14 **Utthita Marichyasana** page 226

19 **Bharadvajasana** page 224

20 **Marichyasana** page 225

21 **Adhomukha Virasana** page 221

22 **Adhomukha Paschimottanasana** page 217

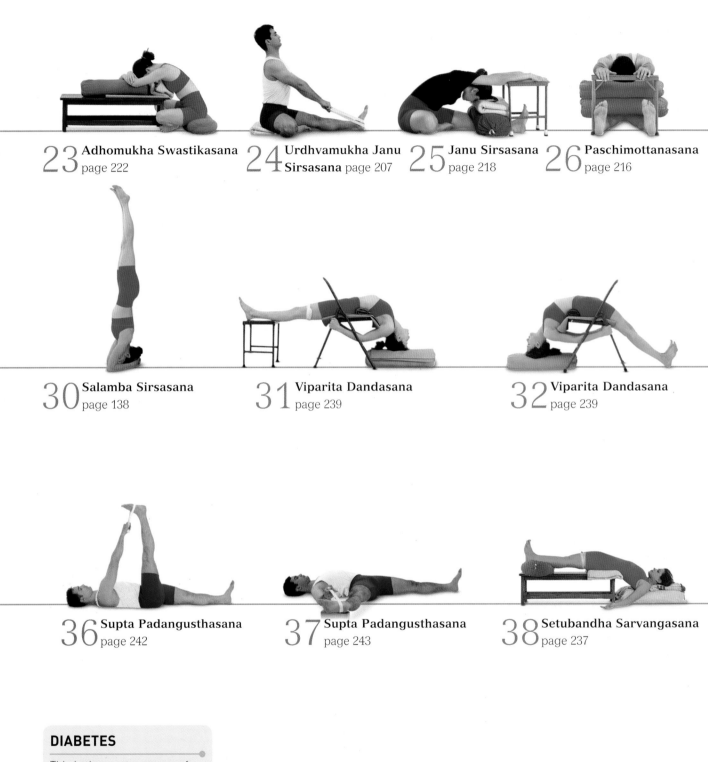

23 **Adhomukha Swastikasana** page 222

24 **Urdhvamukha Janu Sirsasana** page 207

25 **Janu Sirsasana** page 218

26 **Paschimottanasana** page 216

30 **Salamba Sirsasana** page 138

31 **Viparita Dandasana** page 239

32 **Viparita Dandasana** page 239

36 **Supta Padangusthasana** page 242

37 **Supta Padangusthasana** page 243

38 **Setubandha Sarvangasana** page 237

DIABETES

This is the most common of all metabolic disorders. Its symptoms include frequent thirst and urination, excessive hunger, weight loss, and nausea. The condition is caused by insufficient insulin production in the pancreas.

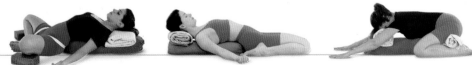

1 **Supta Baddhakonasana** page 244

2 **Supta Virasana** page 246

3 **Adhomukha Virasana** page 220

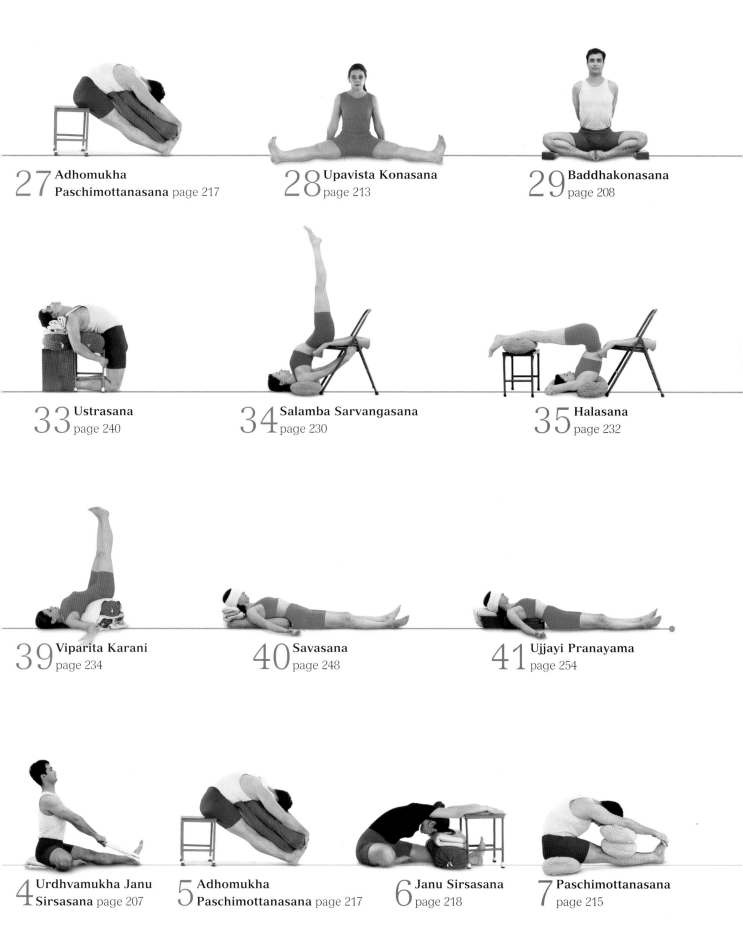

27 **Adhomukha Paschimottanasana** page 217

28 **Upavista Konasana** page 213

29 **Baddhakonasana** page 208

33 **Ustrasana** page 240

34 **Salamba Sarvangasana** page 230

35 **Halasana** page 232

39 **Viparita Karani** page 234

40 **Savasana** page 248

41 **Ujjayi Pranayama** page 254

4 **Urdhvamukha Janu Sirsasana** page 207

5 **Adhomukha Paschimottanasana** page 217

6 **Janu Sirsasana** page 218

7 **Paschimottanasana** page 215

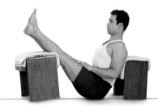

8 **Paripurna Navasana**
page 210

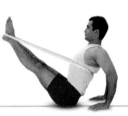

9 **Paripurna Navasana**
page 212

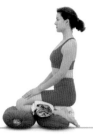

10 **Virasana**
page 206

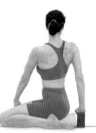

11 **Parsva Virasana**
page 228

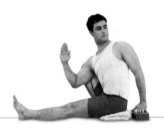

16 **Marichyasana**
page 225

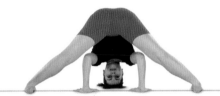

17 **Prasarita Padottanasana**
page 200

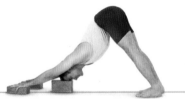

18 **Adhomukha Svanasana**
page 202

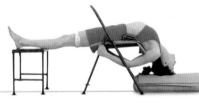

23 **Viparita Dandasana**
page 239

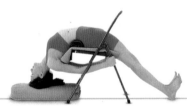

24 **Viparita Dandasana**
page 239

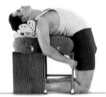

25 **Ustrasana**
page 240

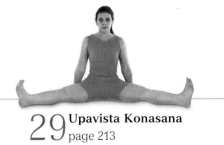

29 **Upavista Konasana**
page 213

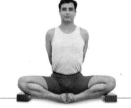

30 **Baddhakonasana**
page 208

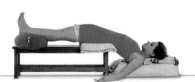

31 **Setubandha Sarvangasana**
page 237

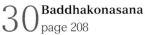

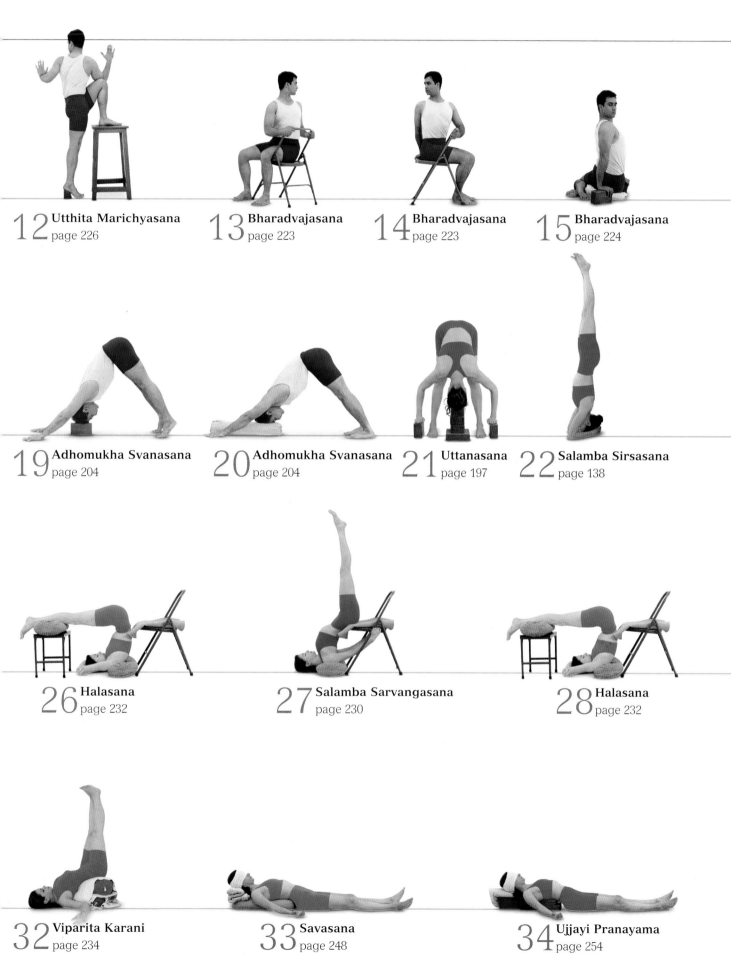

12 Utthita Marichyasana
page 226

13 Bharadvajasana
page 223

14 Bharadvajasana
page 223

15 Bharadvajasana
page 224

19 Adhomukha Svanasana
page 204

20 Adhomukha Svanasana
page 204

21 Uttanasana
page 197

22 Salamba Sirsasana
page 138

26 Halasana
page 232

27 Salamba Sarvangasana
page 230

28 Halasana
page 232

32 Viparita Karani
page 234

33 Savasana
page 248

34 Ujjayi Pranayama
page 254

IMMUNE SYSTEM

The immune system is the defense mechanism of the body and protects us from disease. Its main agent is the blood, a fluid consisting of plasma and red and white corpuscles or blood cells. It is the white corpuscles that inhibit the invasion of the bloodstream by microorganisms. There are two types of immunity: natural and acquired. Yoga strengthens both, and regular practice of the recommended asanas can help to counter the disorders that affect them.

LOW IMMUNE SYSTEM

In this condition, the body's immunity is impaired, resulting in a wide spectrum of illnesses. The symptoms include weight loss, increased susceptibility to infections, fatigue, fevers, and malignant disorders.

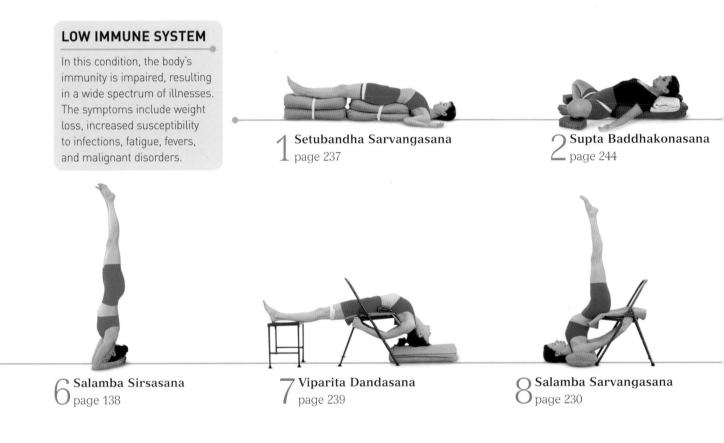

1 **Setubandha Sarvangasana**
page 237

2 **Supta Baddhakonasana**
page 244

6 **Salamba Sirsasana**
page 138

7 **Viparita Dandasana**
page 239

8 **Salamba Sarvangasana**
page 230

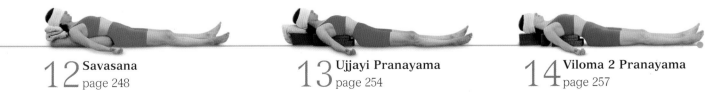

12 **Savasana**
page 248

13 **Ujjayi Pranayama**
page 254

14 **Viloma 2 Pranayama**
page 257

"Your whole body should be symmetrical. Yoga is symmetry."

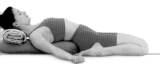

3 **Supta Virasana**
page 246

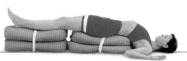

4 **Setubandha Sarvangasana**
page 237

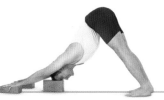

5 **Adhomukha Svanasana**
page 202

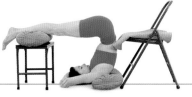

9 **Halasana**
page 232

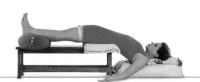

10 **Setubandha Sarvangasana**
page 237

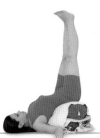

11 **Viparita Karani**
page 234

AIDS

Acquired Immune Deficiency Syndrome, or AIDS, is caused by the Human Immunodeficiency Virus (HIV) which attacks the immune system, and leaves the human body vulnerable to many life-threatening diseases. The following sequence of asanas may help alleviate some of the symptoms of the condition.

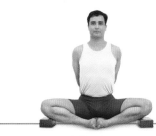

1 **Baddhakonasana**
page 208

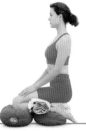

2 **Virasana**
page 206

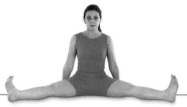

3 **Upavista Konasana**
page 213

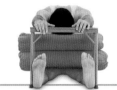

4 **Paschimottanasana**
page 216

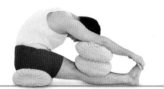

5 **Paschimottanasana**
page 215

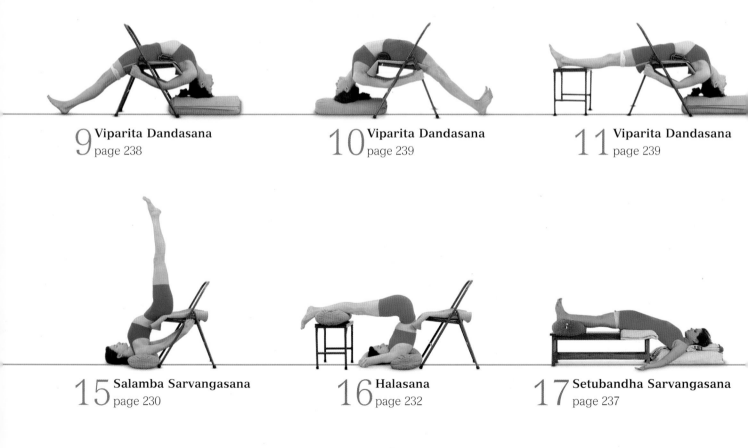

9 **Viparita Dandasana**
page 238

10 **Viparita Dandasana**
page 239

11 **Viparita Dandasana**
page 239

15 **Salamba Sarvangasana**
page 230

16 **Halasana**
page 232

17 **Setubandha Sarvangasana**
page 237

"Yoga is for all of us. To limit yoga to national or cultural boundaries is the denial of universal consciousness."

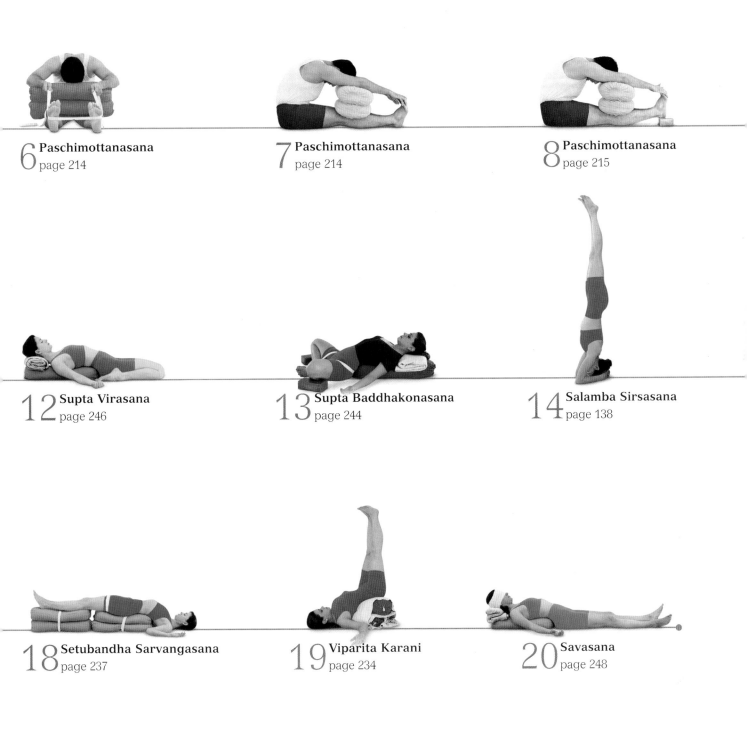

6 **Paschimottanasana**
page 214

7 **Paschimottanasana**
page 214

8 **Paschimottanasana**
page 215

12 **Supta Virasana**
page 246

13 **Supta Baddhakonasana**
page 244

14 **Salamba Sirsasana**
page 138

18 **Setubandha Sarvangasana**
page 237

19 **Viparita Karani**
page 234

20 **Savasana**
page 248

MUSCLES, BONES, AND JOINTS

The human body is composed of bone and muscle. The bones that make up the skeletal frame of the body are attached to each other by joints, which are held in place by strong ligaments and muscles. A muscle contracts or relaxes to move the bones connected to it. Better muscle function means a fitter, stronger body. Practicing yoga strengthens the bones, improves coordination of the muscles, and provides a noninvasive way of treating ailments that affect both.

PHYSICAL FATIGUE

Stressful physical exertion brings on this condition, characterized by exhaustion and a reluctance to exert oneself. If unrelieved by rest, and the removal of stress factors, the condition may lead to chronic fatigue syndrome.

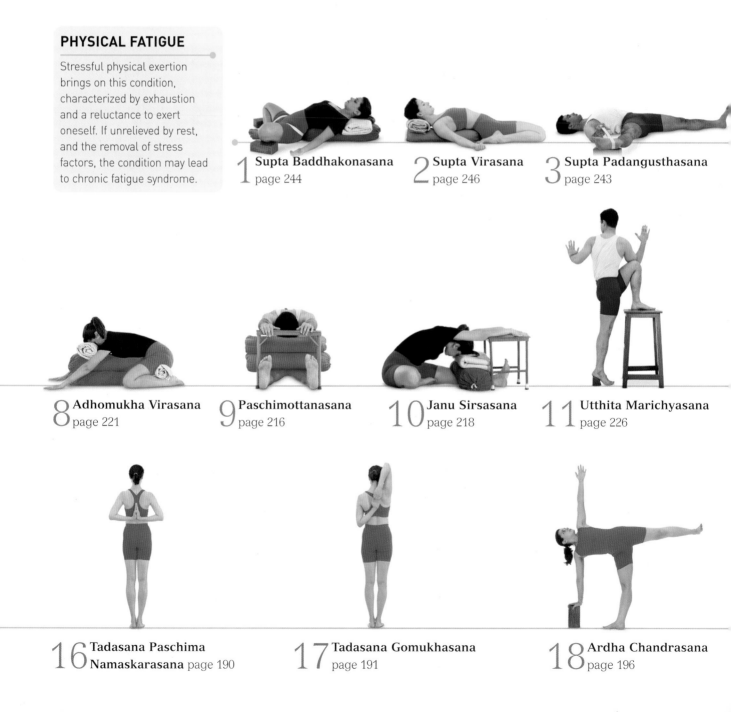

1 **Supta Baddhakonasana** page 244

2 **Supta Virasana** page 246

3 **Supta Padangusthasana** page 243

8 **Adhomukha Virasana** page 221

9 **Paschimottanasana** page 216

10 **Janu Sirsasana** page 218

11 **Utthita Marichyasana** page 226

16 **Tadasana Paschima Namaskarasana** page 190

17 **Tadasana Gomukhasana** page 191

18 **Ardha Chandrasana** page 196

*"Freedom with discipline
is true freedom."*

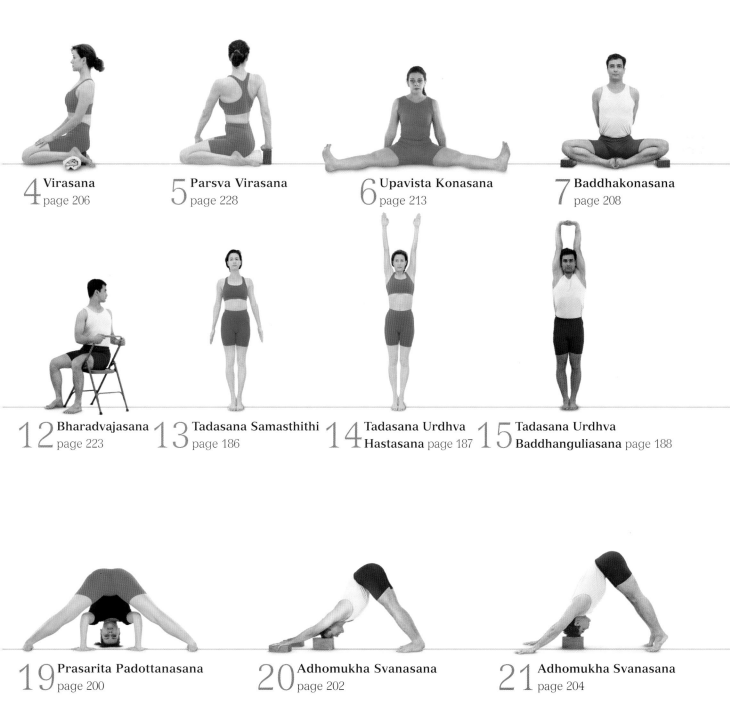

4 **Virasana**
page 206

5 **Parsva Virasana**
page 228

6 **Upavista Konasana**
page 213

7 **Baddhakonasana**
page 208

12 **Bharadvajasana**
page 223

13 **Tadasana Samasthithi**
page 186

14 **Tadasana Urdhva
Hastasana** page 187

15 **Tadasana Urdhva
Baddhanguliasana** page 188

19 **Prasarita Padottanasana**
page 200

20 **Adhomukha Svanasana**
page 202

21 **Adhomukha Svanasana**
page 204

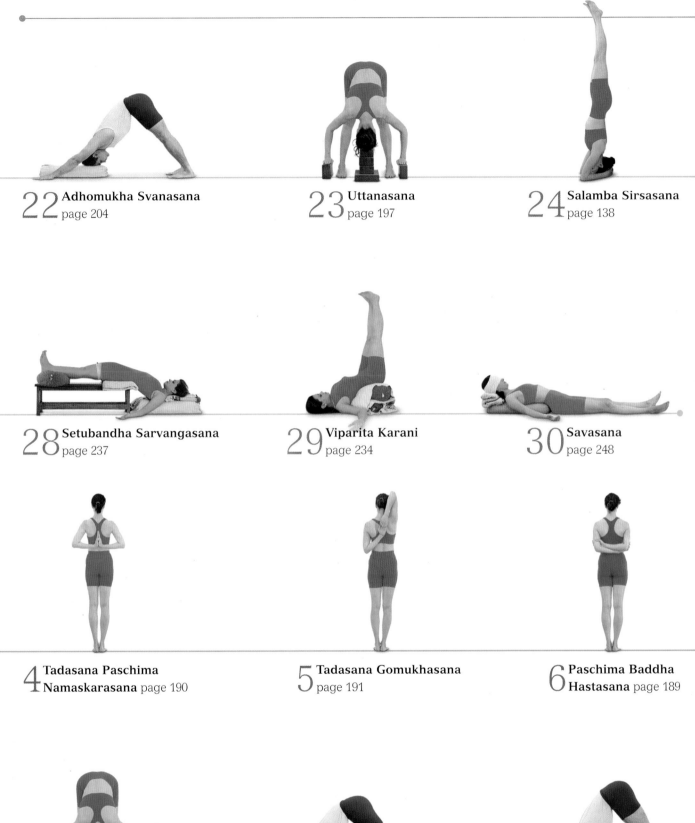

22 Adhomukha Svanasana
page 204

23 Uttanasana
page 197

24 Salamba Sirsasana
page 138

28 Setubandha Sarvangasana
page 237

29 Viparita Karani
page 234

30 Savasana
page 248

4 Tadasana Paschima
Namaskarasana page 190

5 Tadasana Gomukhasana
page 191

6 Paschima Baddha
Hastasana page 189

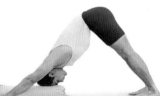

11 Uttanasana
page 197

12 Adhomukha Svanasana
page 204

13 Adhomukha Svanasana
page 204

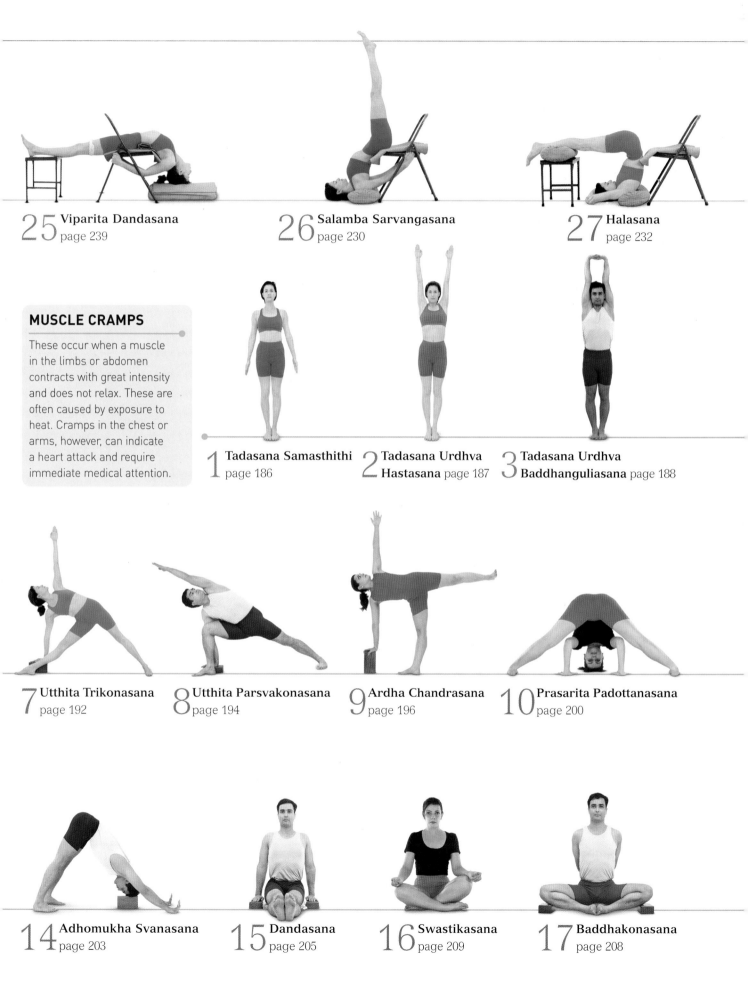

25 **Viparita Dandasana** page 239

26 **Salamba Sarvangasana** page 230

27 **Halasana** page 232

MUSCLE CRAMPS

These occur when a muscle in the limbs or abdomen contracts with great intensity and does not relax. These are often caused by exposure to heat. Cramps in the chest or arms, however, can indicate a heart attack and require immediate medical attention.

1 **Tadasana Samasthithi** page 186

2 **Tadasana Urdhva Hastasana** page 187

3 **Tadasana Urdhva Baddhanguliasana** page 188

7 **Utthita Trikonasana** page 192

8 **Utthita Parsvakonasana** page 194

9 **Ardha Chandrasana** page 196

10 **Prasarita Padottanasana** page 200

14 **Adhomukha Svanasana** page 203

15 **Dandasana** page 205

16 **Swastikasana** page 209

17 **Baddhakonasana** page 208

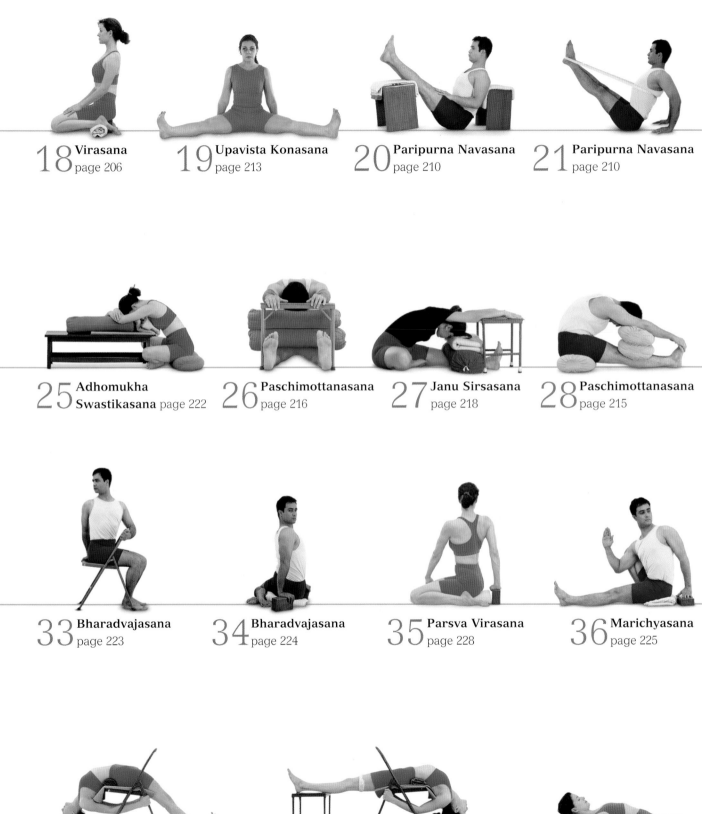

18 **Virasana** page 206

19 **Upavista Konasana** page 213

20 **Paripurna Navasana** page 210

21 **Paripurna Navasana** page 210

25 **Adhomukha Swastikasana** page 222

26 **Paschimottanasana** page 216

27 **Janu Sirsasana** page 218

28 **Paschimottanasana** page 215

33 **Bharadvajasana** page 223

34 **Bharadvajasana** page 224

35 **Parsva Virasana** page 228

36 **Marichyasana** page 225

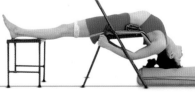

40 **Viparita Dandasana** page 239

41 **Viparita Dandasana** page 239

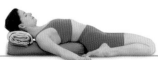

42 **Supta Virasana** page 246

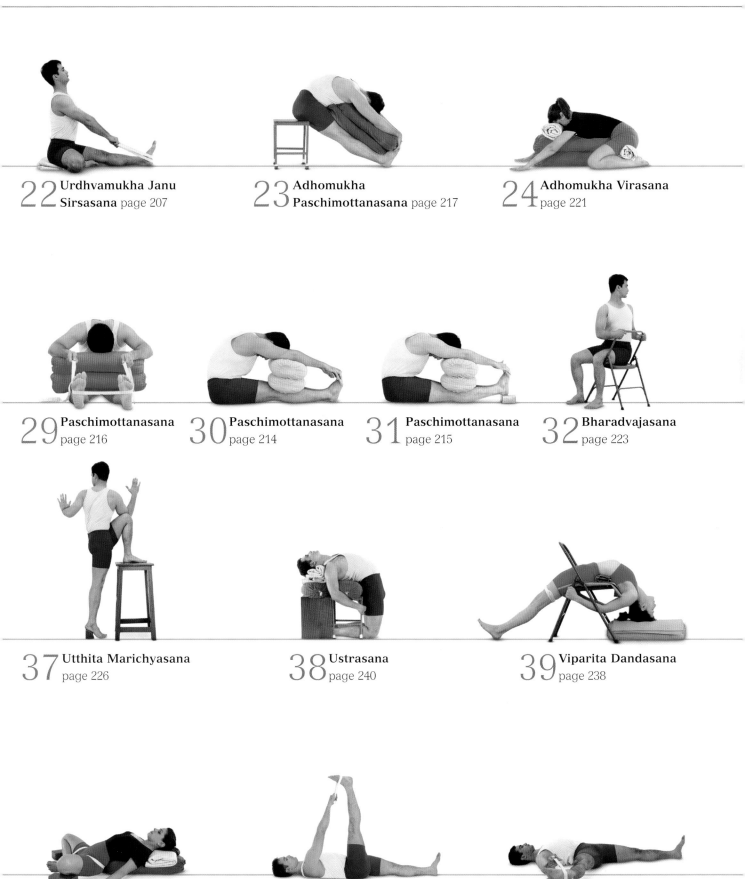

22 **Urdhvamukha Janu Sirsasana** page 207

23 **Adhomukha Paschimottanasana** page 217

24 **Adhomukha Virasana** page 221

29 **Paschimottanasana** page 216

30 **Paschimottanasana** page 214

31 **Paschimottanasana** page 215

32 **Bharadvajasana** page 223

37 **Utthita Marichyasana** page 226

38 **Ustrasana** page 240

39 **Viparita Dandasana** page 238

43 **Supta Baddhakonasana** page 244

44 **Supta Padangusthasana** page 242

45 **Supta Padangusthasana** page 243

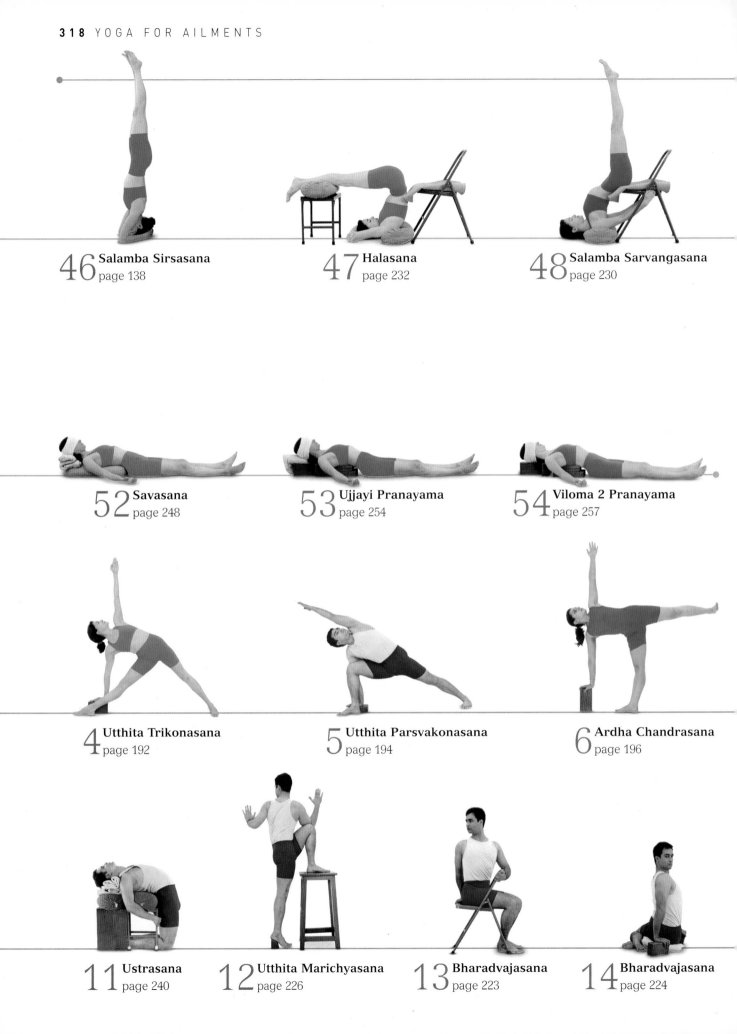

46 **Salamba Sirsasana**
page 138

47 **Halasana**
page 232

48 **Salamba Sarvangasana**
page 230

52 **Savasana**
page 248

53 **Ujjayi Pranayama**
page 254

54 **Viloma 2 Pranayama**
page 257

4 **Utthita Trikonasana**
page 192

5 **Utthita Parsvakonasana**
page 194

6 **Ardha Chandrasana**
page 196

11 **Ustrasana**
page 240

12 **Utthita Marichyasana**
page 226

13 **Bharadvajasana**
page 223

14 **Bharadvajasana**
page 224

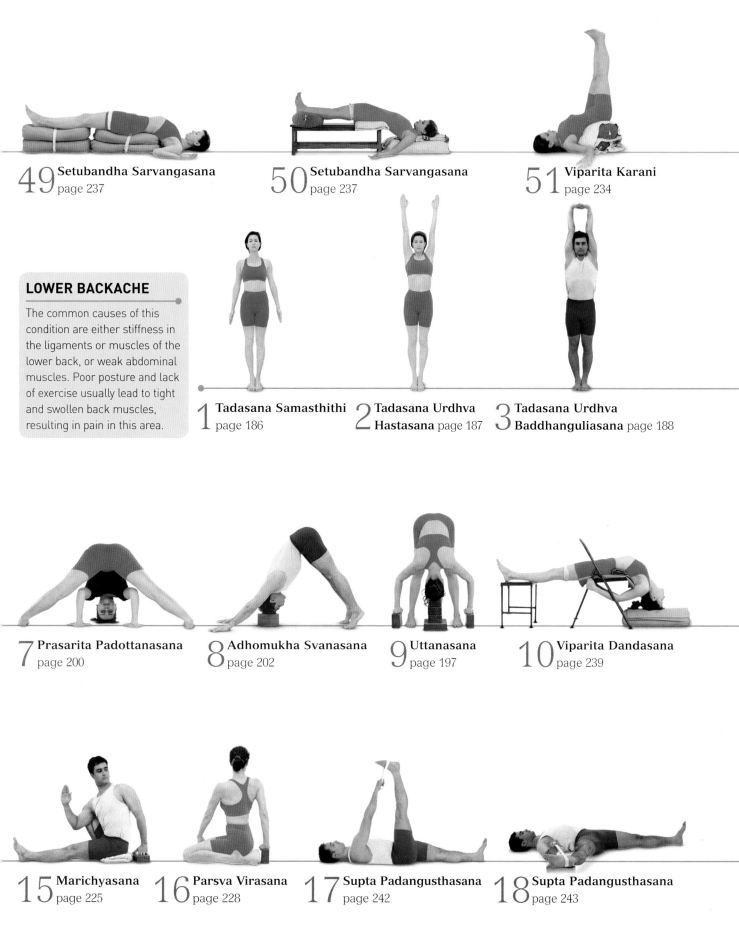

49 Setubandha Sarvangasana
page 237

50 Setubandha Sarvangasana
page 237

51 Viparita Karani
page 234

LOWER BACKACHE

The common causes of this condition are either stiffness in the ligaments or muscles of the lower back, or weak abdominal muscles. Poor posture and lack of exercise usually lead to tight and swollen back muscles, resulting in pain in this area.

1 Tadasana Samasthithi
page 186

2 Tadasana Urdhva
Hastasana page 187

3 Tadasana Urdhva
Baddhanguliasana page 188

7 Prasarita Padottanasana
page 200

8 Adhomukha Svanasana
page 202

9 Uttanasana
page 197

10 Viparita Dandasana
page 239

15 Marichyasana
page 225

16 Parsva Virasana
page 228

17 Supta Padangusthasana
page 242

18 Supta Padangusthasana
page 243

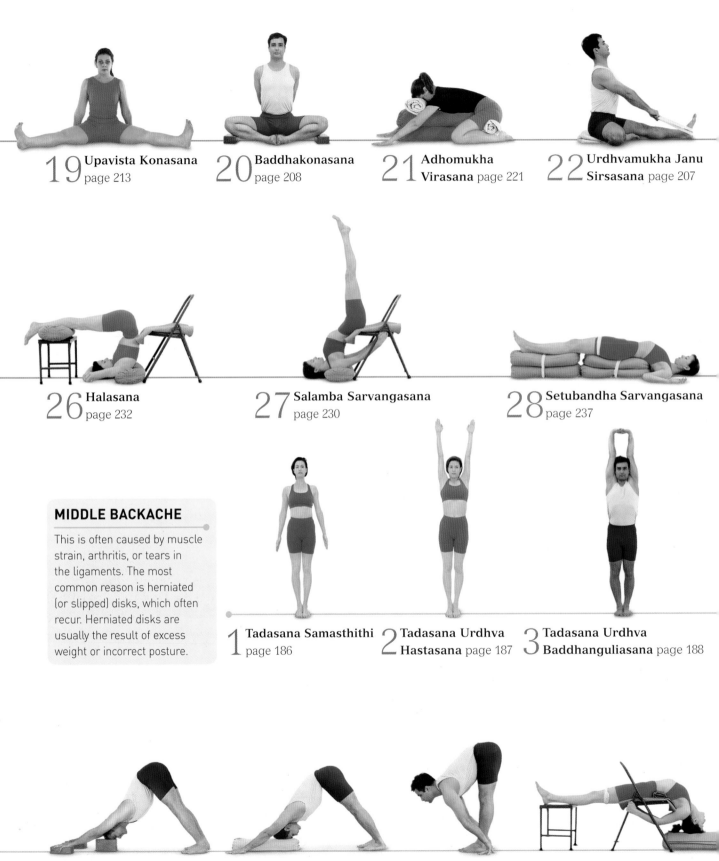

19 **Upavista Konasana**
page 213

20 **Baddhakonasana**
page 208

21 **Adhomukha
Virasana** page 221

22 **Urdhvamukha Janu
Sirsasana** page 207

26 **Halasana**
page 232

27 **Salamba Sarvangasana**
page 230

28 **Setubandha Sarvangasana**
page 237

MIDDLE BACKACHE

This is often caused by muscle strain, arthritis, or tears in the ligaments. The most common reason is herniated (or slipped) disks, which often recur. Herniated disks are usually the result of excess weight or incorrect posture.

1 **Tadasana Samasthithi**
page 186

2 **Tadasana Urdhva
Hastasana** page 187

3 **Tadasana Urdhva
Baddhanguliasana** page 188

8 **Adhomukha Svanasana**
page 202

9 **Adhomukha Svanasana**
page 204

10 **Uttanasana**
page 92

11 **Viparita Dandasana**
page 239

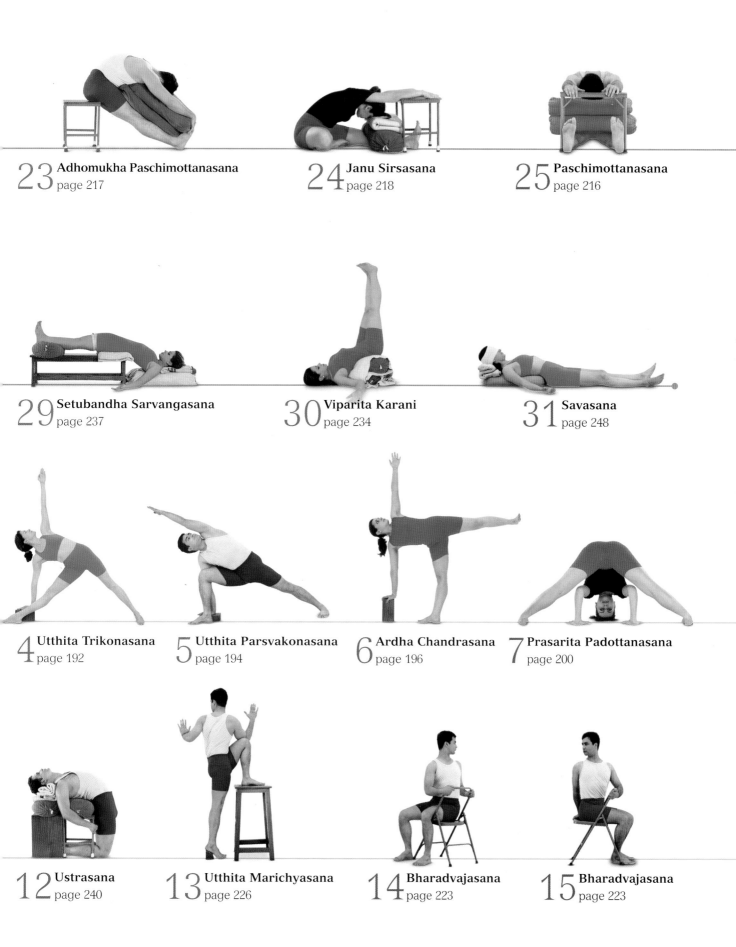

23 **Adhomukha Paschimottanasana**
page 217

24 **Janu Sirsasana**
page 218

25 **Paschimottanasana**
page 216

29 **Setubandha Sarvangasana**
page 237

30 **Viparita Karani**
page 234

31 **Savasana**
page 248

4 **Utthita Trikonasana**
page 192

5 **Utthita Parsvakonasana**
page 194

6 **Ardha Chandrasana**
page 196

7 **Prasarita Padottanasana**
page 200

12 **Ustrasana**
page 240

13 **Utthita Marichyasana**
page 226

14 **Bharadvajasana**
page 223

15 **Bharadvajasana**
page 223

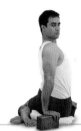

16 **Bharadvajasana**
page 224

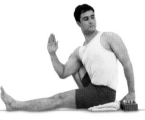

17 **Marichyasana**
page 225

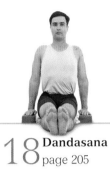

18 **Dandasana**
page 205

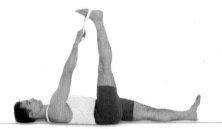

22 **Supta Padangusthasana**
page 242

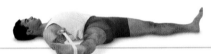

23 **Supta Padangusthasana**
page 243

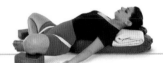

24 **Supta Baddhakonasana**
page 244

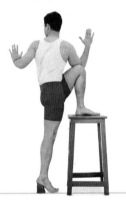

28 **Utthita Marichyasana**
page 226

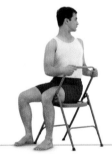

29 **Bharadvajasana**
page 223

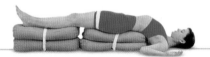

30 **Setubandha Sarvangasana**
page 237

UPPER BACKACHE

Muscle deterioration and pain in the upper back may result from a sedentary lifestyle, excess weight, or a weakening of muscle tone. Other causes include the fusing of vertebrae or the inflammation of muscles and tendons.

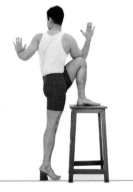

1 **Utthita Marichyasana**
page 226

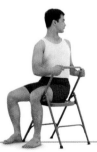

2 **Bharadvajasana**
page 223

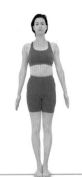

3 **Tadasana Samasthithi**
page 186

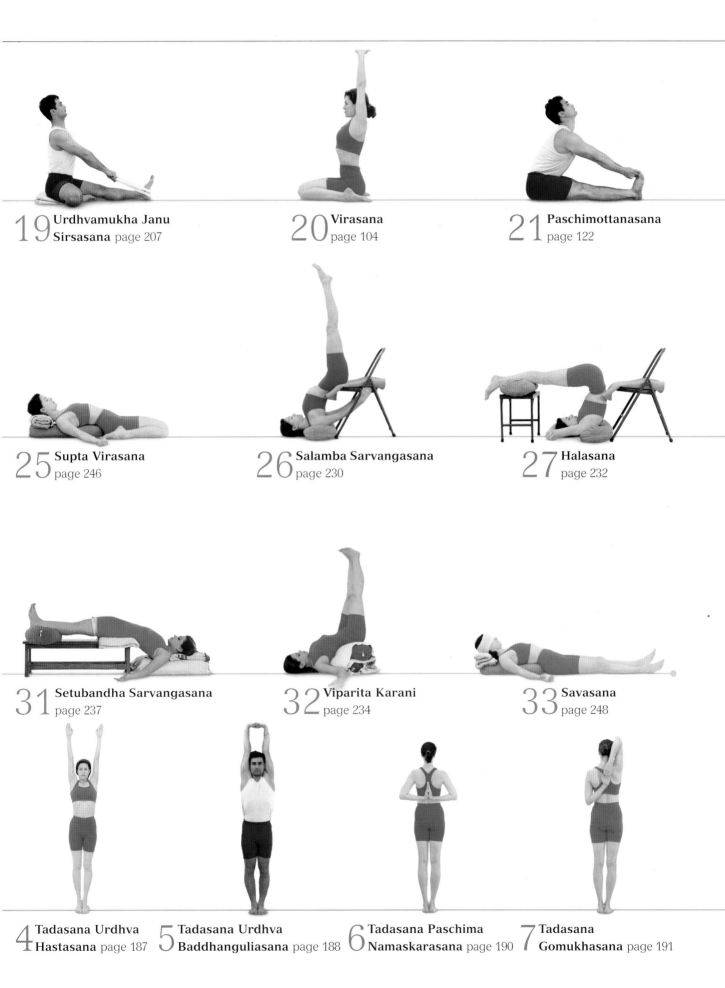

19 **Urdhvamukha Janu Sirsasana** page 207

20 **Virasana** page 104

21 **Paschimottanasana** page 122

25 **Supta Virasana** page 246

26 **Salamba Sarvangasana** page 230

27 **Halasana** page 232

31 **Setubandha Sarvangasana** page 237

32 **Viparita Karani** page 234

33 **Savasana** page 248

4 **Tadasana Urdhva Hastasana** page 187

5 **Tadasana Urdhva Baddhanguliasana** page 188

6 **Tadasana Paschima Namaskarasana** page 190

7 **Tadasana Gomukhasana** page 191

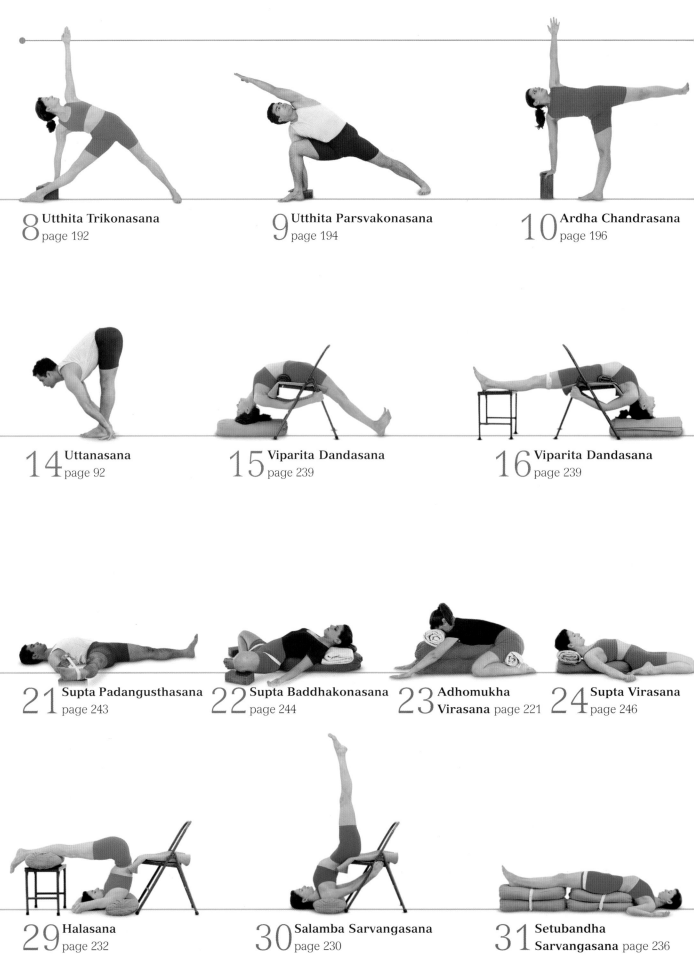

8 **Utthita Trikonasana**
page 192

9 **Utthita Parsvakonasana**
page 194

10 **Ardha Chandrasana**
page 196

14 **Uttanasana**
page 92

15 **Viparita Dandasana**
page 239

16 **Viparita Dandasana**
page 239

21 **Supta Padangusthasana**
page 243

22 **Supta Baddhakonasana**
page 244

23 **Adhomukha Virasana** page 221

24 **Supta Virasana**
page 246

29 **Halasana**
page 232

30 **Salamba Sarvangasana**
page 230

31 **Setubandha Sarvangasana** page 236

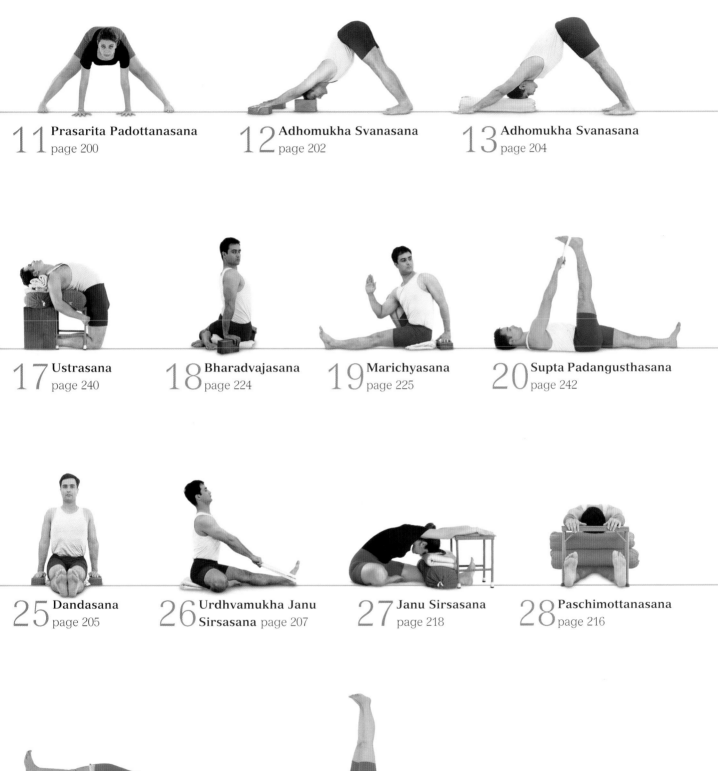

11 **Prasarita Padottanasana**
page 200

12 **Adhomukha Svanasana**
page 202

13 **Adhomukha Svanasana**
page 204

17 **Ustrasana**
page 240

18 **Bharadvajasana**
page 224

19 **Marichyasana**
page 225

20 **Supta Padangusthasana**
page 242

25 **Dandasana**
page 205

26 **Urdhvamukha Janu Sirsasana** page 207

27 **Janu Sirsasana**
page 218

28 **Paschimottanasana**
page 216

32 **Setubandha Sarvangasana**
page 237

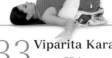

33 **Viparita Karani**
page 234

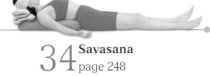

34 **Savasana**
page 248

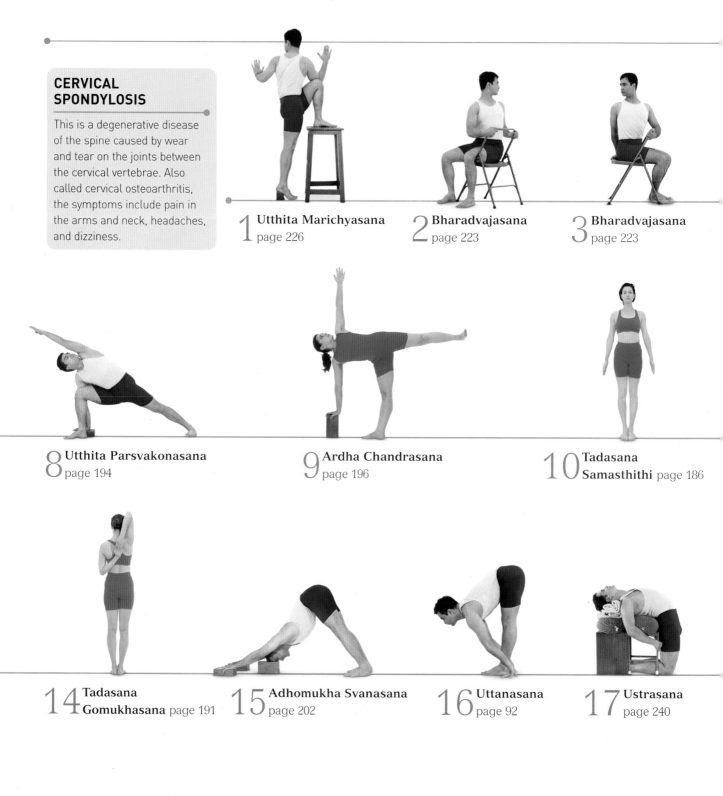

CERVICAL SPONDYLOSIS

This is a degenerative disease of the spine caused by wear and tear on the joints between the cervical vertebrae. Also called cervical osteoarthritis, the symptoms include pain in the arms and neck, headaches, and dizziness.

1 **Utthita Marichyasana** page 226

2 **Bharadvajasana** page 223

3 **Bharadvajasana** page 223

8 **Utthita Parsvakonasana** page 194

9 **Ardha Chandrasana** page 196

10 **Tadasana Samasthithi** page 186

14 **Tadasana Gomukhasana** page 191

15 **Adhomukha Svanasana** page 202

16 **Uttanasana** page 92

17 **Ustrasana** page 240

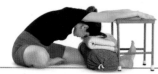

21 **Janu Sirsasana** page 218

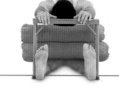

22 **Paschimottanasana** page 216

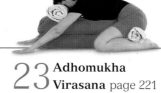

23 **Adhomukha Virasana** page 221

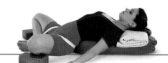

24 **Supta Baddhakonasana** page 244

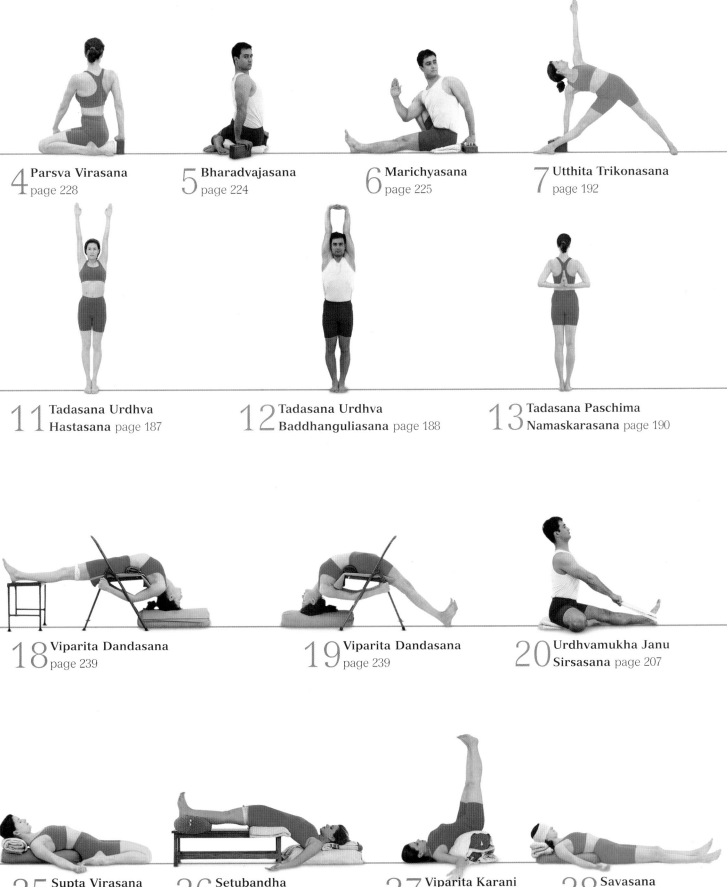

4 **Parsva Virasana**
page 228

5 **Bharadvajasana**
page 224

6 **Marichyasana**
page 225

7 **Utthita Trikonasana**
page 192

11 **Tadasana Urdhva Hastasana** page 187

12 **Tadasana Urdhva Baddhanguliasana** page 188

13 **Tadasana Paschima Namaskarasana** page 190

18 **Viparita Dandasana**
page 239

19 **Viparita Dandasana**
page 239

20 **Urdhvamukha Janu Sirsasana** page 207

25 **Supta Virasana**
page 246

26 **Setubandha Sarvangasana** page 237

27 **Viparita Karani**
page 234

28 **Savasana**
page 248

OSTEOARTHRITIS

SHOULDERS This condition is caused by the erosion of cartilage between joints, causing the bones to press against each other. The narrowing of joint space due to calcification, along with the thickening of tendons in the shoulder joint cause severe pain.

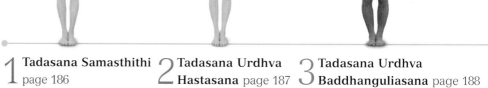

1 **Tadasana Samasthithi** page 186

2 **Tadasana Urdhva Hastasana** page 187

3 **Tadasana Urdhva Baddhanguliasana** page 188

8 **Utthita Parsvakonasana** page 194

9 **Ardha Chandrasana** page 196

10 **Adhomukha Svanasana** page 202

11 **Utthita Marichyasana** page 226

16 **Virasana** page 104

17 **Urdhvamukha Janu Sirsasana** page 207

18 **Janu Sirsasana** page 218

19 **Paschimottanasana** page 214

24 **Salamba Sirsasana** page 138

25 **Ustrasana** page 240

26 **Salamba Sarvangasana** page 230

27 **Halasana** page 232

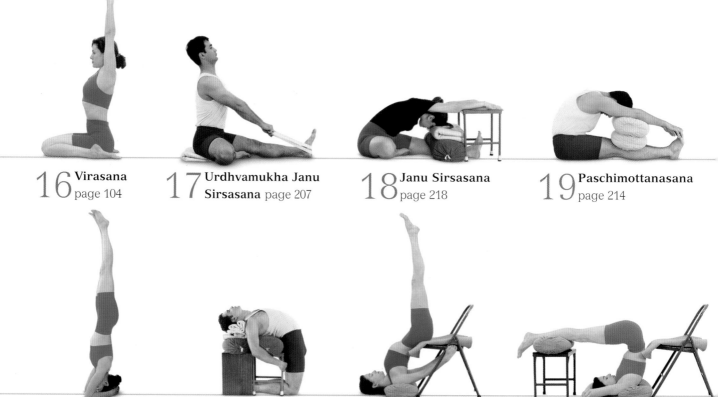

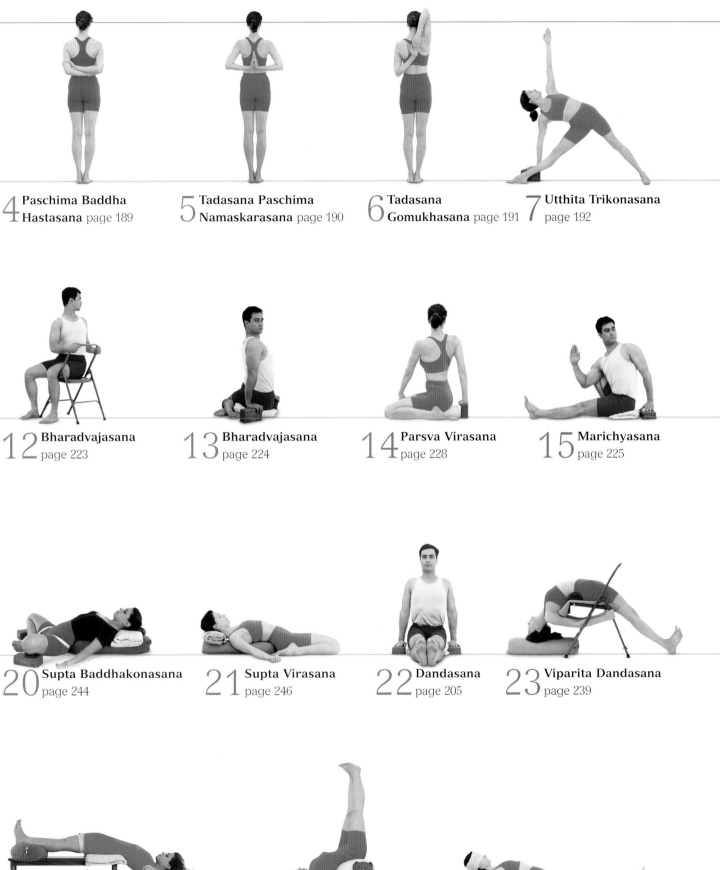

4 **Paschima Baddha Hastasana** page 189

5 **Tadasana Paschima Namaskarasana** page 190

6 **Tadasana Gomukhasana** page 191

7 **Utthita Trikonasana** page 192

12 **Bharadvajasana** page 223

13 **Bharadvajasana** page 224

14 **Parsva Virasana** page 228

15 **Marichyasana** page 225

20 **Supta Baddhakonasana** page 244

21 **Supta Virasana** page 246

22 **Dandasana** page 205

23 **Viparita Dandasana** page 239

28 **Setubandha Sarvangasana** page 237

29 **Viparita Karani** page 234

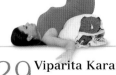

30 **Savasana** page 248

OSTEOARTHRITIS

ELBOWS In this condition, the cartilage between the joints of the elbows wears out, causing inflammation and pain. This can lead to the formation of bone spurs, or the condition of tennis elbow, the latter usually indicated by severe pain in the forearm and elbow.

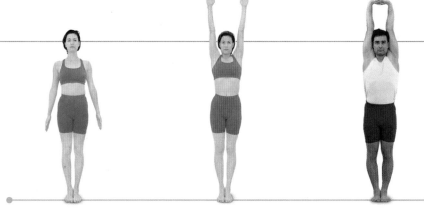

1 **Tadasana Samasthithi** page 186

2 **Tadasana Urdhva Hastasana** page 187

3 **Tadasana Urdhva Baddhanguliasana** page 188

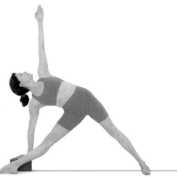

7 **Utthita Trikonasana** page 192

8 **Utthita Parsvakonasana** page 194

9 **Ardha Chandrasana** page 196

14 **Urdhvamukha Janu Sirsasana** page 207

15 **Janu Sirsasana** page 114

16 **Paschimottanasana** page 122

17 **Supta Baddhakonasana** page 244

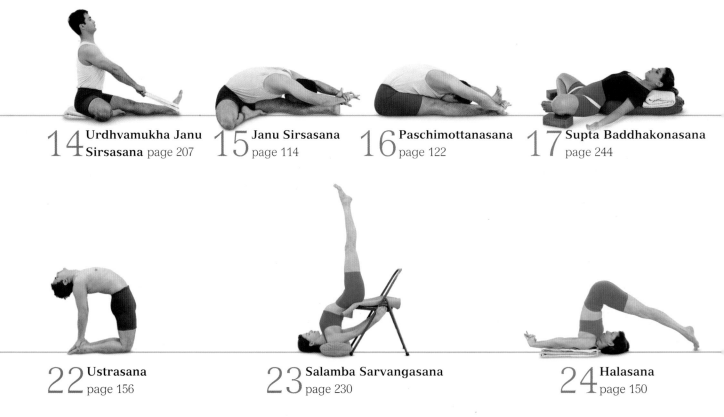

22 **Ustrasana** page 156

23 **Salamba Sarvangasana** page 230

24 **Halasana** page 150

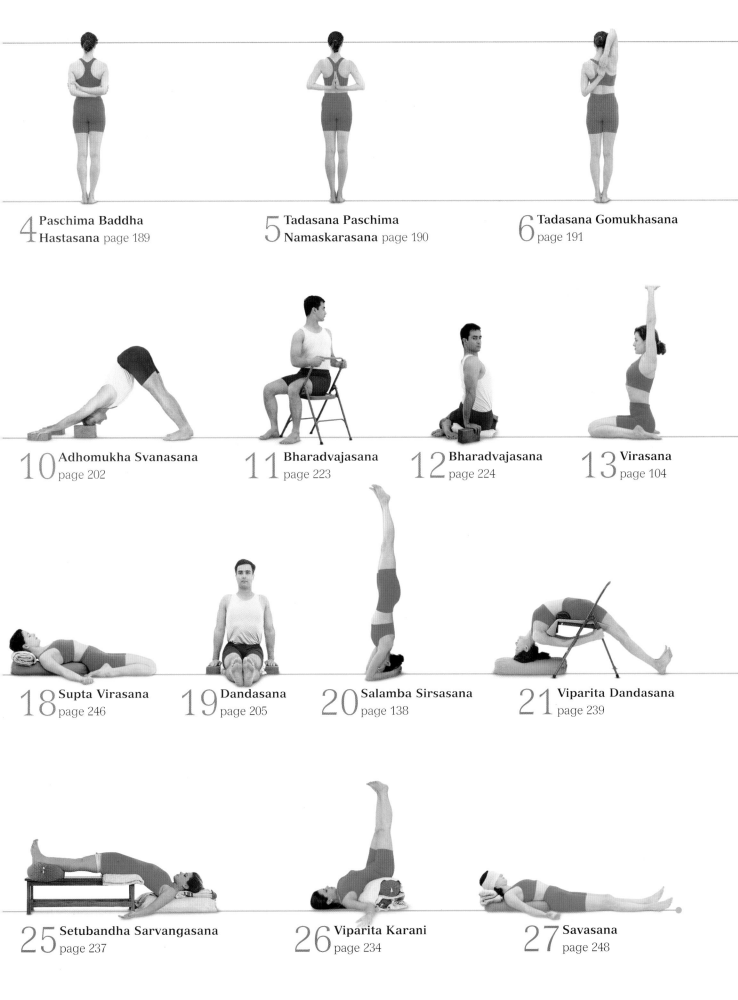

4 **Paschima Baddha Hastasana** page 189

5 **Tadasana Paschima Namaskarasana** page 190

6 **Tadasana Gomukhasana** page 191

10 **Adhomukha Svanasana** page 202

11 **Bharadvajasana** page 223

12 **Bharadvajasana** page 224

13 **Virasana** page 104

18 **Supta Virasana** page 246

19 **Dandasana** page 205

20 **Salamba Sirsasana** page 138

21 **Viparita Dandasana** page 239

25 **Setubandha Sarvangasana** page 237

26 **Viparita Karani** page 234

27 **Savasana** page 248

OSTEOARTHRITIS

WRISTS AND FINGERS In the wrist, this condition is usually the result of an old injury and is characterized by restricted movement and pain in the joint. In the fingers, osteoarthritis is most common at the base of the thumb.

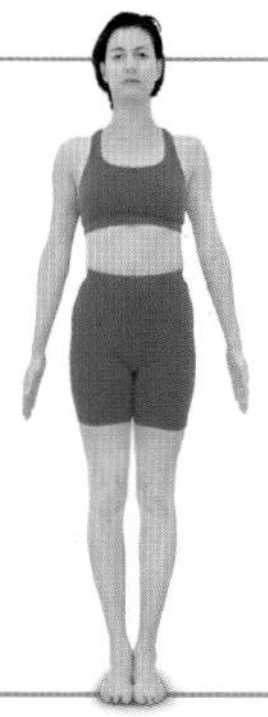

1 **Tadasana Samasthithi** page 186

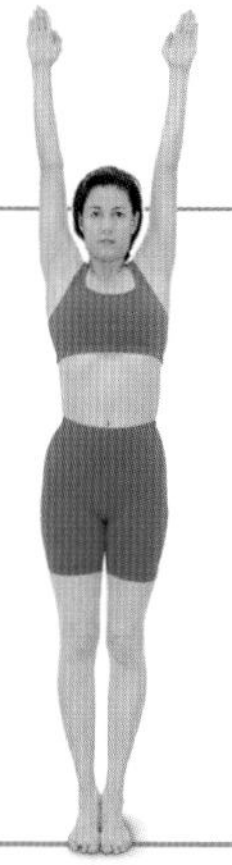

2 **Tadasana Urdhva Hastasana** page 187

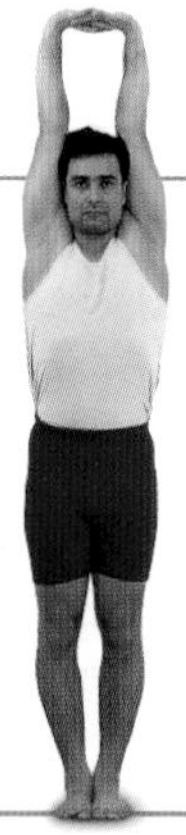

3 **Tadasana Urdhva Baddhanguliasana** page 188

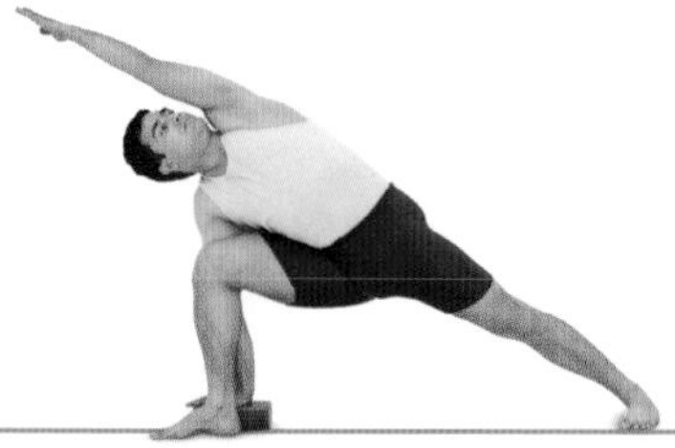

8 **Utthita Parsvakonasana** page 194

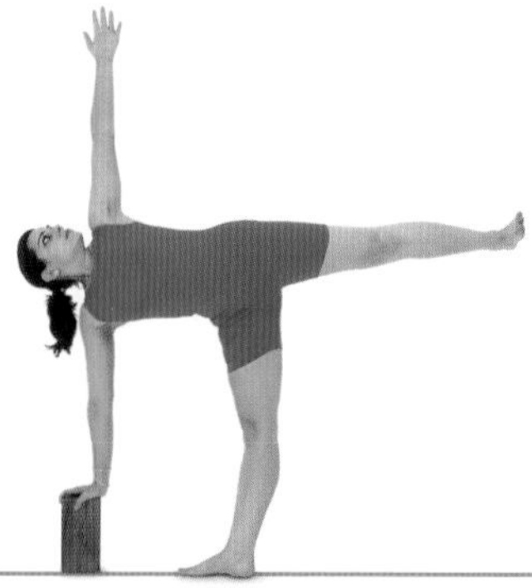

9 **Ardha Chandrasana** page 196

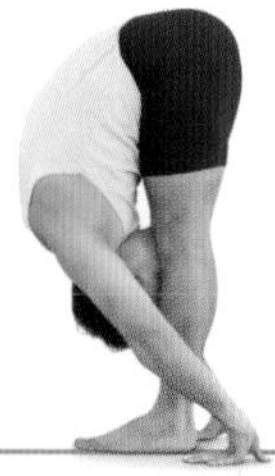

10 **Uttanasana** page 92

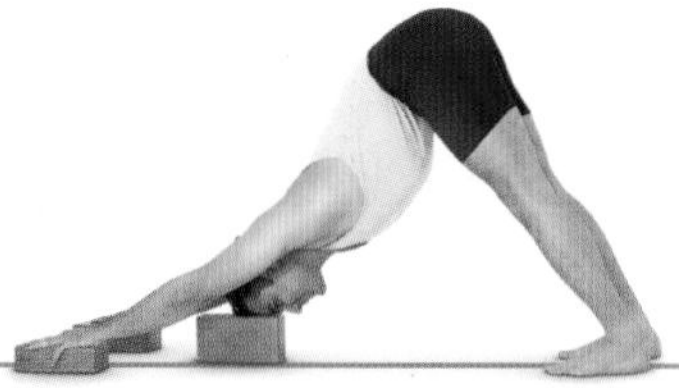

11 **Adhomukha Svanasana** page 202

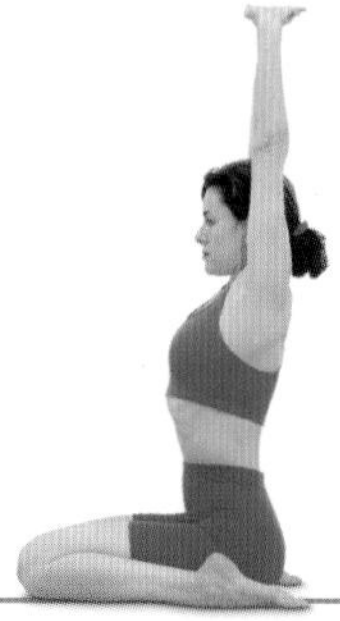

16 **Virasana** page 104

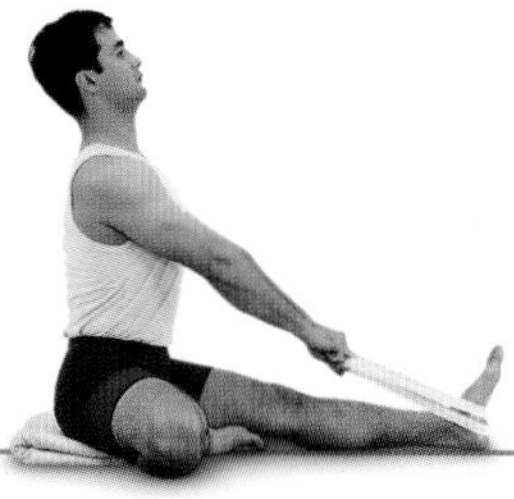

17 **Urdhvamukha Janu Sirsasana** page 207

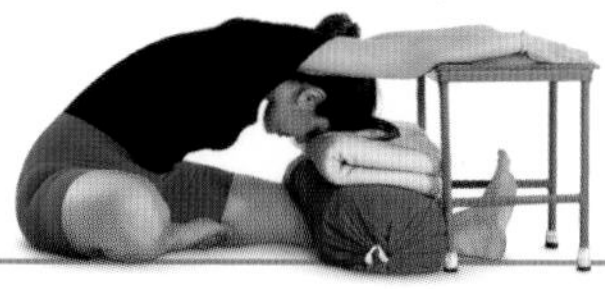

18 **Janu Sirsasana** page 218

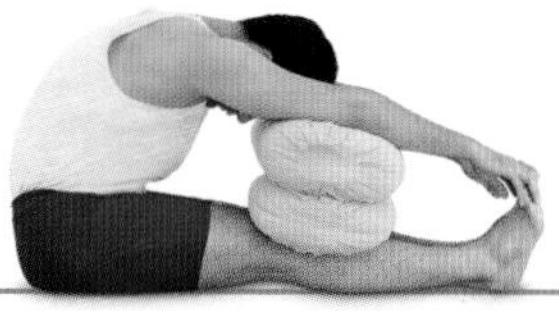

19 **Paschimottanasana** page 214

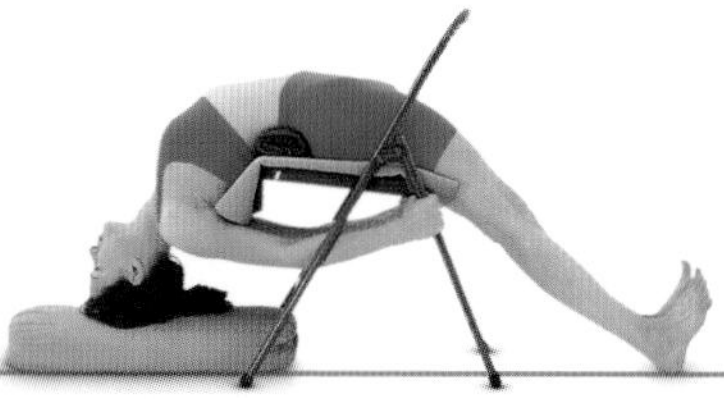

24 **Viparita Dandasana** page 239

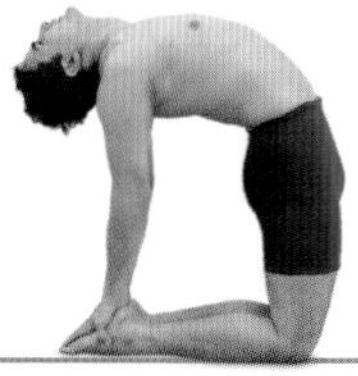

25 **Ustrasana** page 156

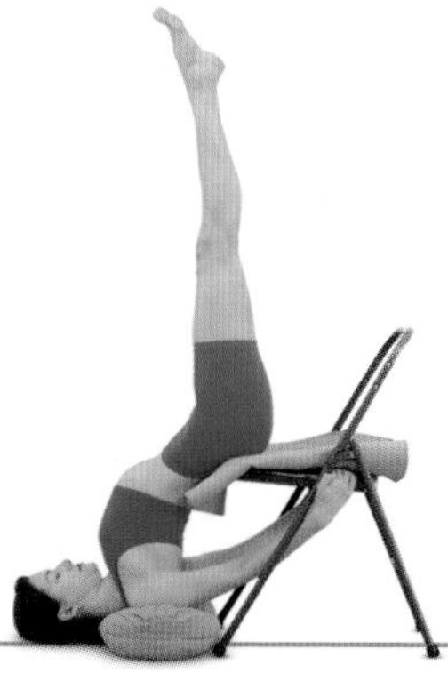

26 **Salamba Sarvangasana** page 230

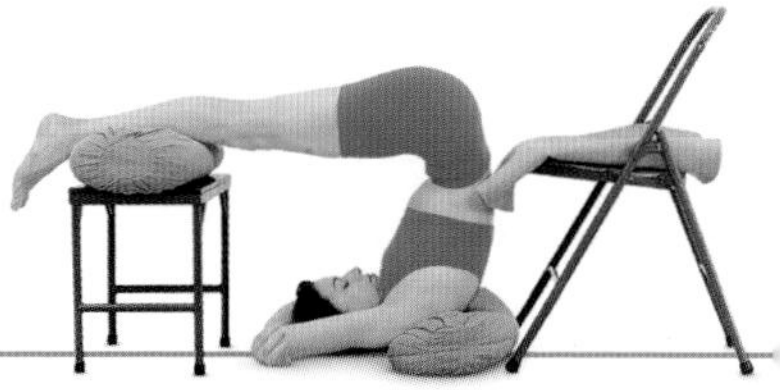

27 **Halasana** page 232

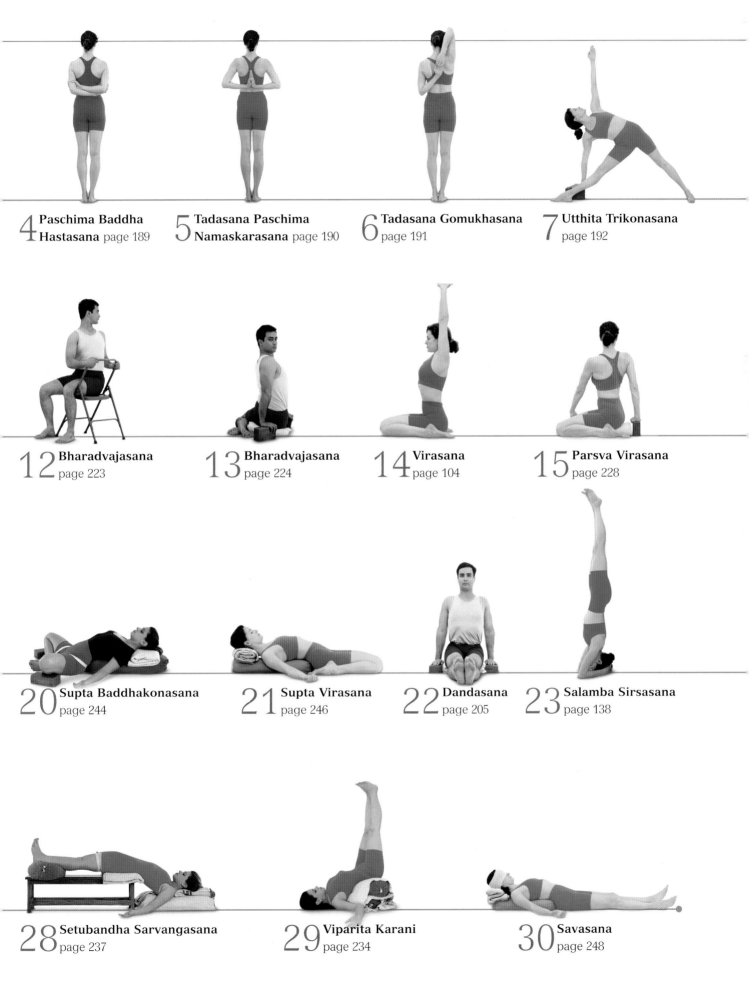

4 **Paschima Baddha Hastasana** page 189

5 **Tadasana Paschima Namaskarasana** page 190

6 **Tadasana Gomukhasana** page 191

7 **Utthita Trikonasana** page 192

12 **Bharadvajasana** page 223

13 **Bharadvajasana** page 224

14 **Virasana** page 104

15 **Parsva Virasana** page 228

20 **Supta Baddhakonasana** page 244

21 **Supta Virasana** page 246

22 **Dandasana** page 205

23 **Salamba Sirsasana** page 138

28 **Setubandha Sarvangasana** page 237

29 **Viparita Karani** page 234

30 **Savasana** page 248

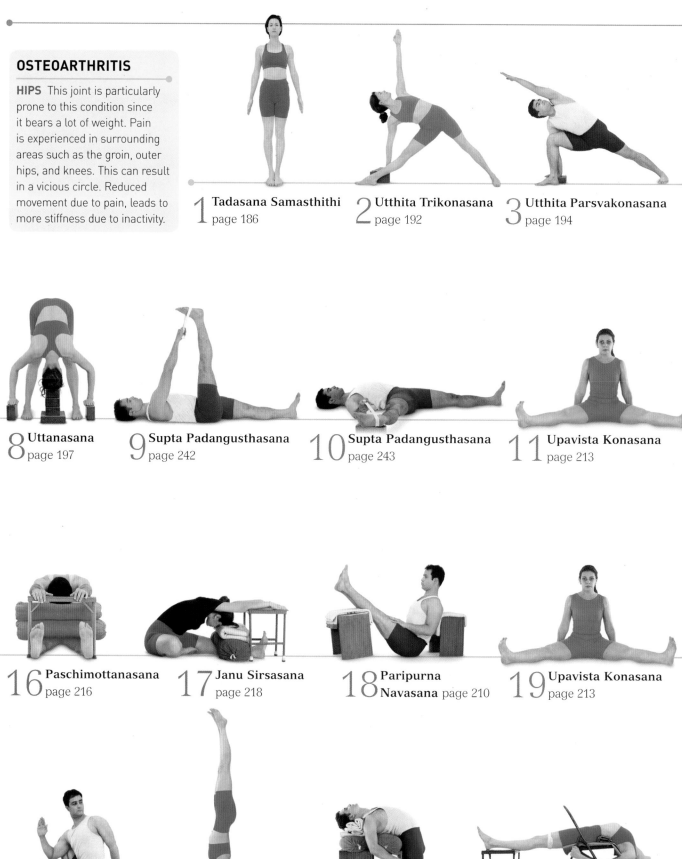

OSTEOARTHRITIS

HIPS This joint is particularly prone to this condition since it bears a lot of weight. Pain is experienced in surrounding areas such as the groin, outer hips, and knees. This can result in a vicious circle. Reduced movement due to pain, leads to more stiffness due to inactivity.

1 **Tadasana Samasthithi** page 186

2 **Utthita Trikonasana** page 192

3 **Utthita Parsvakonasana** page 194

8 **Uttanasana** page 197

9 **Supta Padangusthasana** page 242

10 **Supta Padangusthasana** page 243

11 **Upavista Konasana** page 213

16 **Paschimottanasana** page 216

17 **Janu Sirsasana** page 218

18 **Paripurna Navasana** page 210

19 **Upavista Konasana** page 213

24 **Marichyasana** page 225

25 **Salamba Sirsasana** page 138

26 **Ustrasana** page 240

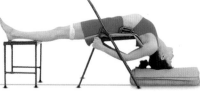

27 **Viparita Dandasana** page 239

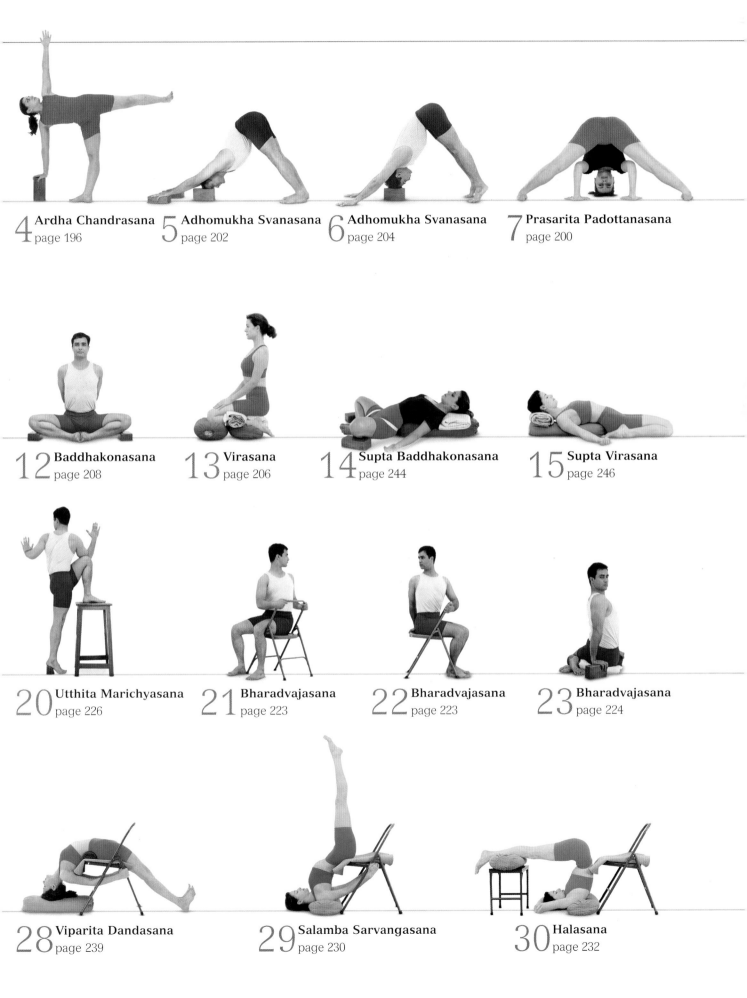

4 **Ardha Chandrasana**
page 196

5 **Adhomukha Svanasana**
page 202

6 **Adhomukha Svanasana**
page 204

7 **Prasarita Padottanasana**
page 200

12 **Baddhakonasana**
page 208

13 **Virasana**
page 206

14 **Supta Baddhakonasana**
page 244

15 **Supta Virasana**
page 246

20 **Utthita Marichyasana**
page 226

21 **Bharadvajasana**
page 223

22 **Bharadvajasana**
page 223

23 **Bharadvajasana**
page 224

28 **Viparita Dandasana**
page 239

29 **Salamba Sarvangasana**
page 230

30 **Halasana**
page 232

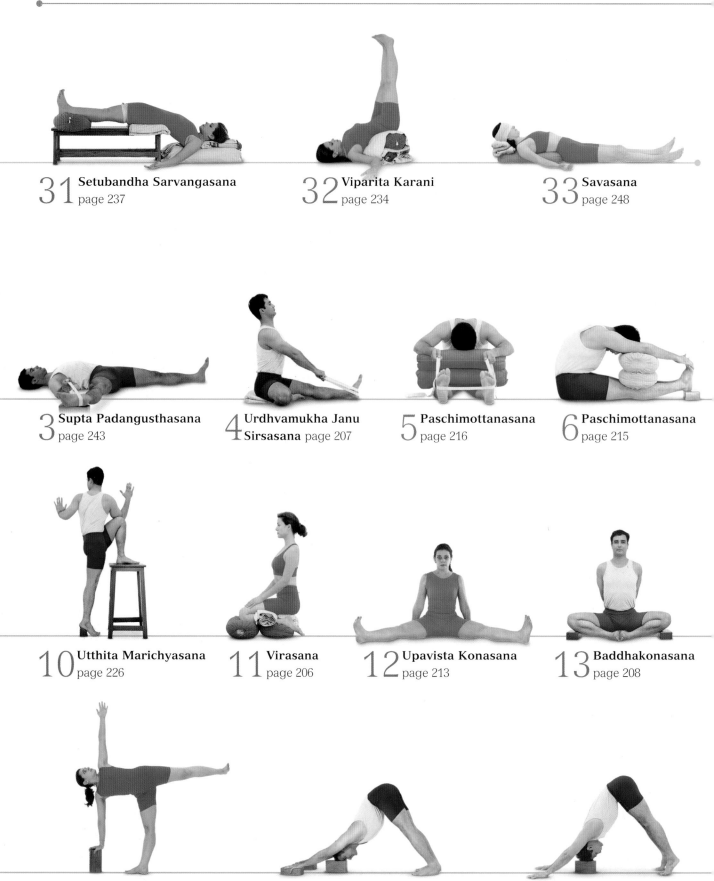

31 **Setubandha Sarvangasana**
page 237

32 **Viparita Karani**
page 234

33 **Savasana**
page 248

3 **Supta Padangusthasana**
page 243

4 **Urdhvamukha Janu Sirsasana** page 207

5 **Paschimottanasana**
page 216

6 **Paschimottanasana**
page 215

10 **Utthita Marichyasana**
page 226

11 **Virasana**
page 206

12 **Upavista Konasana**
page 213

13 **Baddhakonasana**
page 208

17 **Ardha Chandrasana**
page 196

18 **Adhomukha Svanasana**
page 202

19 **Adhomukha Svanasana**
page 204

OSTEOARTHRITIS

KNEES A decrease in the synovial fluid that lubricates the knee joint leads to this condition. The cartilage in the area becomes rough and tends to flake off. The knee looks swollen, and the joint loses flexibility and the ability to stretch and bend.

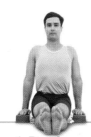

1 **Dandasana**
page 205

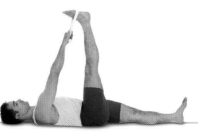

2 **Supta Padangusthasana**
page 242

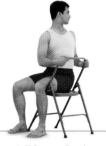

7 **Janu Sirsasana**
page 218

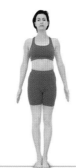

8 **Paripurna Navasana**
page 210

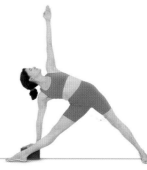

9 **Paripurna Navasana**
page 212

14 **Bharadvajasana**
page 223

15 **Tadasana Samasthithi**
page 186

16 **Utthita Trikonasana**
page 192

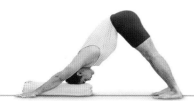

20 **Adhomukha Svanasana**
page 204

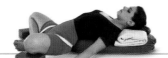

21 **Supta Baddhakonasana**
page 244

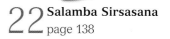

22 **Salamba Sirsasana**
page 138

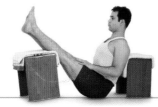
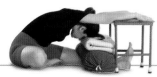
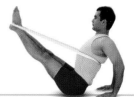

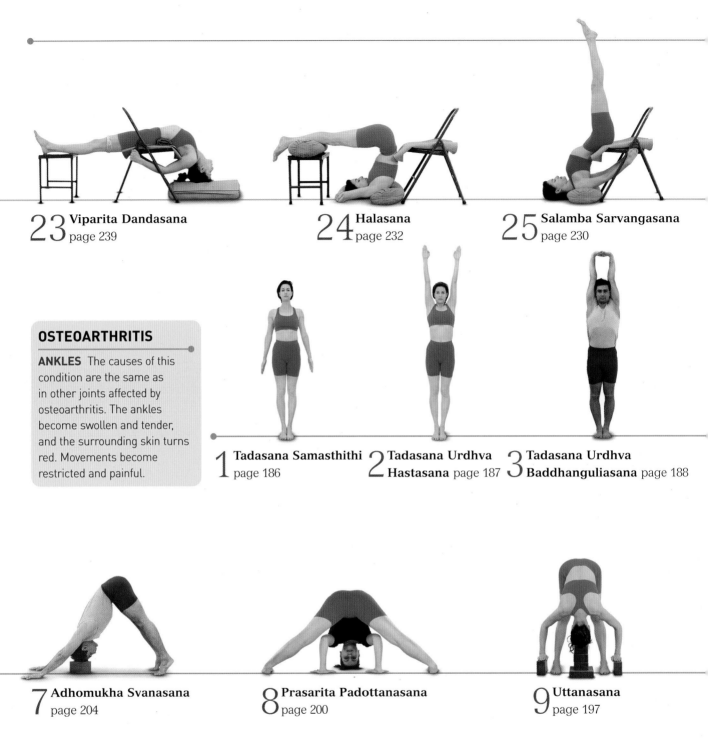

23 **Viparita Dandasana** page 239

24 **Halasana** page 232

25 **Salamba Sarvangasana** page 230

OSTEOARTHRITIS

ANKLES The causes of this condition are the same as in other joints affected by osteoarthritis. The ankles become swollen and tender, and the surrounding skin turns red. Movements become restricted and painful.

1 **Tadasana Samasthithi** page 186

2 **Tadasana Urdhva Hastasana** page 187

3 **Tadasana Urdhva Baddhanguliasana** page 188

7 **Adhomukha Svanasana** page 204

8 **Prasarita Padottanasana** page 200

9 **Uttanasana** page 197

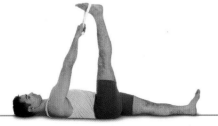

14 **Supta Padangusthasana** page 242

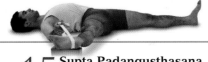

15 **Supta Padangusthasana** page 243

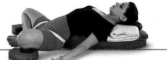

16 **Supta Baddhakonasana** page 244

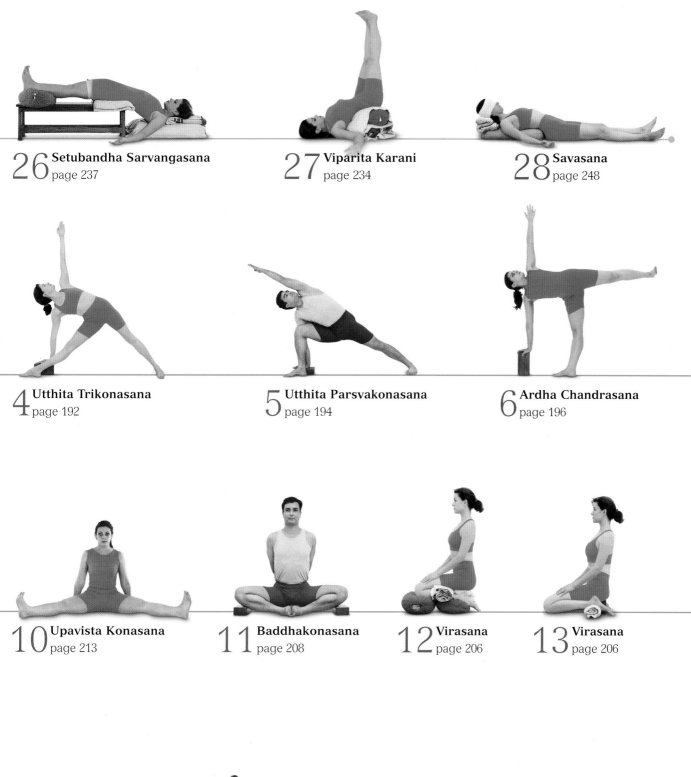

26 Setubandha Sarvangasana
page 237

27 Viparita Karani
page 234

28 Savasana
page 248

4 Utthita Trikonasana
page 192

5 Utthita Parsvakonasana
page 194

6 Ardha Chandrasana
page 196

10 Upavista Konasana
page 213

11 Baddhakonasana
page 208

12 Virasana
page 206

13 Virasana
page 206

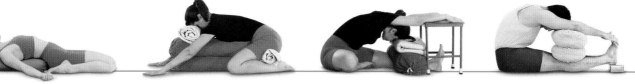

17 Supta Virasana
page 246

18 Adhomukha Virasana
page 221

19 Janu Sirsasana
page 218

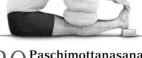

20 Paschimottanasana
page 215

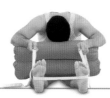

21 **Paschimottanasana**
page 216

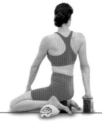

22 **Dandasana**
page 205

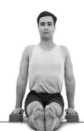

23 **Salamba Sirsasana**
page 138

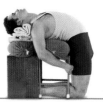

24 **Ustrasana**
page 240

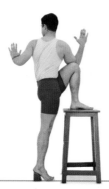

28 **Utthita Marichyasana**
page 226

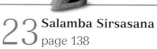

29 **Parsva Virasana**
page 228

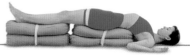

30 **Setubandha Sarvangasana**
page 237

RHEUMATOID ARTHRITIS

This is a chronic, systemic, inflammatory condition, which leads to the eventual disability of the joints. The symptoms are stiffness in the mornings, fatigue, burning, and swelling of the joints, and the appearance of rheumatoid nodules.

1 **Savasana**
page 248

2 **Supta Baddhakonasana**
page 244

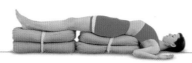

6 **Setubandha Sarvangasana**
page 237

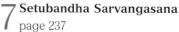

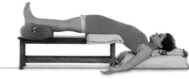

7 **Setubandha Sarvangasana**
page 237

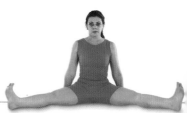

8 **Upavista Konasana**
page 213

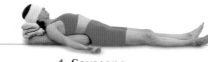

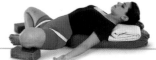

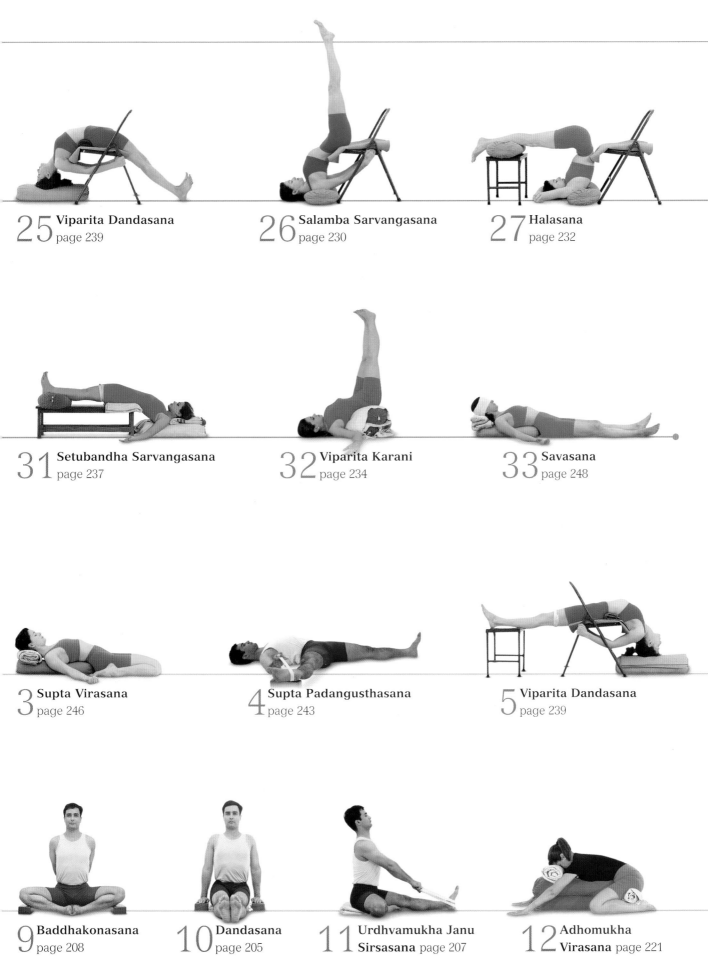

25 **Viparita Dandasana** page 239

26 **Salamba Sarvangasana** page 230

27 **Halasana** page 232

31 **Setubandha Sarvangasana** page 237

32 **Viparita Karani** page 234

33 **Savasana** page 248

3 **Supta Virasana** page 246

4 **Supta Padangusthasana** page 243

5 **Viparita Dandasana** page 239

9 **Baddhakonasana** page 208

10 **Dandasana** page 205

11 **Urdhvamukha Janu Sirsasana** page 207

12 **Adhomukha Virasana** page 221

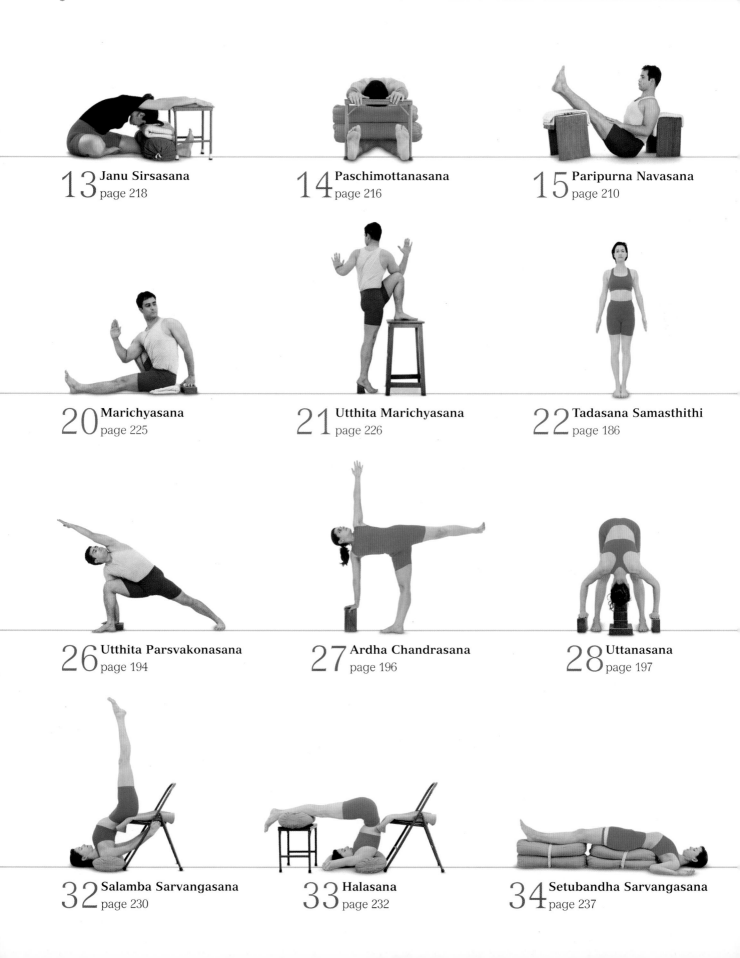

13 **Janu Sirsasana**
page 218

14 **Paschimottanasana**
page 216

15 **Paripurna Navasana**
page 210

20 **Marichyasana**
page 225

21 **Utthita Marichyasana**
page 226

22 **Tadasana Samasthithi**
page 186

26 **Utthita Parsvakonasana**
page 194

27 **Ardha Chandrasana**
page 196

28 **Uttanasana**
page 197

32 **Salamba Sarvangasana**
page 230

33 **Halasana**
page 232

34 **Setubandha Sarvangasana**
page 237

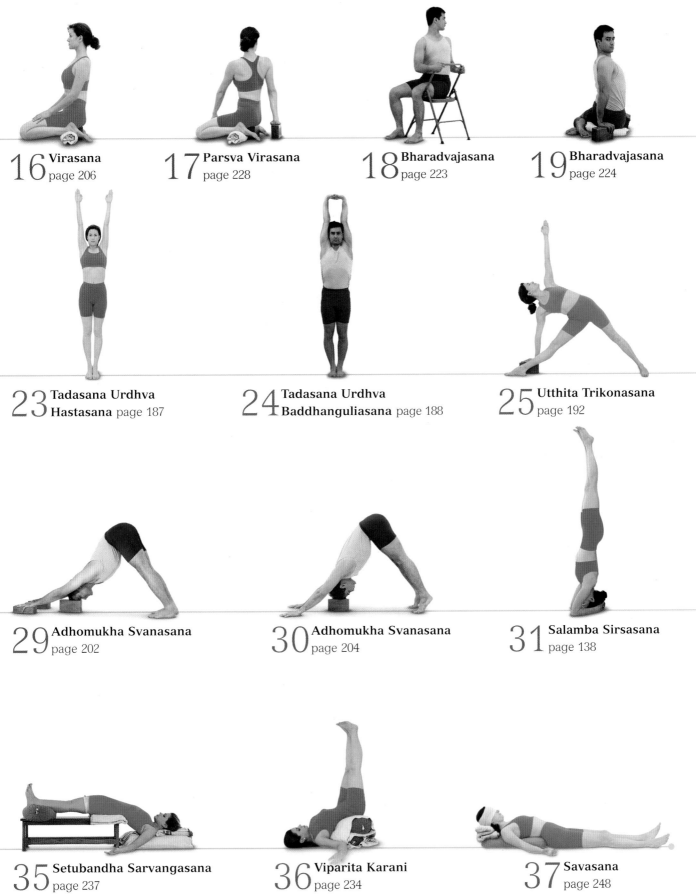

16 **Virasana**
page 206

17 **Parsva Virasana**
page 228

18 **Bharadvajasana**
page 223

19 **Bharadvajasana**
page 224

23 **Tadasana Urdhva Hastasana** page 187

24 **Tadasana Urdhva Baddhanguliasana** page 188

25 **Utthita Trikonasana**
page 192

29 **Adhomukha Svanasana**
page 202

30 **Adhomukha Svanasana**
page 204

31 **Salamba Sirsasana**
page 138

35 **Setubandha Sarvangasana**
page 237

36 **Viparita Karani**
page 234

37 **Savasana**
page 248

SKIN

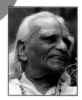

The skin, the largest organ of the body, is part of the sensory system. It is the principal organ of the sense of touch and it serves to protect the internal organs. The skin also regulates body temperature. It consists of a vascular layer called the dermis, and an external covering called the epidermis. The sweat glands, hair follicles, and sebaceous glands are embedded in the dermis.

ACNE

This is a skin disorder caused by inflammation of the sebaceous glands or hair follicles. Acne, appearing as boils, pimples, pustules, spots, or whiteheads, is sometimes triggered by anxiety. It usually affects adolescents, but may persist in later age.

1 **Tadasana Samasthithi** page 186

2 **Tadasana Urdhva Hastasana** page 187

3 **Tadasana Urdhva Baddhanguliasana** page 188

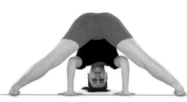

8 **Prasarita Padottanasana** page 200

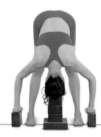

9 **Uttanasana** page 197

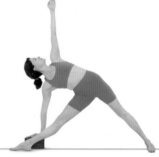

10 **Utthita Trikonasana** page 192

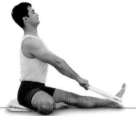

14 **Urdhvamukha Janu Sirsasana** page 207

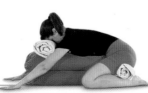

15 **Adhomukha Virasana** page 221

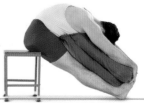

16 **Adhomukha Paschimottanasana** page 217

"Disorders of the skin are common, and yoga asanas offer a healthy and effective form of treatment. Keep your brain calm and quiet. Let your body be active."

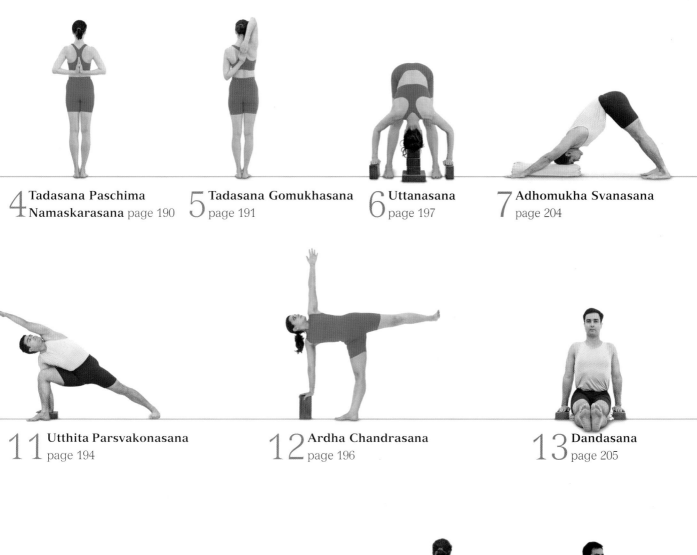

4 **Tadasana Paschima Namaskarasana** page 190

5 **Tadasana Gomukhasana** page 191

6 **Uttanasana** page 197

7 **Adhomukha Svanasana** page 204

11 **Utthita Parsvakonasana** page 194

12 **Ardha Chandrasana** page 196

13 **Dandasana** page 205

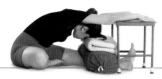

17 **Janu Sirsasana** page 218

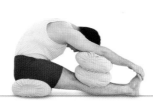

18 **Paschimottanasana** page 215

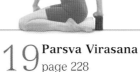

19 **Parsva Virasana** page 228

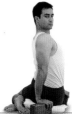

20 **Bharadvajasana** page 224

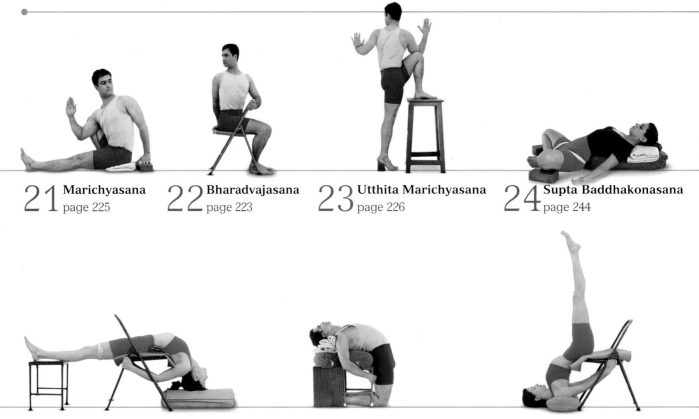

21 **Marichyasana**
page 225

22 **Bharadvajasana**
page 223

23 **Utthita Marichyasana**
page 226

24 **Supta Baddhakonasana**
page 244

29 **Viparita Dandasana**
page 239

30 **Ustrasana**
page 240

31 **Salamba Sarvangasana**
page 230

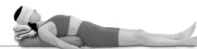

35 **Savasana**
page 248

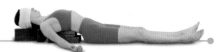

36 **Ujjayi Pranayama**
page 254

37 **Viloma 2 Pranayama**
page 257

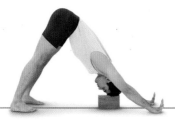

4 **Adhomukha Svanasana**
page 203

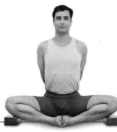

5 **Baddhakonasana**
page 208

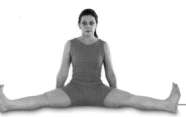

6 **Upavista Konasana**
page 213

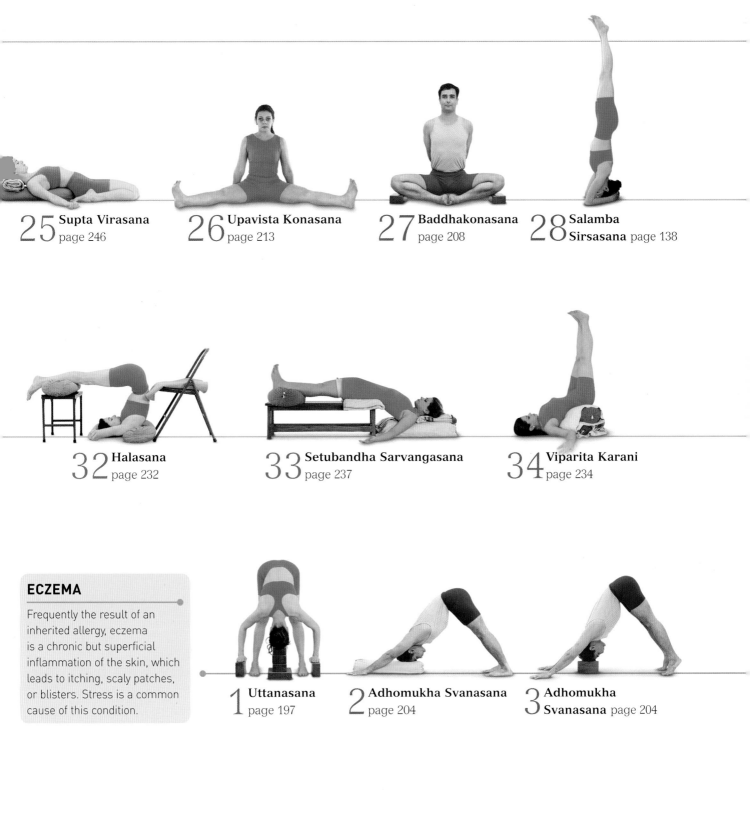

25 **Supta Virasana** page 246

26 **Upavista Konasana** page 213

27 **Baddhakonasana** page 208

28 **Salamba Sirsasana** page 138

32 **Halasana** page 232

33 **Setubandha Sarvangasana** page 237

34 **Viparita Karani** page 234

ECZEMA

Frequently the result of an inherited allergy, eczema is a chronic but superficial inflammation of the skin, which leads to itching, scaly patches, or blisters. Stress is a common cause of this condition.

1 **Uttanasana** page 197

2 **Adhomukha Svanasana** page 204

3 **Adhomukha Svanasana** page 204

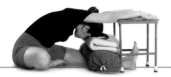

7 **Janu Sirsasana** page 218

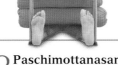

8 **Paschimottanasana** page 216

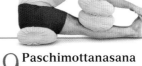

9 **Paschimottanasana** page 215

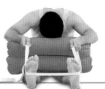

10 **Paschimottanasana** page 216

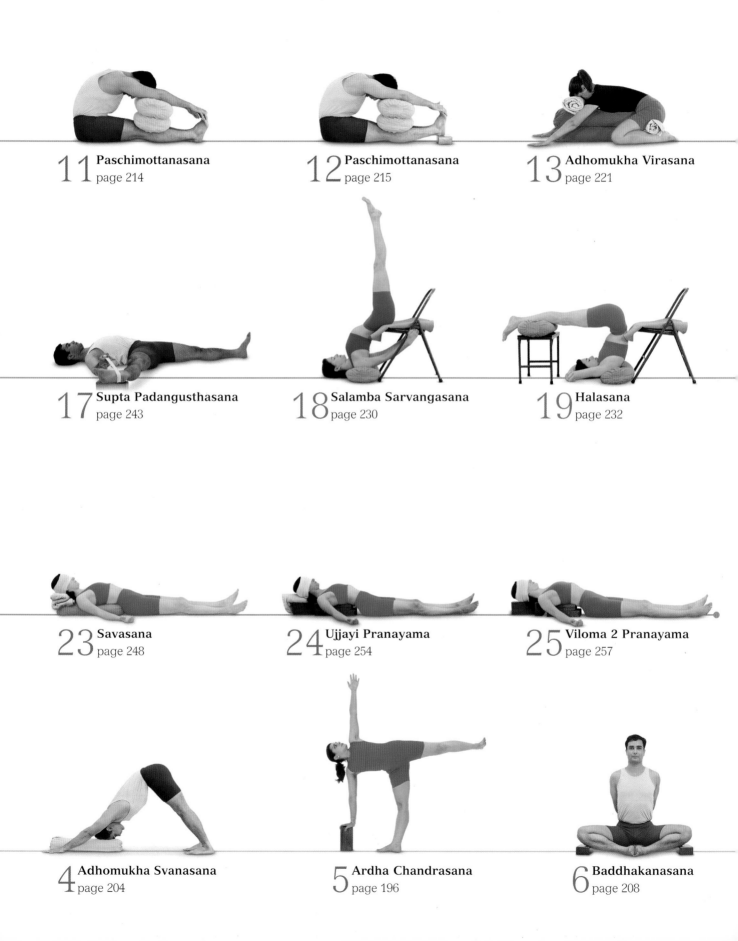

11 **Paschimottanasana**
page 214

12 **Paschimottanasana**
page 215

13 **Adhomukha Virasana**
page 221

17 **Supta Padangusthasana**
page 243

18 **Salamba Sarvangasana**
page 230

19 **Halasana**
page 232

23 **Savasana**
page 248

24 **Ujjayi Pranayama**
page 254

25 **Viloma 2 Pranayama**
page 257

4 **Adhomukha Svanasana**
page 204

5 **Ardha Chandrasana**
page 196

6 **Baddhakanasana**
page 208

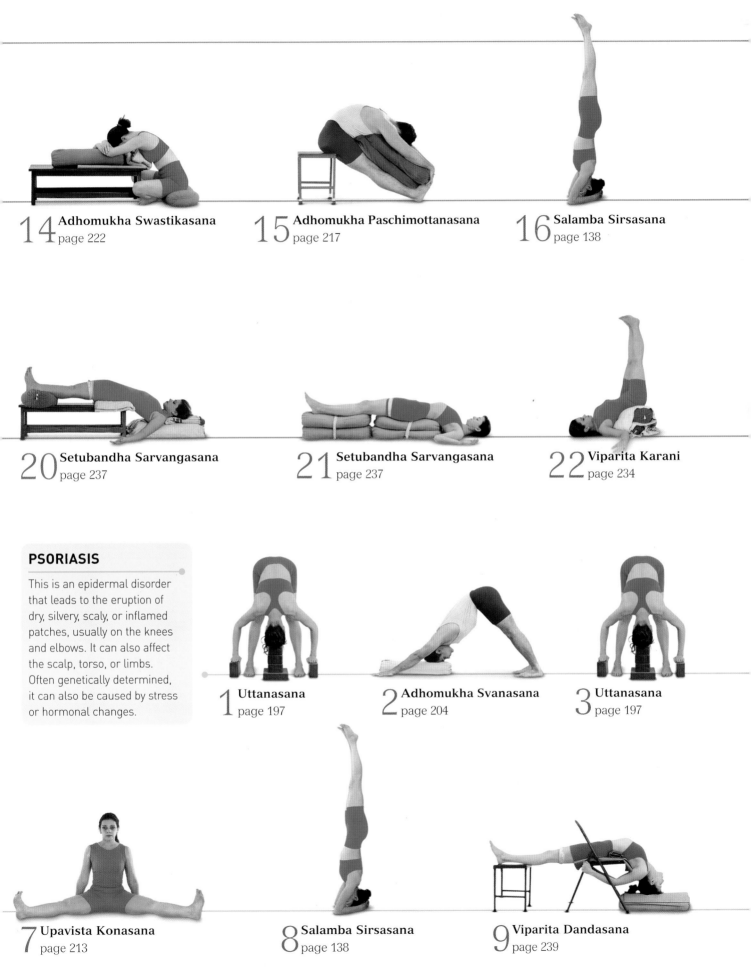

14 **Adhomukha Swastikasana**
page 222

15 **Adhomukha Paschimottanasana**
page 217

16 **Salamba Sirsasana**
page 138

20 **Setubandha Sarvangasana**
page 237

21 **Setubandha Sarvangasana**
page 237

22 **Viparita Karani**
page 234

PSORIASIS

This is an epidermal disorder that leads to the eruption of dry, silvery, scaly, or inflamed patches, usually on the knees and elbows. It can also affect the scalp, torso, or limbs. Often genetically determined, it can also be caused by stress or hormonal changes.

1 **Uttanasana**
page 197

2 **Adhomukha Svanasana**
page 204

3 **Uttanasana**
page 197

7 **Upavista Konasana**
page 213

8 **Salamba Sirsasana**
page 138

9 **Viparita Dandasana**
page 239

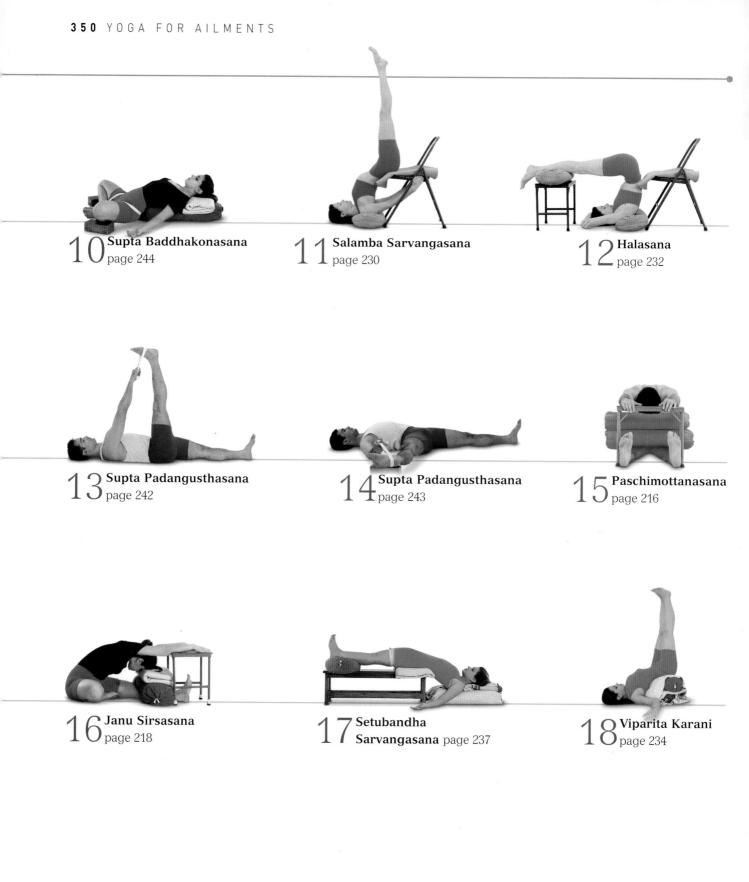

10 **Supta Baddhakonasana**
page 244

11 **Salamba Sarvangasana**
page 230

12 **Halasana**
page 232

13 **Supta Padangusthasana**
page 242

14 **Supta Padangusthasana**
page 243

15 **Paschimottanasana**
page 216

16 **Janu Sirsasana**
page 218

17 **Setubandha Sarvangasana** page 237

18 **Viparita Karani**
page 234

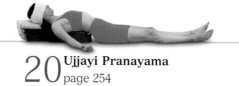

19 **Savasana**
page 248

20 **Ujjayi Pranayama**
page 254

BRAIN AND NERVOUS SYSTEM

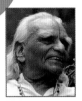

The main engine of the nervous system is the central nervous system, composed of the brain and the spinal cord, the body's information-gathering, storage, and control center. Within this, the sympathetic and the parasympathetic nervous systems control the involuntary functions of the organs, glands, and other parts of the body. Regular practice of the recommended sequences of asanas relieves pressure on the brain and the entire nervous system.

HEADACHE AND EYE STRAIN

This is characterized by severe, piercing pain around the eyes and temples. Usually, the pain increases rapidly within 15 minutes of inception, but the episode itself can last for up to 2 hours.

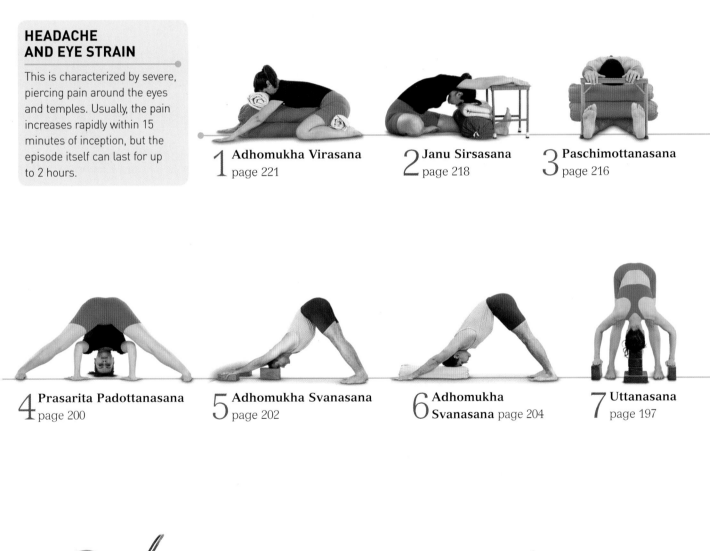

1 **Adhomukha Virasana** page 221

2 **Janu Sirsasana** page 218

3 **Paschimottanasana** page 216

4 **Prasarita Padottanasana** page 200

5 **Adhomukha Svanasana** page 202

6 **Adhomukha Svanasana** page 204

7 **Uttanasana** page 197

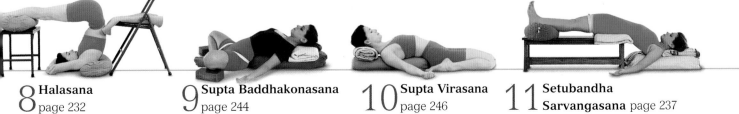

8 **Halasana** page 232

9 **Supta Baddhakonasana** page 244

10 **Supta Virasana** page 246

11 **Setubandha Sarvangasana** page 237

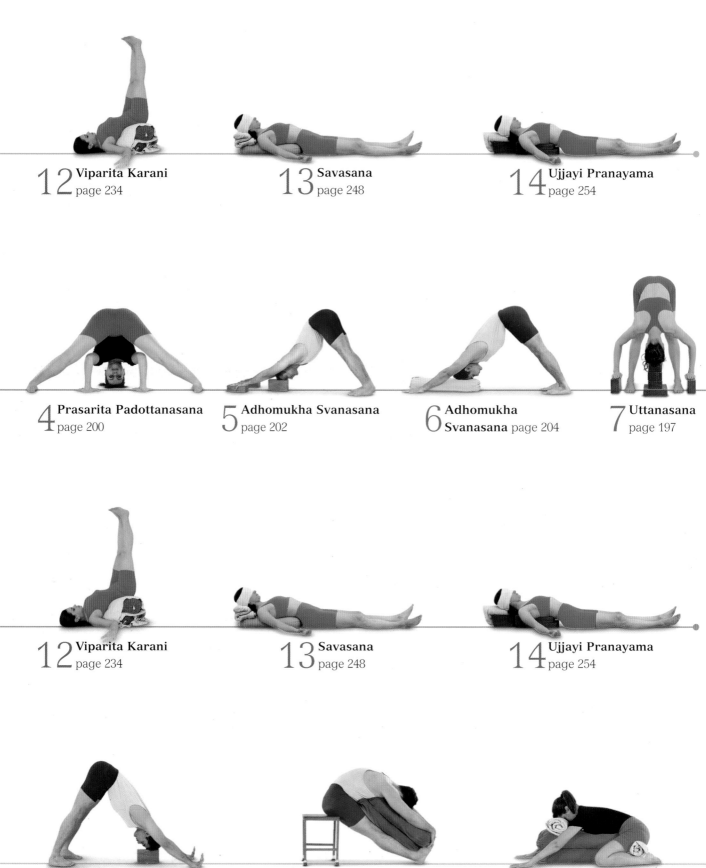

12 **Viparita Karani**
page 234

13 **Savasana**
page 248

14 **Ujjayi Pranayama**
page 254

4 **Prasarita Padottanasana**
page 200

5 **Adhomukha Svanasana**
page 202

6 **Adhomukha Svanasana** page 204

7 **Uttanasana**
page 197

12 **Viparita Karani**
page 234

13 **Savasana**
page 248

14 **Ujjayi Pranayama**
page 254

4 **Adhomukha Svanasana**
page 203

5 **Adhomukha Paschimottanasana**
page 217

6 **Adhomukha Virasana**
page 221

STRESS-RELATED HEADACHE

This condition usually takes the form of a dull ache at the back of the skull due to the tautness of the muscles of the scalp and neck. It can also occur as a dull, throbbing pain of moderate intensity, usually following a stressful event.

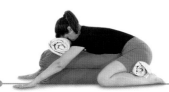

1 **Adhomukha Virasana** page 221

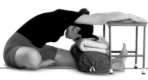

2 **Janu Sirsasana** page 218

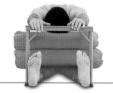

3 **Paschimottanasana** page 216

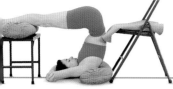

8 **Halasana** page 232

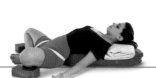

9 **Supta Baddhakonasana** page 244

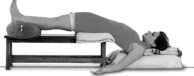

10 **Supta Virasana** page 246

11 **Setubandha Sarvangasana** page 237

MEMORY IMPAIRMENT

The aging process is often associated with mild loss of memory. However, it is important to distinguish between this and the onset of serious progressive dementia, such as Alzheimer's disease.

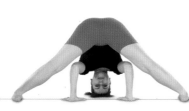

1 **Prasarita Padottanasana** page 200

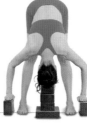

2 **Uttanasana** page 197

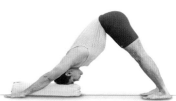

3 **Adhomukha Svanasana** page 204

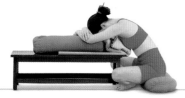

7 **Adhomukha Swastikasana** page 222

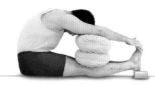

8 **Paschimottanasana** page 215

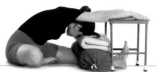

9 **Janu Sirsasana** page 218

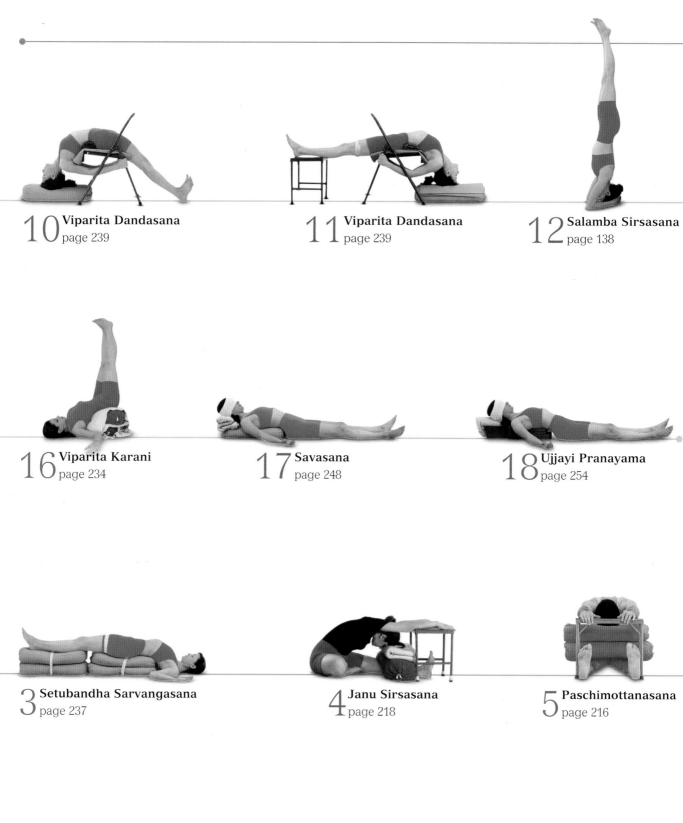

10 **Viparita Dandasana**
page 239

11 **Viparita Dandasana**
page 239

12 **Salamba Sirsasana**
page 138

16 **Viparita Karani**
page 234

17 **Savasana**
page 248

18 **Ujjayi Pranayama**
page 254

3 **Setubandha Sarvangasana**
page 237

4 **Janu Sirsasana**
page 218

5 **Paschimottanasana**
page 216

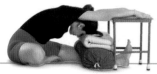

9 **Janu Sirsasana**
page 218

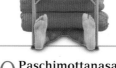

10 **Paschimottanasana**
page 216

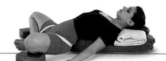

11 **Supta Baddhakonasana**
page 244

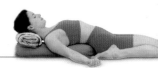

12 **Supta Virasana**
page 246

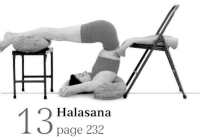

13 **Halasana**
page 232

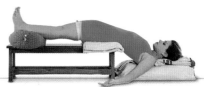

14 **Salamba Sarvangasana**
page 230

Setubandha Sarvangasana
15 page 237

MIGRAINE

This condition is associated with periodic, throbbing headaches, often accompanied by nausea and vomiting. The pain can be at the front, back, or sides of the skull. The attack can be preceded by sensitivity to light, partial loss of vision, and numbness in the lips.

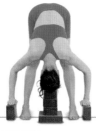

1 **Adhomukha Virasana**
page 221

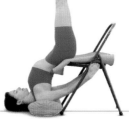

2 **Adhomukha Swastikasana**
page 222

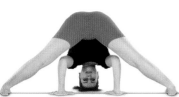

6 **Prasarita Padottanasana**
page 200

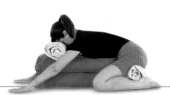

7 **Uttanasana**
page 197

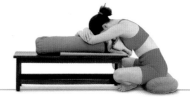

Halasana
8 page 232

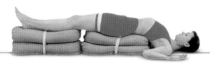

13 **Setubandha Sarvangasana**
page 237

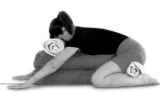

14 **Adhomukha Virasana**
page 221

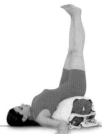

Viparita Karani
15 page 234

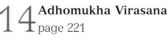
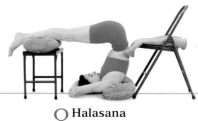

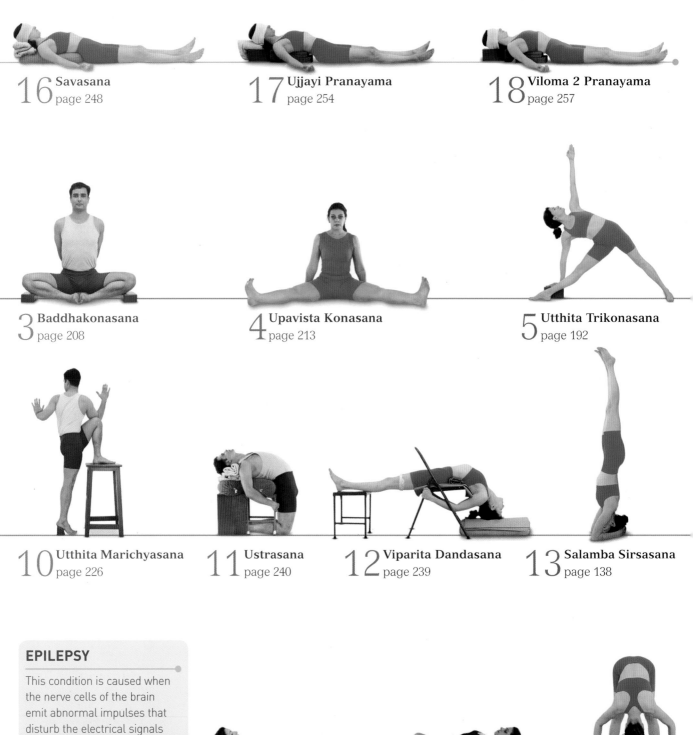

16 **Savasana**
page 248

17 **Ujjayi Pranayama**
page 254

18 **Viloma 2 Pranayama**
page 257

3 **Baddhakonasana**
page 208

4 **Upavista Konasana**
page 213

5 **Utthita Trikonasana**
page 192

10 **Utthita Marichyasana**
page 226

11 **Ustrasana**
page 240

12 **Viparita Dandasana**
page 239

13 **Salamba Sirsasana**
page 138

EPILEPSY

This condition is caused when the nerve cells of the brain emit abnormal impulses that disturb the electrical signals by which the brain controls the body. Epileptic seizures occur irregularly. The causes include head injuries, brain infections, and inherited predisposition.

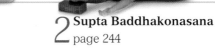

1 **Supta Virasana**
page 246

2 **Supta Baddhakonasana**
page 244

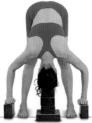

3 **Uttanasana**
page 197

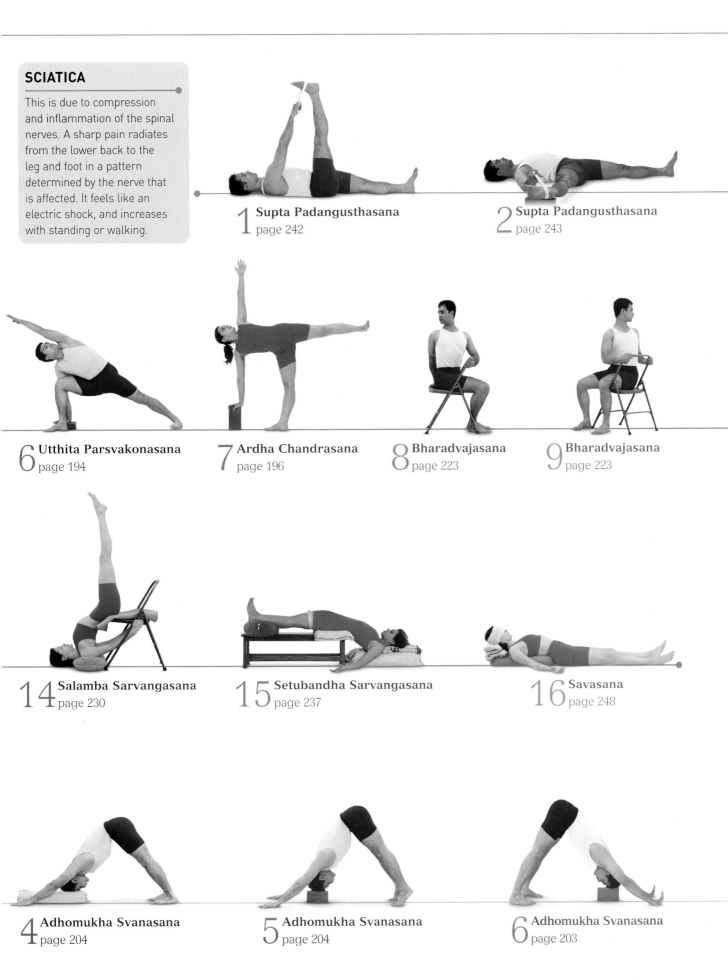

SCIATICA

This is due to compression and inflammation of the spinal nerves. A sharp pain radiates from the lower back to the leg and foot in a pattern determined by the nerve that is affected. It feels like an electric shock, and increases with standing or walking.

1 **Supta Padangusthasana** page 242

2 **Supta Padangusthasana** page 243

6 **Utthita Parsvakonasana** page 194

7 **Ardha Chandrasana** page 196

8 **Bharadvajasana** page 223

9 **Bharadvajasana** page 223

14 **Salamba Sarvangasana** page 230

15 **Setubandha Sarvangasana** page 237

16 **Savasana** page 248

4 **Adhomukha Svanasana** page 204

5 **Adhomukha Svanasana** page 204

6 **Adhomukha Svanasana** page 203

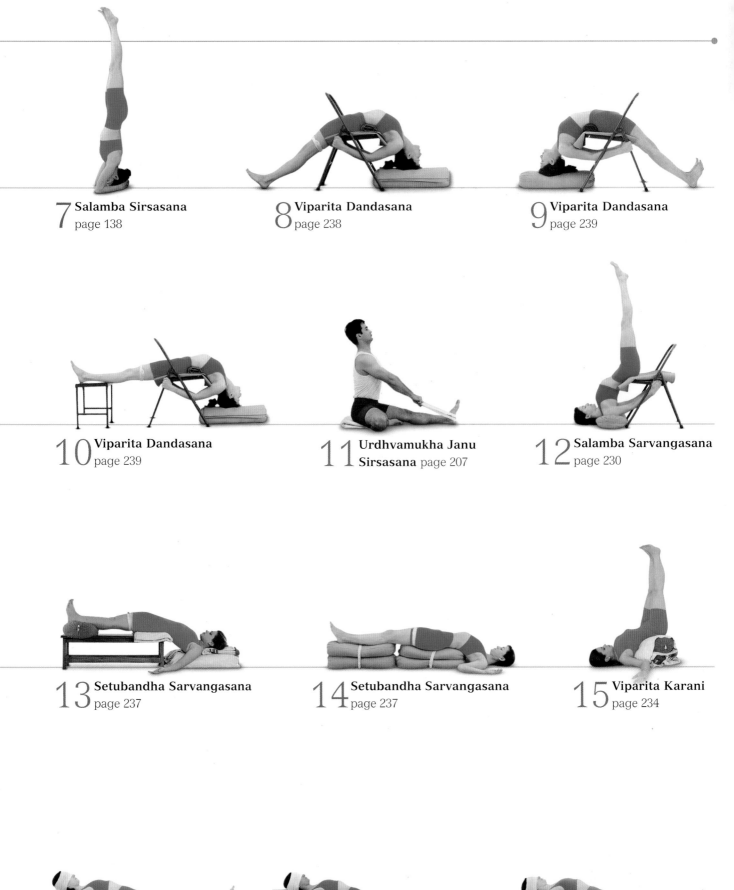

7 **Salamba Sirsasana**
page 138

8 **Viparita Dandasana**
page 238

9 **Viparita Dandasana**
page 239

10 **Viparita Dandasana**
page 239

11 **Urdhvamukha Janu Sirsasana** page 207

12 **Salamba Sarvangasana**
page 230

13 **Setubandha Sarvangasana**
page 237

14 **Setubandha Sarvangasana**
page 237

15 **Viparita Karani**
page 234

16 **Savasana**
page 248

17 **Ujjayi Pranayama**
page 254

18 **Viloma 2 Pranayama**
page 257

MIND AND EMOTIONS

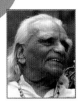

The tensions of daily life have an impact on our emotions. In yogic science, the secretions of the hormonal system are believed to influence the mind and the nervous system. Strong emotions are linked to hormonal imbalances which leave us vulnerable to infection and ill health. The following sequences of asanas work on the endocrine glands and the sympathetic and central nervous systems, to pacify the nerves, reduce the respiratory rate, and calm a stressed body and mind.

IRRITABILITY

Short bursts of impatience and overreaction to daily events are the result of stress factors, which arise from major life changes such as divorce or bereavement, and from sleep deprivation, work-related anxieties, or allergies. These asanas help reduce stress.

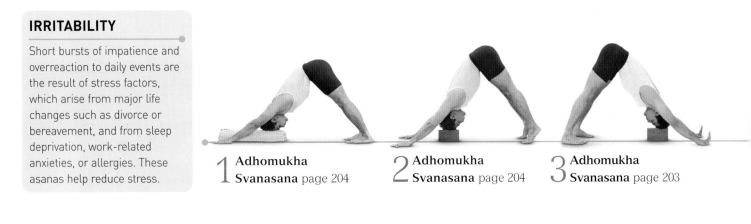

1 **Adhomukha Svanasana** page 204

2 **Adhomukha Svanasana** page 204

3 **Adhomukha Svanasana** page 203

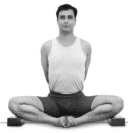
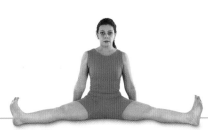
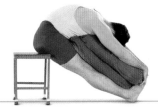

4 **Baddhakonasana** page 208

5 **Upavista Konasana** page 213

6 **Adhomukha Paschimottanasana** page 217

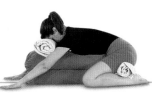
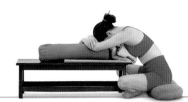
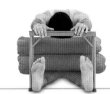
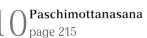

7 **Adhomukha Virasana** page 221

8 **Adhomukha Swastikasana** page 222

9 **Paschimottanasana** page 216

10 **Paschimottanasana** page 215

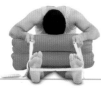

11 **Paschimottanasana**
page 216

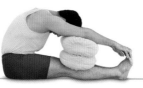

12 **Paschimottanasana**
page 214

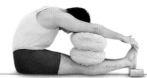

13 **Paschimottanasana**
page 215

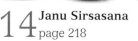

14 **Janu Sirsasana**
page 218

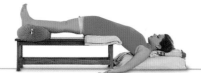

19 **Setubandha Sarvangasana**
page 237

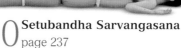

20 **Setubandha Sarvangasana**
page 237

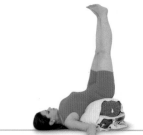

21 **Viparita Karani**
page 234

MENTAL FATIGUE

This condition is characterized by forgetfulness, irritability, boredom, confusion, lack of concentration, and depression. Its causes include lack of sleep, emotional loss, or stress in the workplace. The potential seriousness of this condition is often underestimated.

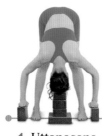

1 **Uttanasana**
page 197

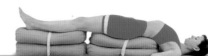

2 **Adhomukha Svanasana**
page 202

3 **Adhomukha Svanasana**
page 204

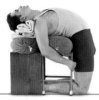

8 **Ustrasana**
page 240

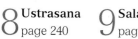

9 **Salamba Sirsasana**
page 138

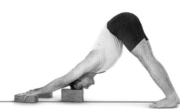

10 **Adhomukha Virasana**
page 221

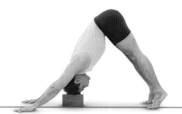

11 **Adhomukha Paschimottanasana**
page 217

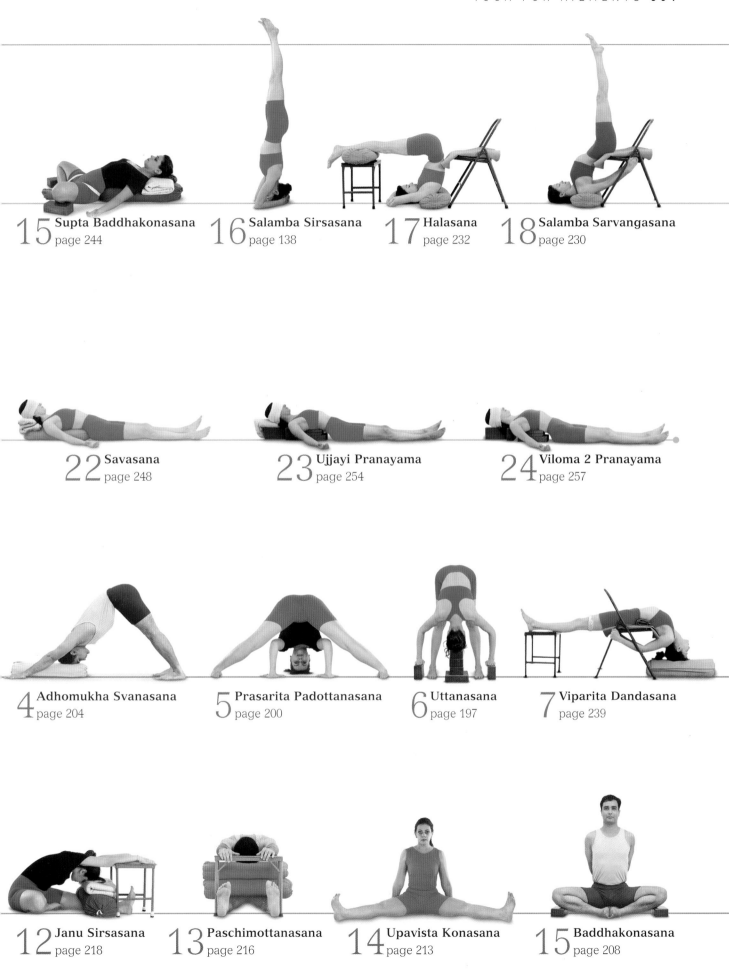

15 **Supta Baddhakonasana** page 244

16 **Salamba Sirsasana** page 138

17 **Halasana** page 232

18 **Salamba Sarvangasana** page 230

22 **Savasana** page 248

23 **Ujjayi Pranayama** page 254

24 **Viloma 2 Pranayama** page 257

4 **Adhomukha Svanasana** page 204

5 **Prasarita Padottanasana** page 200

6 **Uttanasana** page 197

7 **Viparita Dandasana** page 239

12 **Janu Sirsasana** page 218

13 **Paschimottanasana** page 216

14 **Upavista Konasana** page 213

15 **Baddhakonasana** page 208

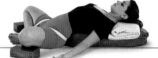

16 **Supta Baddhakonasana**
page 244

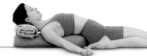

17 **Supta Virasana**
page 246

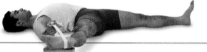

18 **Supta Padangusthasana**
page 243

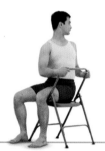

22 **Bharadvajasana**
page 223

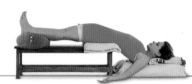

23 **Setubandha Sarvangasana**
page 237

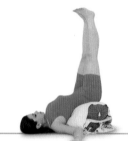

24 **Viparita Karani**
page 234

INSOMNIA

Periodic wakefulness, difficulty in falling asleep, or waking up too early, are symptoms of insomnia. They can be transient and pass with the life crises that cause them, or they can be chronic, associated with medical or psychiatric conditions, or long-term medication.

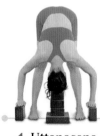

1 **Uttanasana**
page 197

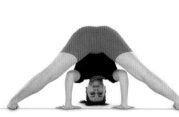

2 **Prasarita Padottanasana**
page 200

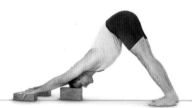

3 **Adhomukha Svanasana**
page 202

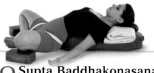

8 **Supta Baddhakonasana**
page 244

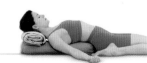

9 **Supta Virasana**
page 246

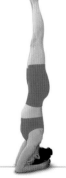

10 **Salamba Sirsasana**
page 138

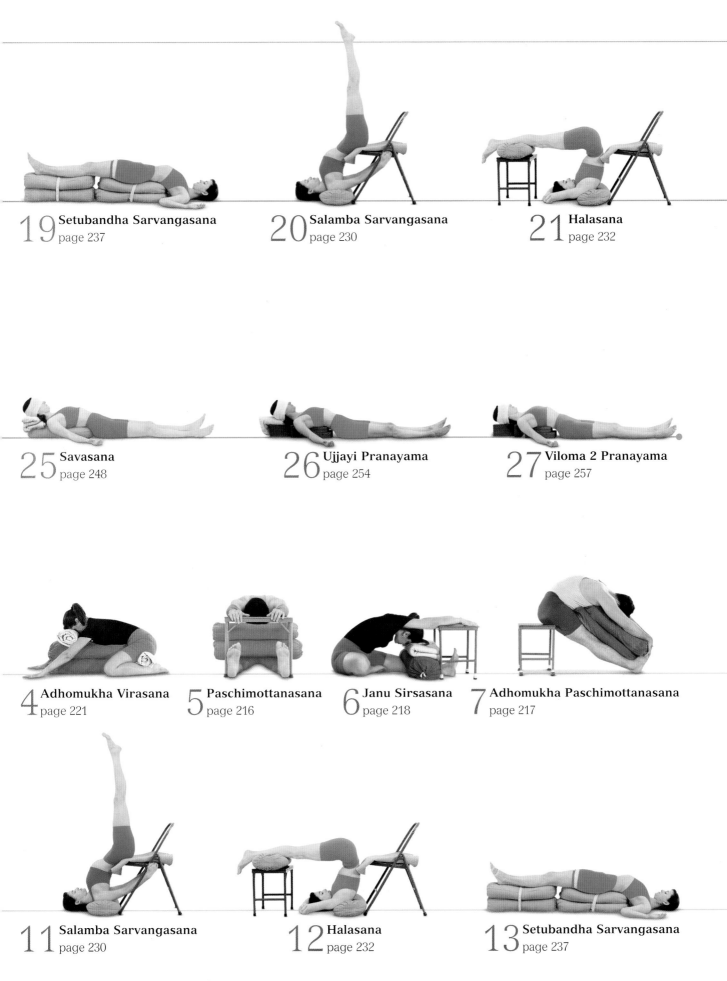

19 **Setubandha Sarvangasana**
page 237

20 **Salamba Sarvangasana**
page 230

21 **Halasana**
page 232

25 **Savasana**
page 248

26 **Ujjayi Pranayama**
page 254

27 **Viloma 2 Pranayama**
page 257

4 **Adhomukha Virasana**
page 221

5 **Paschimottanasana**
page 216

6 **Janu Sirsasana**
page 218

7 **Adhomukha Paschimottanasana**
page 217

11 **Salamba Sarvangasana**
page 230

12 **Halasana**
page 232

13 **Setubandha Sarvangasana**
page 237

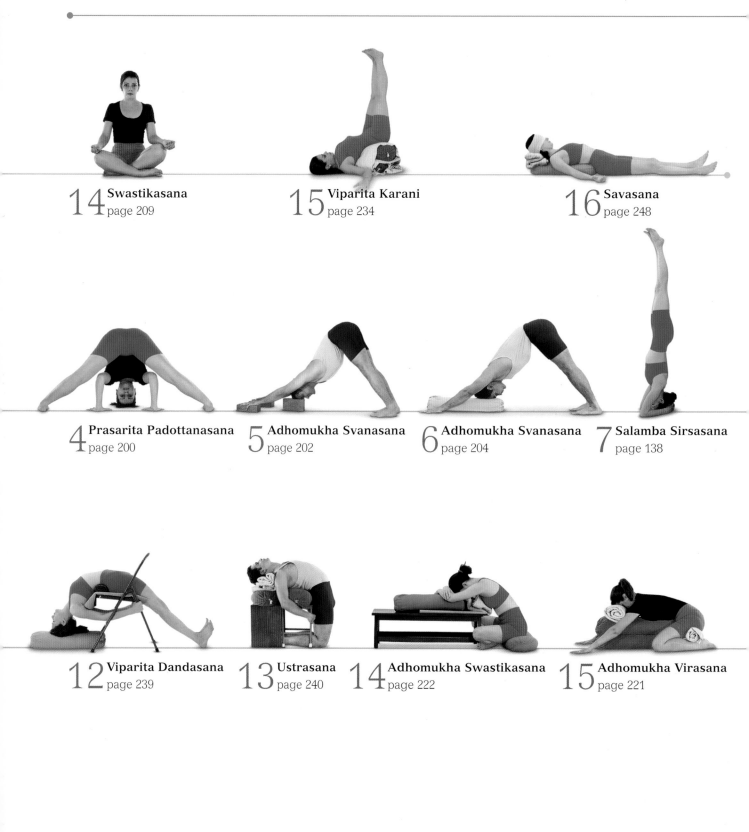

14 **Swastikasana**
page 209

15 **Viparita Karani**
page 234

16 **Savasana**
page 248

4 **Prasarita Padottanasana**
page 200

5 **Adhomukha Svanasana**
page 202

6 **Adhomukha Svanasana**
page 204

7 **Salamba Sirsasana**
page 138

12 **Viparita Dandasana**
page 239

13 **Ustrasana**
page 240

14 **Adhomukha Swastikasana**
page 222

15 **Adhomukha Virasana**
page 221

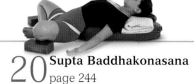

20 **Supta Baddhakonasana**
page 244

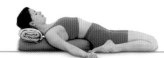

21 **Supta Virasana**
page 246

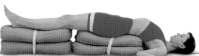

22 **Setubandha Sarvangasana**
page 237

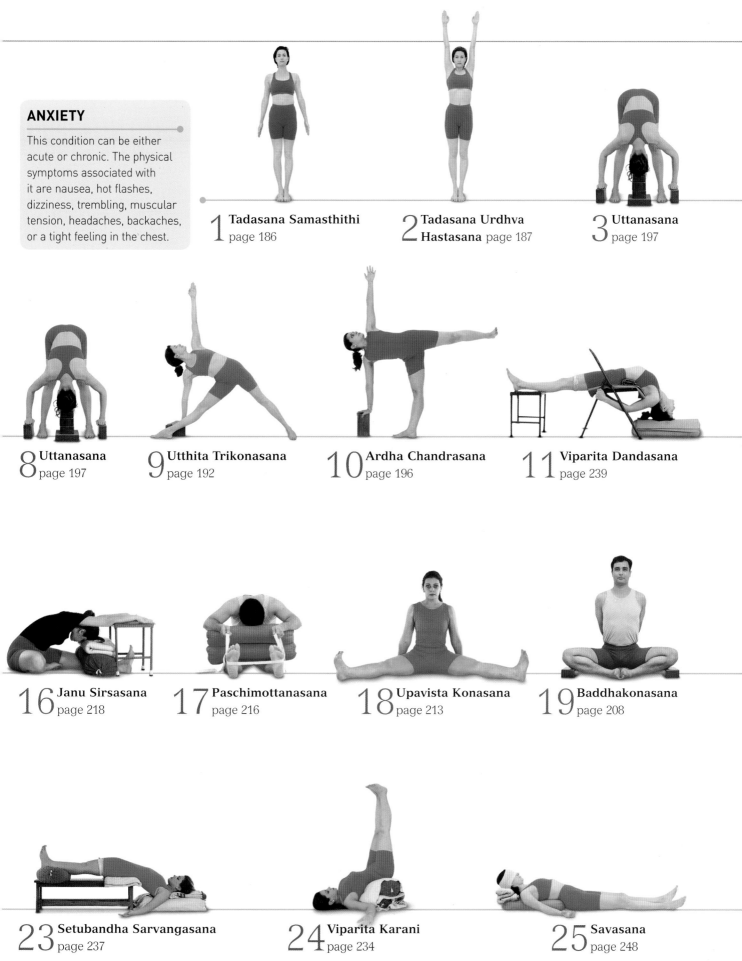

ANXIETY

This condition can be either acute or chronic. The physical symptoms associated with it are nausea, hot flashes, dizziness, trembling, muscular tension, headaches, backaches, or a tight feeling in the chest.

1 **Tadasana Samasthithi** page 186

2 **Tadasana Urdhva Hastasana** page 187

3 **Uttanasana** page 197

8 **Uttanasana** page 197

9 **Utthita Trikonasana** page 192

10 **Ardha Chandrasana** page 196

11 **Viparita Dandasana** page 239

16 **Janu Sirsasana** page 218

17 **Paschimottanasana** page 216

18 **Upavista Konasana** page 213

19 **Baddhakonasana** page 208

23 **Setubandha Sarvangasana** page 237

24 **Viparita Karani** page 234

25 **Savasana** page 248

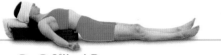

26 **Ujjayi Pranayama**
page 254

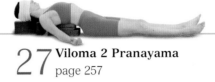

27 **Viloma 2 Pranayama**
page 257

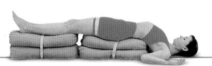

3 **Setubandha Sarvangasana**
page 237

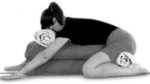

4 **Adhomukha Virasana**
page 221

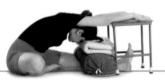

5 **Janu Sirsasana**
page 218

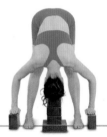

6 **Uttanasana**
page 197

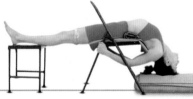

10 **Viparita Dandasana**
page 239

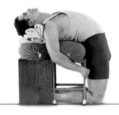

11 **Ustrasana**
page 240

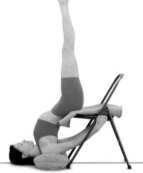

12 **Salamba Sarvangasana**
page 230

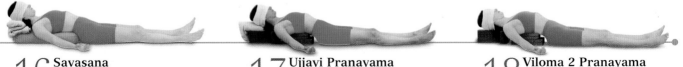

16 **Savasana**
page 248

17 **Ujjayi Pranayama**
page 254

18 **Viloma 2 Pranayama**
page 257

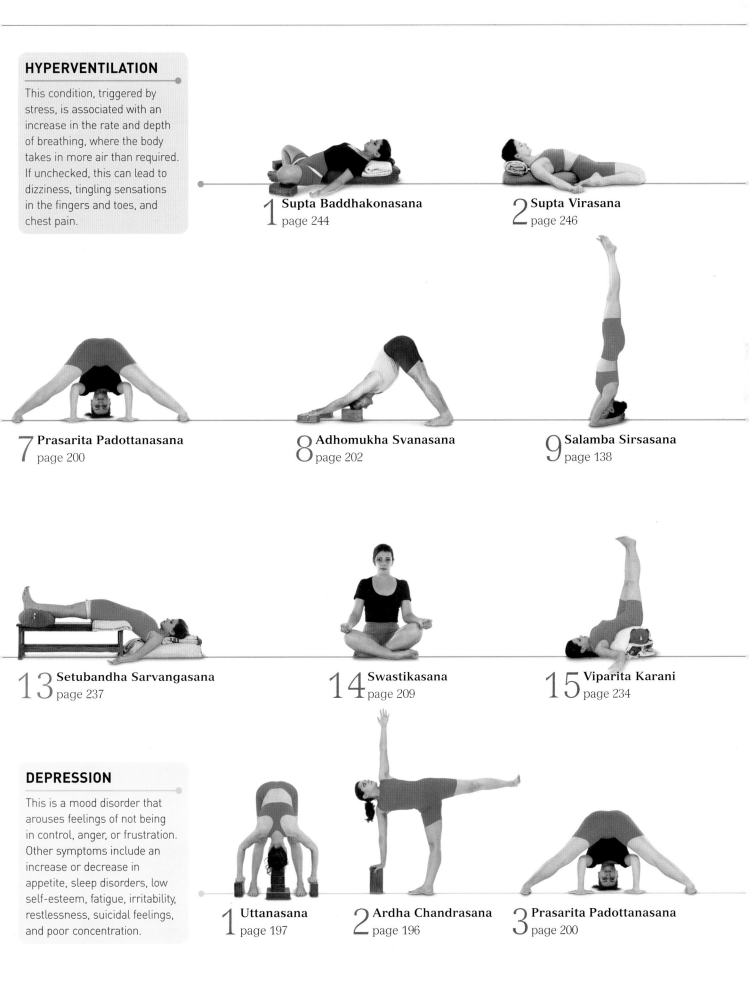

HYPERVENTILATION

This condition, triggered by stress, is associated with an increase in the rate and depth of breathing, where the body takes in more air than required. If unchecked, this can lead to dizziness, tingling sensations in the fingers and toes, and chest pain.

1 **Supta Baddhakonasana**
page 244

2 **Supta Virasana**
page 246

7 **Prasarita Padottanasana**
page 200

8 **Adhomukha Svanasana**
page 202

9 **Salamba Sirsasana**
page 138

13 **Setubandha Sarvangasana**
page 237

14 **Swastikasana**
page 209

15 **Viparita Karani**
page 234

DEPRESSION

This is a mood disorder that arouses feelings of not being in control, anger, or frustration. Other symptoms include an increase or decrease in appetite, sleep disorders, low self-esteem, fatigue, irritability, restlessness, suicidal feelings, and poor concentration.

1 **Uttanasana**
page 197

2 **Ardha Chandrasana**
page 196

3 **Prasarita Padottanasana**
page 200

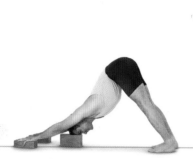

4 **Adhomukha Svanasana**
page 202

5 **Salamba Sirsasana**
page 138

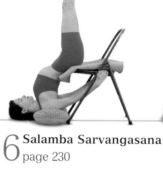

6 **Salamba Sarvangasana**
page 230

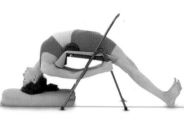

7 **Viparita Dandasana**
page 239

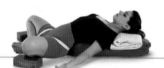

12 **Supta Baddhakonasana**
page 244

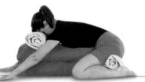

13 **Adhomukha Virasana** page 221

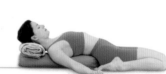

14 **Supta Virasana**
page 246

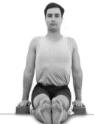

15 **Dandasana**
page 205

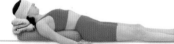

20 **Savasana**
page 248

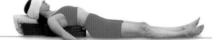

21 **Ujjayi Pranayama**
page 254

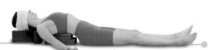

22 **Viloma 2 Pranayama**
page 257

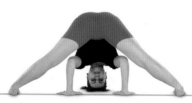

4 **Prasarita Padottanasana**
page 200

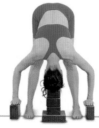

5 **Uttanasana**
page 197

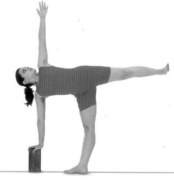

6 **Ardha Chandrasana**
page 196

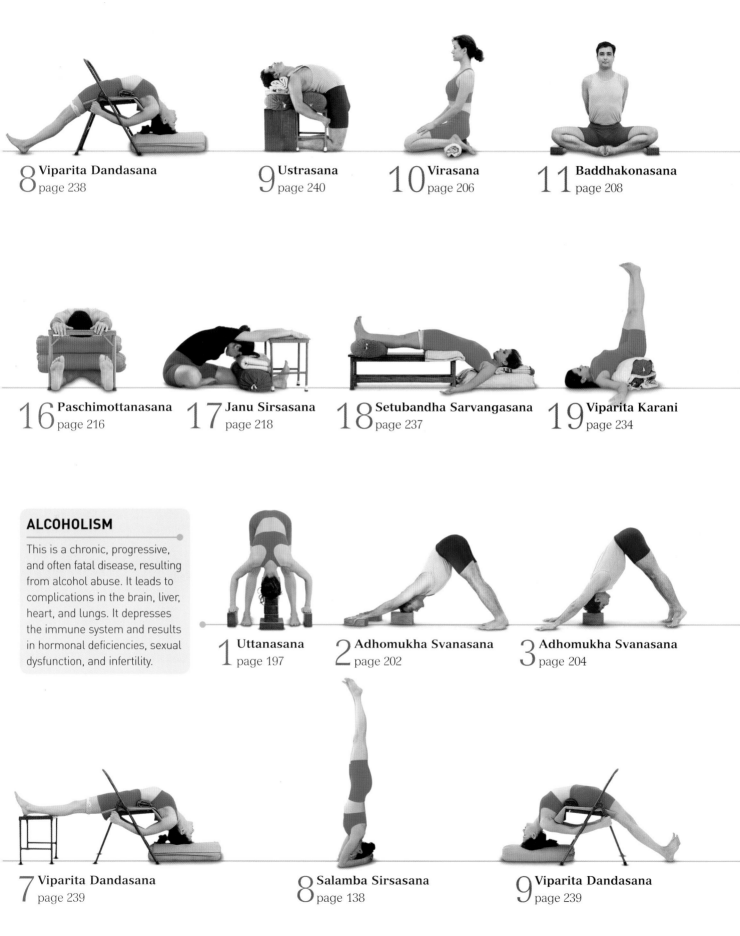

8 **Viparita Dandasana**
page 238

9 **Ustrasana**
page 240

10 **Virasana**
page 206

11 **Baddhakonasana**
page 208

16 **Paschimottanasana**
page 216

17 **Janu Sirsasana**
page 218

18 **Setubandha Sarvangasana**
page 237

19 **Viparita Karani**
page 234

ALCOHOLISM

This is a chronic, progressive, and often fatal disease, resulting from alcohol abuse. It leads to complications in the brain, liver, heart, and lungs. It depresses the immune system and results in hormonal deficiencies, sexual dysfunction, and infertility.

1 **Uttanasana**
page 197

2 **Adhomukha Svanasana**
page 202

3 **Adhomukha Svanasana**
page 204

7 **Viparita Dandasana**
page 239

8 **Salamba Sirsasana**
page 138

9 **Viparita Dandasana**
page 239

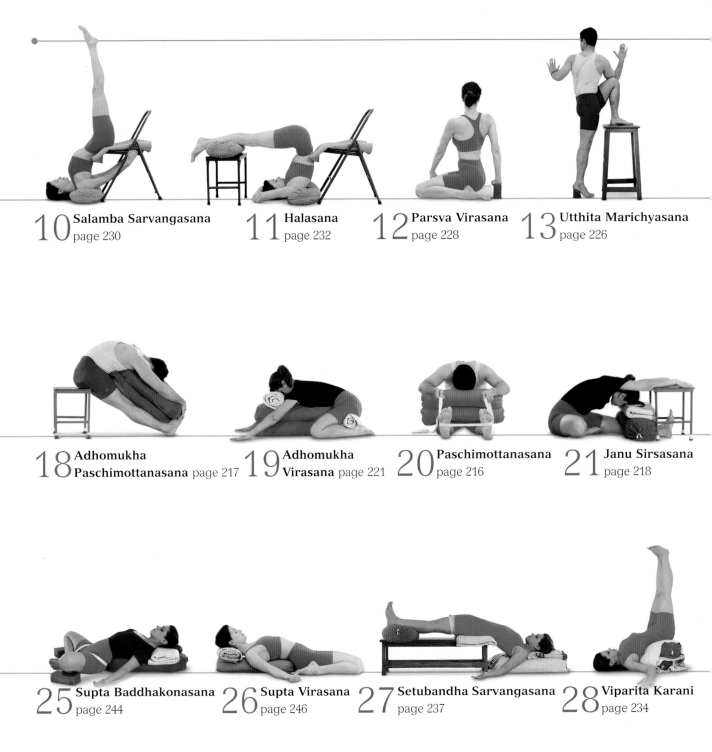

10 **Salamba Sarvangasana** page 230

11 **Halasana** page 232

12 **Parsva Virasana** page 228

13 **Utthita Marichyasana** page 226

18 **Adhomukha Paschimottanasana** page 217

19 **Adhomukha Virasana** page 221

20 **Paschimottanasana** page 216

21 **Janu Sirsasana** page 218

25 **Supta Baddhakonasana** page 244

26 **Supta Virasana** page 246

27 **Setubandha Sarvangasana** page 237

28 **Viparita Karani** page 234

BULIMIA

Binge eating followed by purging with self-induced vomiting and the compulsive use of laxatives, are common warning signs of this condition. Its causes include low body image and a feeling of not being in control. It is often associated with anorexia (*see page* 373).

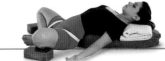

1 **Supta Baddhakonasana** page 244

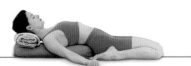

2 **Supta Virasana** page 246

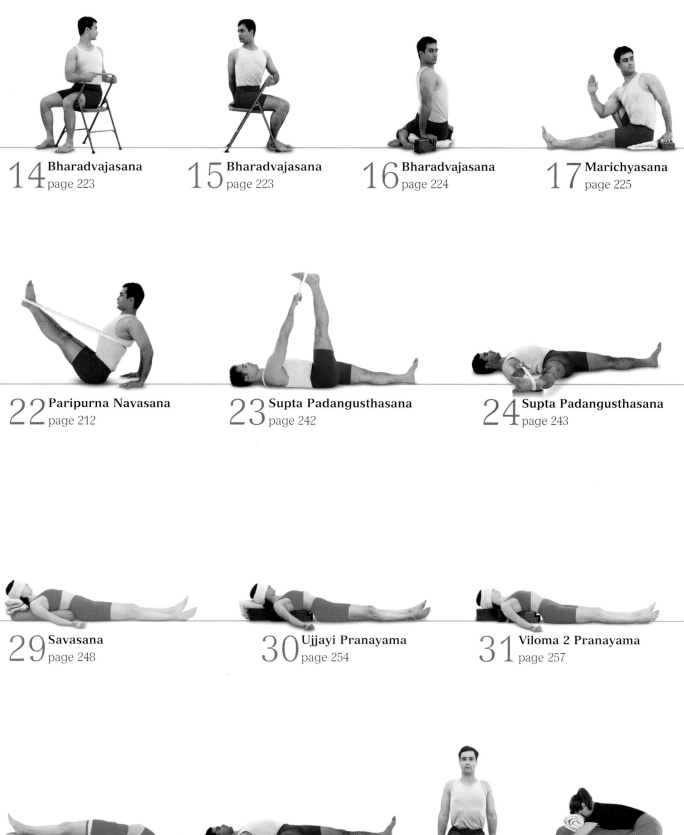

14 **Bharadvajasana**
page 223

15 **Bharadvajasana**
page 223

16 **Bharadvajasana**
page 224

17 **Marichyasana**
page 225

22 **Paripurna Navasana**
page 212

23 **Supta Padangusthasana**
page 242

24 **Supta Padangusthasana**
page 243

29 **Savasana**
page 248

30 **Ujjayi Pranayama**
page 254

31 **Viloma 2 Pranayama**
page 257

3 **Setubandha Sarvangasana**
page 237

4 **Supta Padangusthasana**
page 243

5 **Dandasana**
page 205

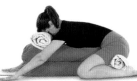

6 **Adhomukha Virasana**
page 221

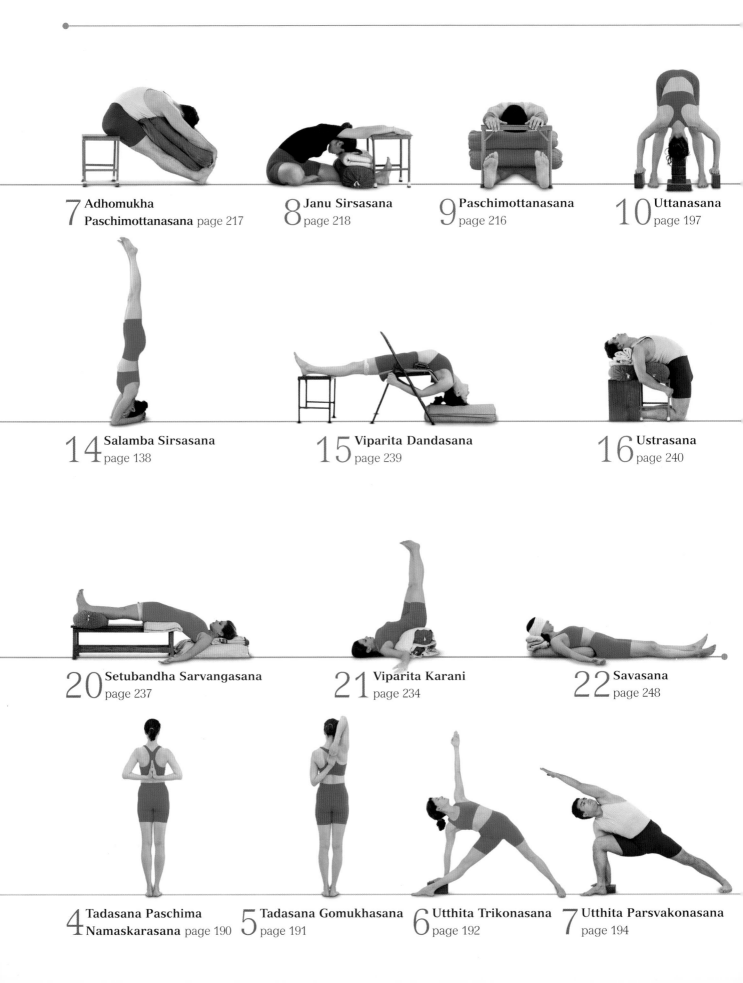

7 **Adhomukha Paschimottanasana** page 217

8 **Janu Sirsasana** page 218

9 **Paschimottanasana** page 216

10 **Uttanasana** page 197

14 **Salamba Sirsasana** page 138

15 **Viparita Dandasana** page 239

16 **Ustrasana** page 240

20 **Setubandha Sarvangasana** page 237

21 **Viparita Karani** page 234

22 **Savasana** page 248

4 **Tadasana Paschima Namaskarasana** page 190

5 **Tadasana Gomukhasana** page 191

6 **Utthita Trikonasana** page 192

7 **Utthita Parsvakonasana** page 194

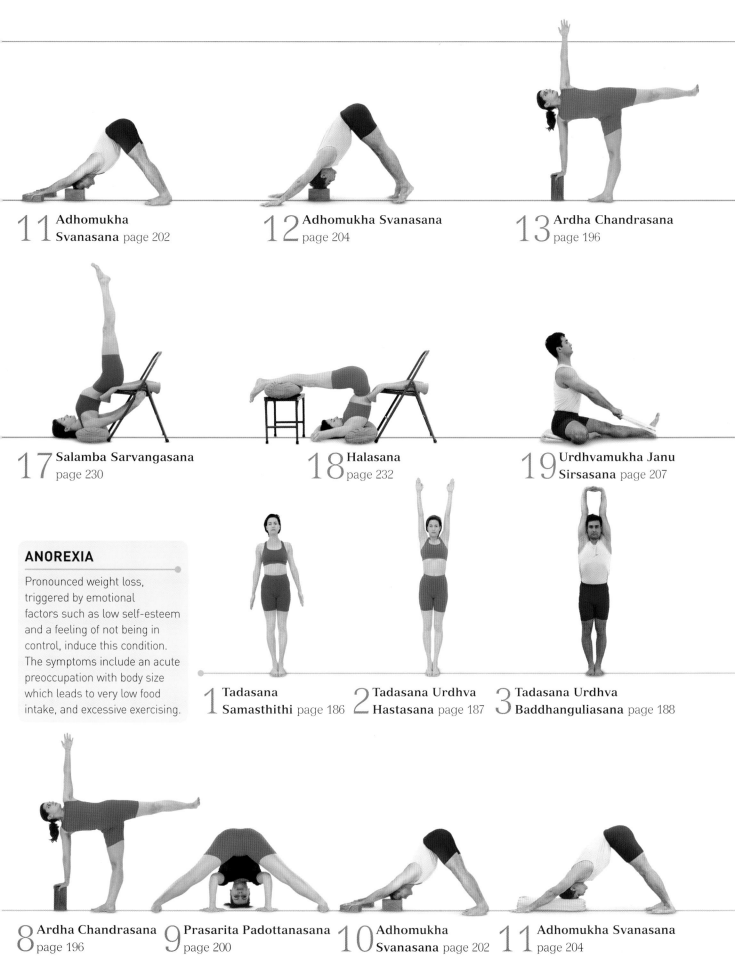

11 **Adhomukha Svanasana** page 202

12 **Adhomukha Svanasana** page 204

13 **Ardha Chandrasana** page 196

17 **Salamba Sarvangasana** page 230

18 **Halasana** page 232

19 **Urdhvamukha Janu Sirsasana** page 207

ANOREXIA

Pronounced weight loss, triggered by emotional factors such as low self-esteem and a feeling of not being in control, induce this condition. The symptoms include an acute preoccupation with body size which leads to very low food intake, and excessive exercising.

1 **Tadasana Samasthithi** page 186

2 **Tadasana Urdhva Hastasana** page 187

3 **Tadasana Urdhva Baddhanguliasana** page 188

8 **Ardha Chandrasana** page 196

9 **Prasarita Padottanasana** page 200

10 **Adhomukha Svanasana** page 202

11 **Adhomukha Svanasana** page 204

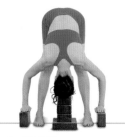

12 **Uttanasana**
page 197

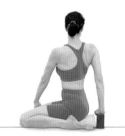

13 **Parsva Virasana**
page 228

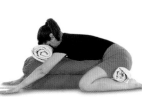

14 **Adhomukha Virasana**
page 221

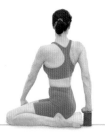

15 **Parsva Virasana**
page 228

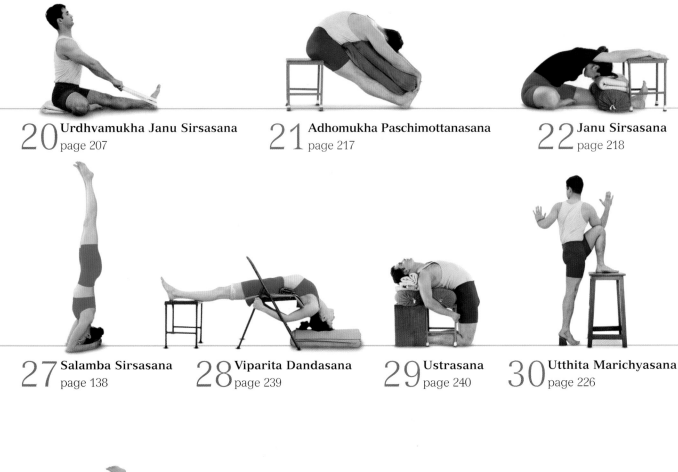

20 **Urdhvamukha Janu Sirsasana**
page 207

21 **Adhomukha Paschimottanasana**
page 217

22 **Janu Sirsasana**
page 218

27 **Salamba Sirsasana**
page 138

28 **Viparita Dandasana**
page 239

29 **Ustrasana**
page 240

30 **Utthita Marichyasana**
page 226

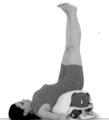

34 **Viparita Karani**
page 234

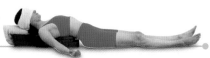

35 **Savasana**
page 248

36 **Ujjayi Pranayama**
page 254

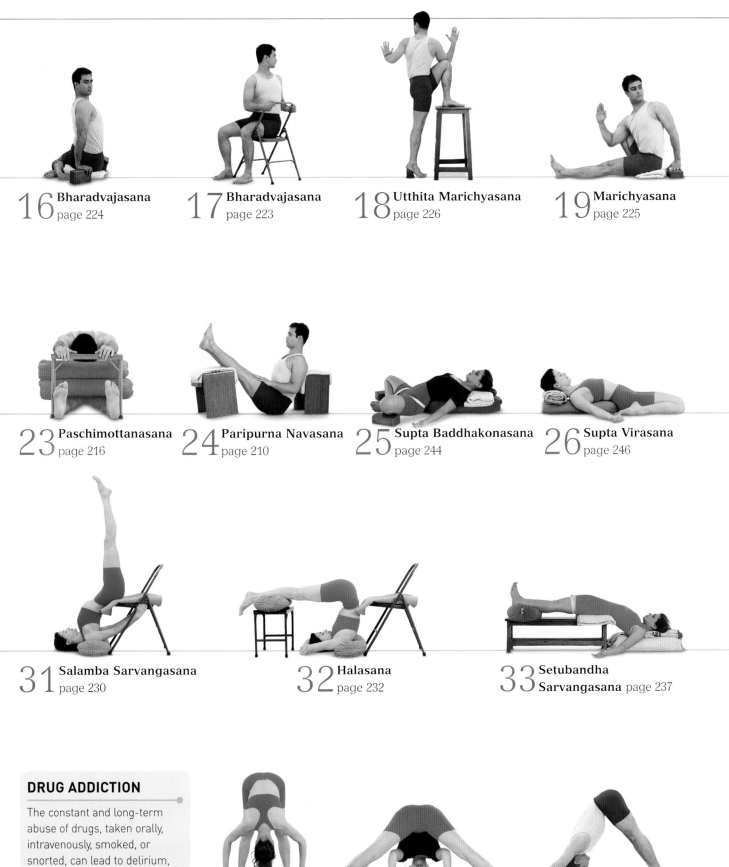

16 **Bharadvajasana**
page 224

17 **Bharadvajasana**
page 223

18 **Utthita Marichyasana**
page 226

19 **Marichyasana**
page 225

23 **Paschimottanasana**
page 216

24 **Paripurna Navasana**
page 210

25 **Supta Baddhakonasana**
page 244

26 **Supta Virasana**
page 246

31 **Salamba Sarvangasana**
page 230

32 **Halasana**
page 232

33 **Setubandha
Sarvangasana** page 237

DRUG ADDICTION

The constant and long-term abuse of drugs, taken orally, intravenously, smoked, or snorted, can lead to delirium, depersonalization, panic attacks, severe paranoia, and impaired memory. Heavy doses can even be fatal.

1 **Uttanasana**
page 197

2 **Prasarita Padottanasana**
page 200

3 **Adhomukha Svanasana**
page 204

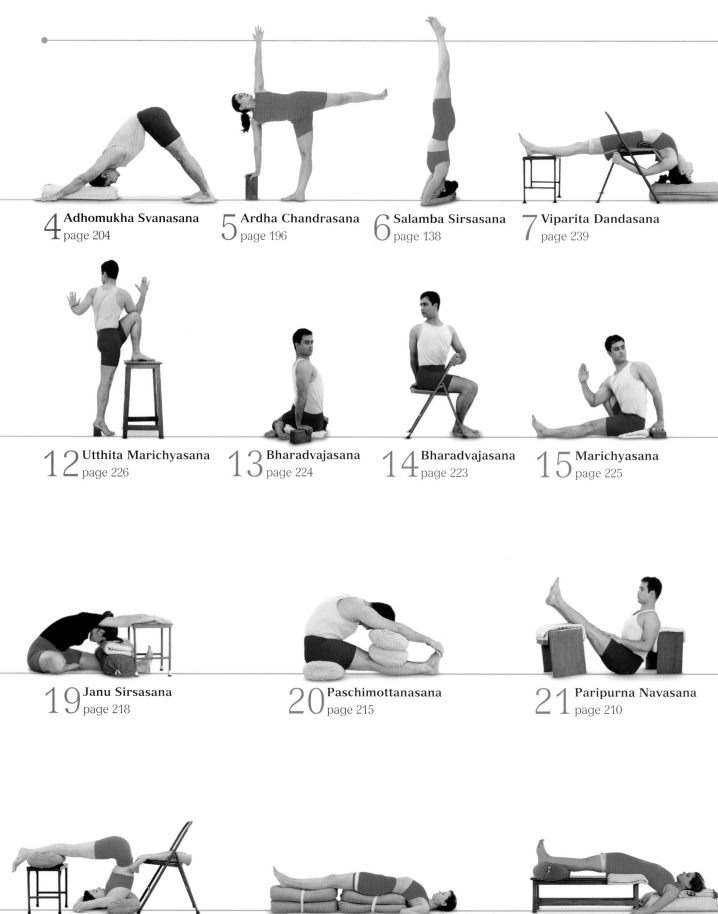

4 **Adhomukha Svanasana** page 204

5 **Ardha Chandrasana** page 196

6 **Salamba Sirsasana** page 138

7 **Viparita Dandasana** page 239

12 **Utthita Marichyasana** page 226

13 **Bharadvajasana** page 224

14 **Bharadvajasana** page 223

15 **Marichyasana** page 225

19 **Janu Sirsasana** page 218

20 **Paschimottanasana** page 215

21 **Paripurna Navasana** page 210

25 **Halasana** page 232

26 **Setubandha Sarvangasana** page 237

27 **Setubandha Sarvangasana** page 237

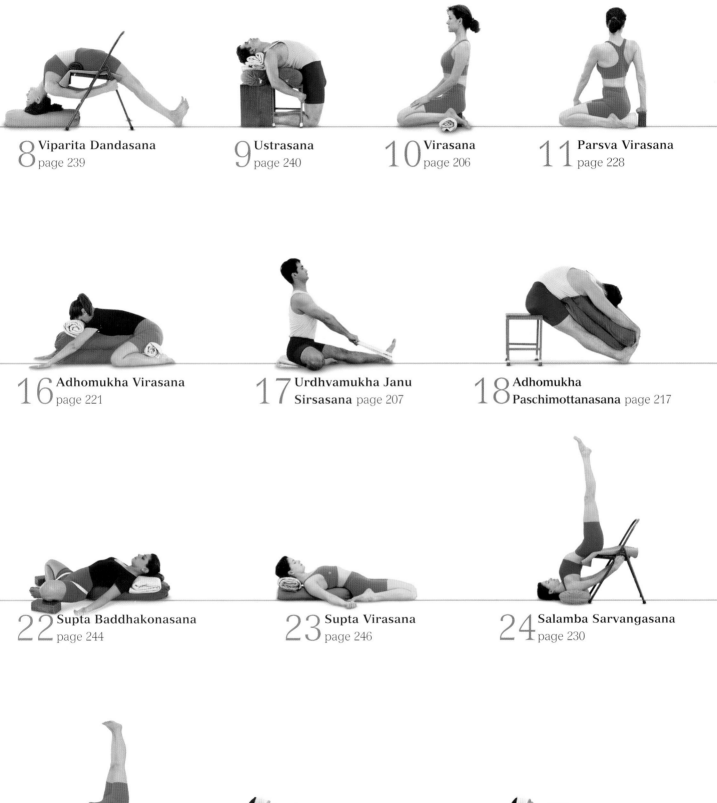

8 **Viparita Dandasana**
page 239

9 **Ustrasana**
page 240

10 **Virasana**
page 206

11 **Parsva Virasana**
page 228

16 **Adhomukha Virasana**
page 221

17 **Urdhvamukha Janu Sirsasana** page 207

18 **Adhomukha Paschimottanasana** page 217

22 **Supta Baddhakonasana**
page 244

23 **Supta Virasana**
page 246

24 **Salamba Sarvangasana**
page 230

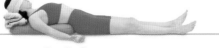

28 **Viparita Karani**
page 234

29 **Savasana**
page 248

30 **Ujjayi Pranayama**
page 254

WOMEN'S HEALTH

Practicing yoga can help prevent or reduce the severity of many ailments that specifically affect women, by providing a form of treatment directed at the basic causes. For instance, yoga can help correct gynecological factors that lead to hypertension, diabetes, indigestion, degeneration in the bones and joints, hernia, and varicose veins. Yoga also helps regulate menstrual disorders, thyroid imbalance, the effects of osteoporosis, and the side effects of menopause.

MENSTRUATION

Menstruation is not an ailment, but it can sometimes cause discomfort. When menstruating, avoid inversions and standing poses, but practice forward bends, along with the following sequences, since they control the flow of blood and check excess discharge. The following sequence tones your system.

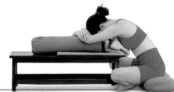

1 **Supta Baddhakonasana**
page 244

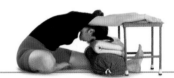

2 **Supta Virasana**
page 246

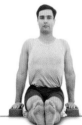

6 **Dandasana**
page 205

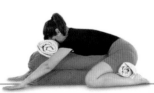

7 **Adhomukha Virasana**
page 221

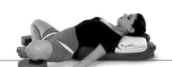

8 **Adhomukha Swastikasana**
page 222

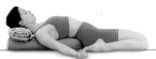

9 **Janu Sirsasana**
page 218

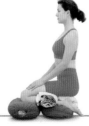

13 **Virasana**
page 206

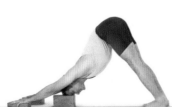

14 **Adhomukha Svanasana**
page 202

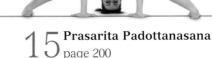

15 **Prasarita Padottanasana**
page 200

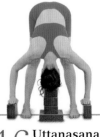

16 **Uttanasana**
page 197

"Spiritual yoga uses the intellect of the heart as well as the head."

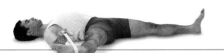

3 Supta Padangusthasana
page 243

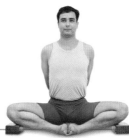

4 Baddhakonasana
page 208

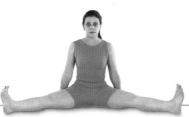

5 Upavista Konasana
page 213

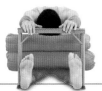

10 Paschimottanasana
page 216

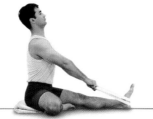

11 Urdhvamukha Janu
Sirsasana page 207

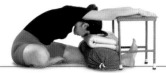

12 Janu Sirsasana
page 218

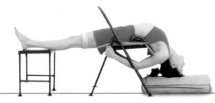

17 Viparita Dandasana
page 239

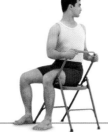

18 Bharadvajasana
page 223

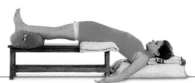

19 Setubandha Sarvangasana
page 237

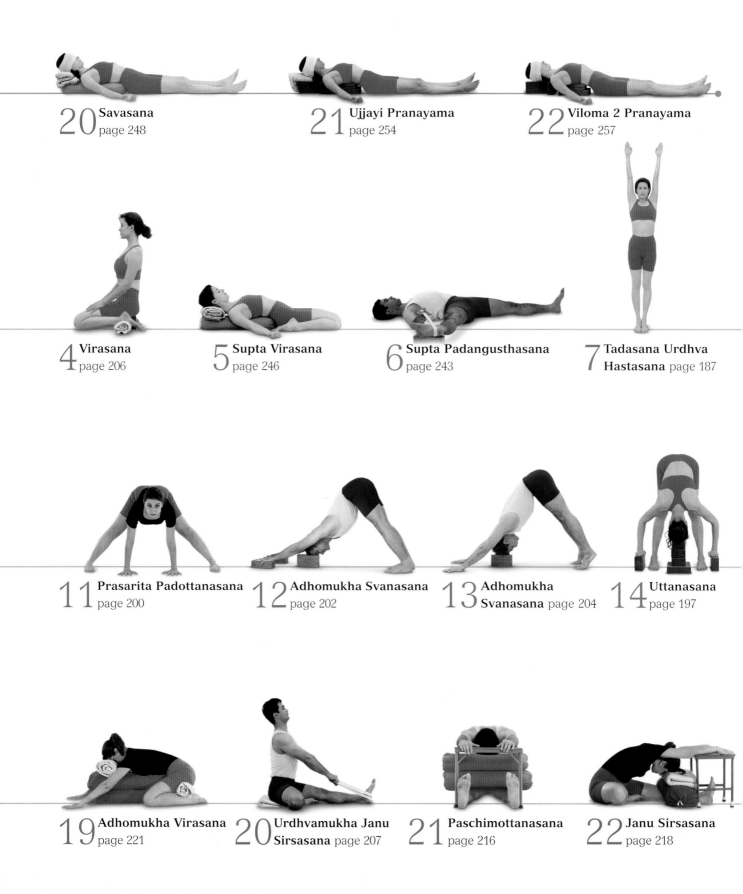

20 **Savasana** page 248

21 **Ujjayi Pranayama** page 254

22 **Viloma 2 Pranayama** page 257

4 **Virasana** page 206

5 **Supta Virasana** page 246

6 **Supta Padangusthasana** page 243

7 **Tadasana Urdhva Hastasana** page 187

11 **Prasarita Padottanasana** page 200

12 **Adhomukha Svanasana** page 202

13 **Adhomukha Svanasana** page 204

14 **Uttanasana** page 197

19 **Adhomukha Virasana** page 221

20 **Urdhvamukha Janu Sirsasana** page 207

21 **Paschimottanasana** page 216

22 **Janu Sirsasana** page 218

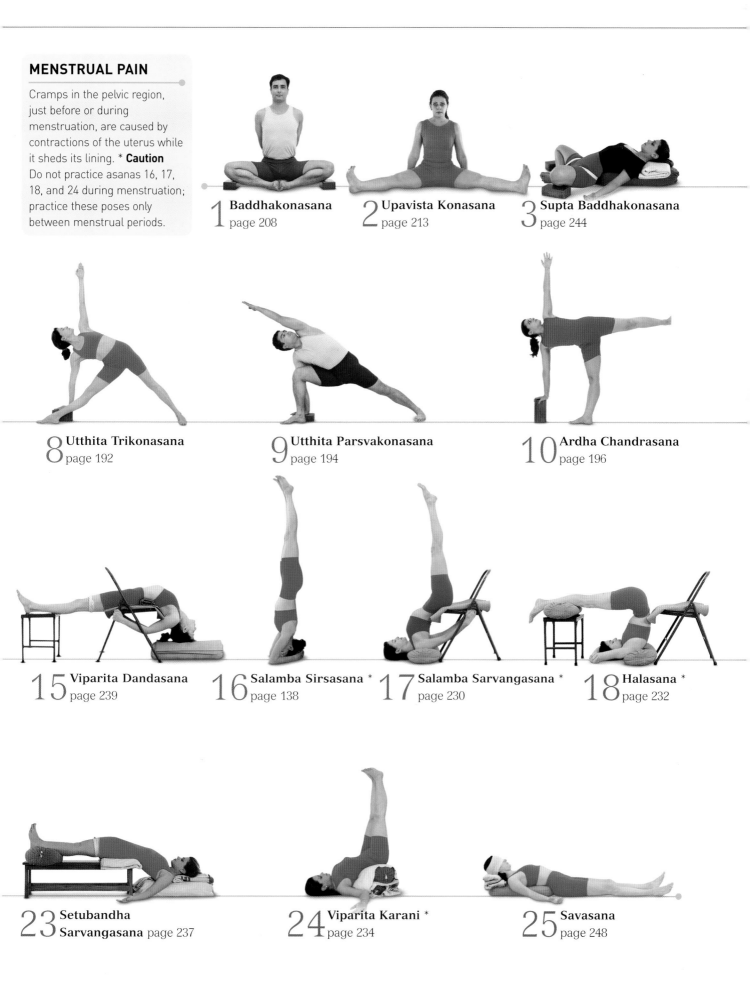

MENSTRUAL PAIN

Cramps in the pelvic region, just before or during menstruation, are caused by contractions of the uterus while it sheds its lining. * **Caution** Do not practice asanas 16, 17, 18, and 24 during menstruation; practice these poses only between menstrual periods.

1 **Baddhakonasana** page 208

2 **Upavista Konasana** page 213

3 **Supta Baddhakonasana** page 244

8 **Utthita Trikonasana** page 192

9 **Utthita Parsvakonasana** page 194

10 **Ardha Chandrasana** page 196

15 **Viparita Dandasana** page 239

16 **Salamba Sirsasana** * page 138

17 **Salamba Sarvangasana** * page 230

18 **Halasana** * page 232

23 **Setubandha Sarvangasana** page 237

24 **Viparita Karani** * page 234

25 **Savasana** page 248

PREMENSTRUAL SYNDROME

This is a condition that occurs 3–4 days before menstruation, and is relieved by its onset. The symptoms of premenstrual syndrome include mood swings, abdominal cramps, lower backache, and aching legs.

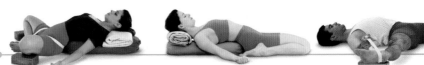

1 **Supta Baddhakonasana**
page 244

2 **Supta Virasana**
page 246

3 **Supta Padangusthasana**
page 243

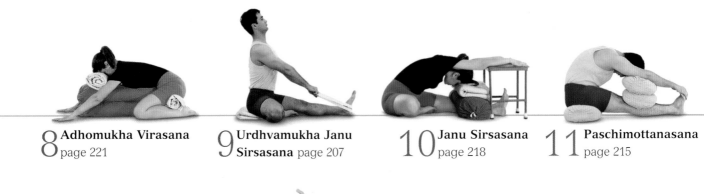

8 **Adhomukha Virasana**
page 221

9 **Urdhvamukha Janu Sirsasana** page 207

10 **Janu Sirsasana**
page 218

11 **Paschimottanasana**
page 215

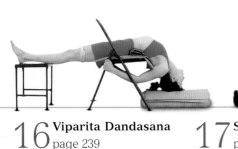

16 **Viparita Dandasana**
page 239

17 **Salamba Sarvangasana**
page 230

18 **Halasana**
page 232

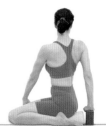

19 **Parsva Virasana**
page 228

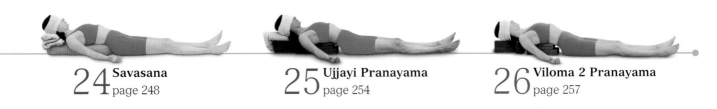

24 **Savasana**
page 248

25 **Ujjayi Pranayama**
page 254

26 **Viloma 2 Pranayama**
page 257

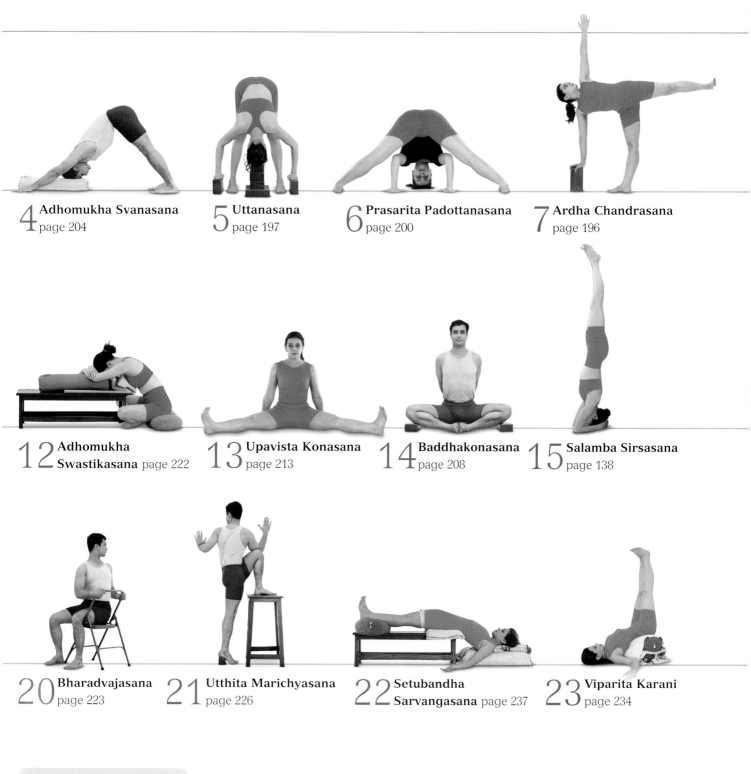

4 **Adhomukha Svanasana**
page 204

5 **Uttanasana**
page 197

6 **Prasarita Padottanasana**
page 200

7 **Ardha Chandrasana**
page 196

12 **Adhomukha Swastikasana** page 222

13 **Upavista Konasana**
page 213

14 **Baddhakonasana**
page 208

15 **Salamba Sirsasana**
page 138

20 **Bharadvajasana**
page 223

21 **Utthita Marichyasana**
page 226

22 **Setubandha Sarvangasana** page 237

23 **Viparita Karani**
page 234

MENOPAUSE

The cessation of the menstrual cycle, usually between the ages of 45–55, can occur abruptly or after a series of irregular periods. Menopause triggers hormonal changes and may cause sweating, hot flashes, depression, insomnia, and mood swings.

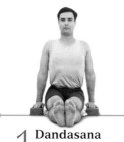

1 **Dandasana**
page 205

2 **Upavista Konasana**
page 213

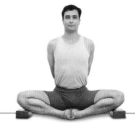

3 **Baddhakonasana**
page 208

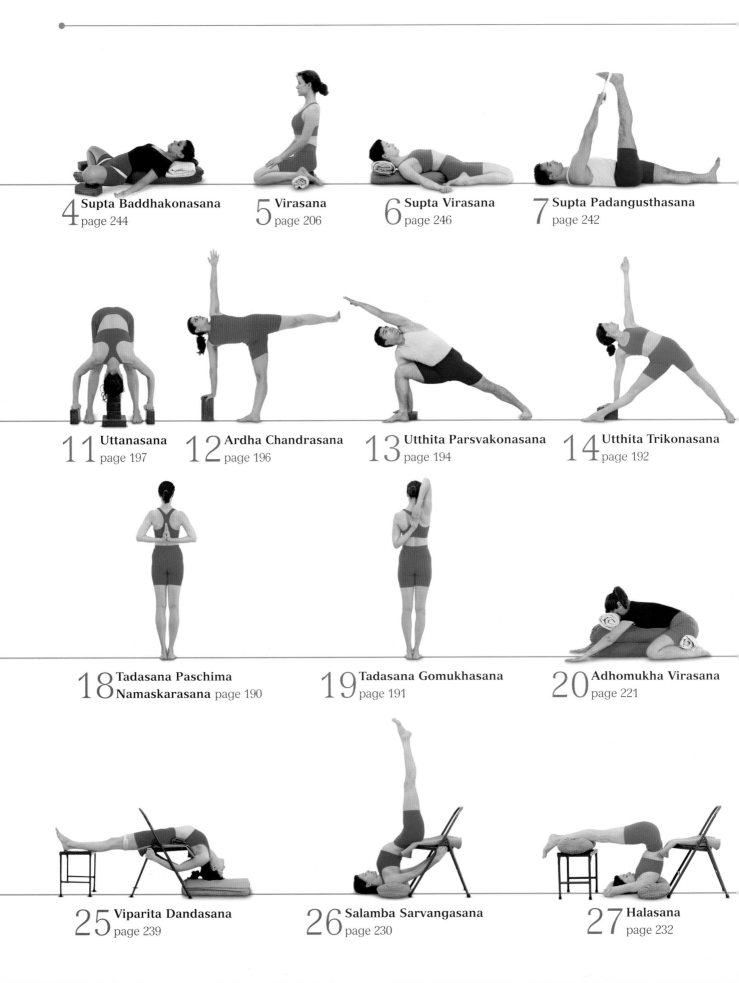

4 **Supta Baddhakonasana**
page 244

5 **Virasana**
page 206

6 **Supta Virasana**
page 246

7 **Supta Padangusthasana**
page 242

11 **Uttanasana**
page 197

12 **Ardha Chandrasana**
page 196

13 **Utthita Parsvakonasana**
page 194

14 **Utthita Trikonasana**
page 192

18 **Tadasana Paschima Namaskarasana** page 190

19 **Tadasana Gomukhasana**
page 191

20 **Adhomukha Virasana**
page 221

25 **Viparita Dandasana**
page 239

26 **Salamba Sarvangasana**
page 230

27 **Halasana**
page 232

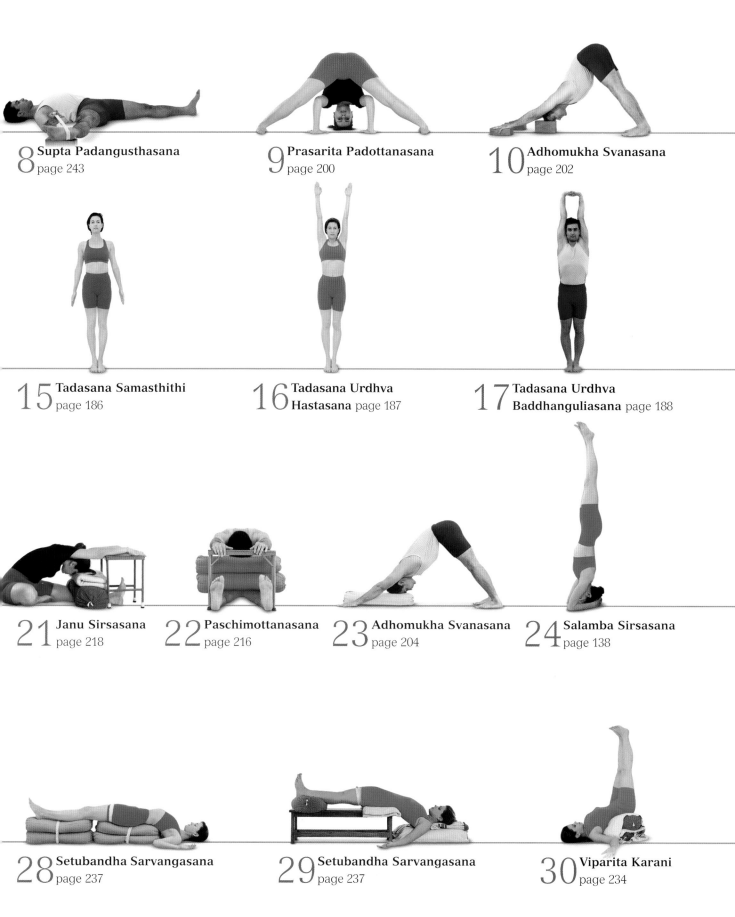

8 **Supta Padangusthasana**
page 243

9 **Prasarita Padottanasana**
page 200

10 **Adhomukha Svanasana**
page 202

15 **Tadasana Samasthithi**
page 186

16 **Tadasana Urdhva
Hastasana** page 187

17 **Tadasana Urdhva
Baddhanguliasana** page 188

21 **Janu Sirsasana**
page 218

22 **Paschimottanasana**
page 216

23 **Adhomukha Svanasana**
page 204

24 **Salamba Sirsasana**
page 138

28 **Setubandha Sarvangasana**
page 237

29 **Setubandha Sarvangasana**
page 237

30 **Viparita Karani**
page 234

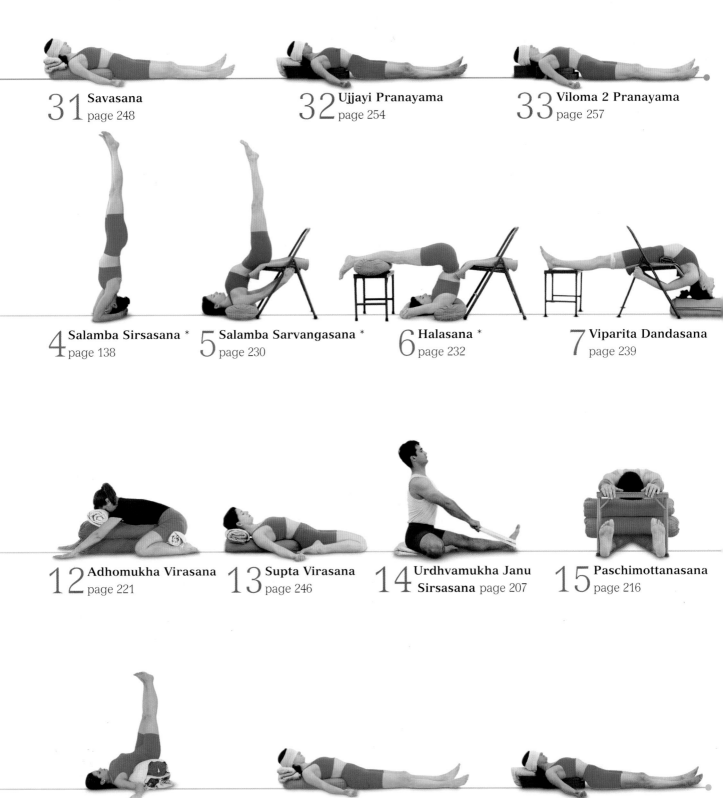

31 **Savasana**
page 248

32 **Ujjayi Pranayama**
page 254

33 **Viloma 2 Pranayama**
page 257

4 **Salamba Sirsasana** *
page 138

5 **Salamba Sarvangasana** *
page 230

6 **Halasana** *
page 232

7 **Viparita Dandasana**
page 239

12 **Adhomukha Virasana**
page 221

13 **Supta Virasana**
page 246

14 **Urdhvamukha Janu Sirsasana** page 207

15 **Paschimottanasana**
page 216

19 **Viparita Karani** *
page 234

20 **Savasana**
page 248

21 **Ujjayi Pranayama**
page 254

METRORRHAGIA

This condition is characterized by irregular and heavy bleeding between menstrual periods. The causes include uterine cysts and fibroids, miscarriage, uterine inflammation, or displacement of the uterus. * **Caution** Avoid practicing asanas 4, 5, 6, 8, and 19 if bleeding continues, but practice them regularly when there is no bleeding.

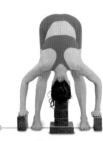
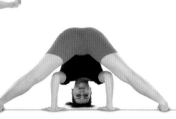

1 **Uttanasana**
page 197

2 **Ardha Chandrasana**
page 196

3 **Prasarita Padottanasana**
page 200

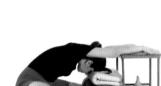
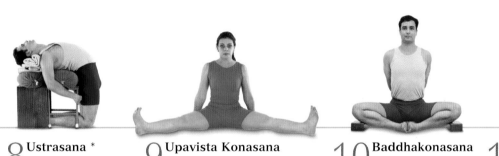

8 **Ustrasana** *
page 240

9 **Upavista Konasana**
page 213

10 **Baddhakonasana**
page 208

11 **Supta Baddhakonasana**
page 244

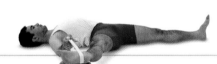
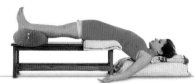

16 **Janu Sirsasana**
page 218

17 **Supta Padangusthasana**
page 243

18 **Setubandha Sarvangasana** page 237

LEUKORRHEA

Excess white discharge from the vagina can cause acute discomfort and embarrassment. It is usually caused by stress, the presence of a foreign body in the vagina, or an infection.

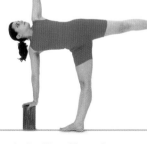
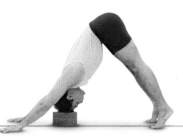

1 **Ardha Chandrasana**
page 196

2 **Uttanasana**
page 197

3 **Adhomukha Svanasana**
page 204

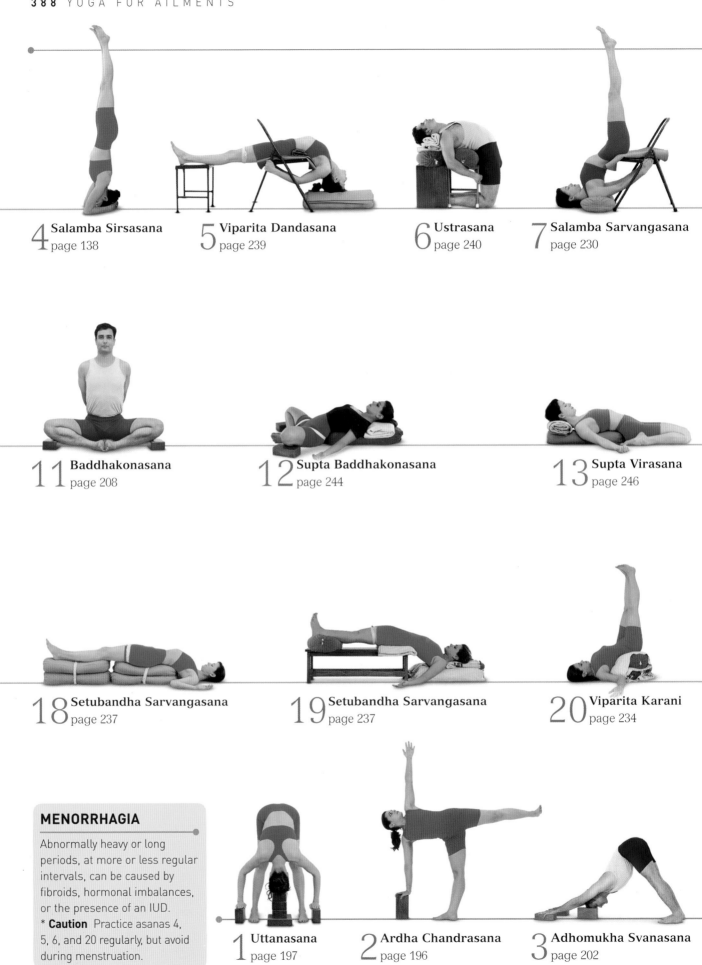

4 **Salamba Sirsasana**
page 138

5 **Viparita Dandasana**
page 239

6 **Ustrasana**
page 240

7 **Salamba Sarvangasana**
page 230

11 **Baddhakonasana**
page 208

12 **Supta Baddhakonasana**
page 244

13 **Supta Virasana**
page 246

18 **Setubandha Sarvangasana**
page 237

19 **Setubandha Sarvangasana**
page 237

20 **Viparita Karani**
page 234

MENORRHAGIA

Abnormally heavy or long periods, at more or less regular intervals, can be caused by fibroids, hormonal imbalances, or the presence of an IUD.

* Caution Practice asanas 4, 5, 6, and 20 regularly, but avoid during menstruation.

1 **Uttanasana**
page 197

2 **Ardha Chandrasana**
page 196

3 **Adhomukha Svanasana**
page 202

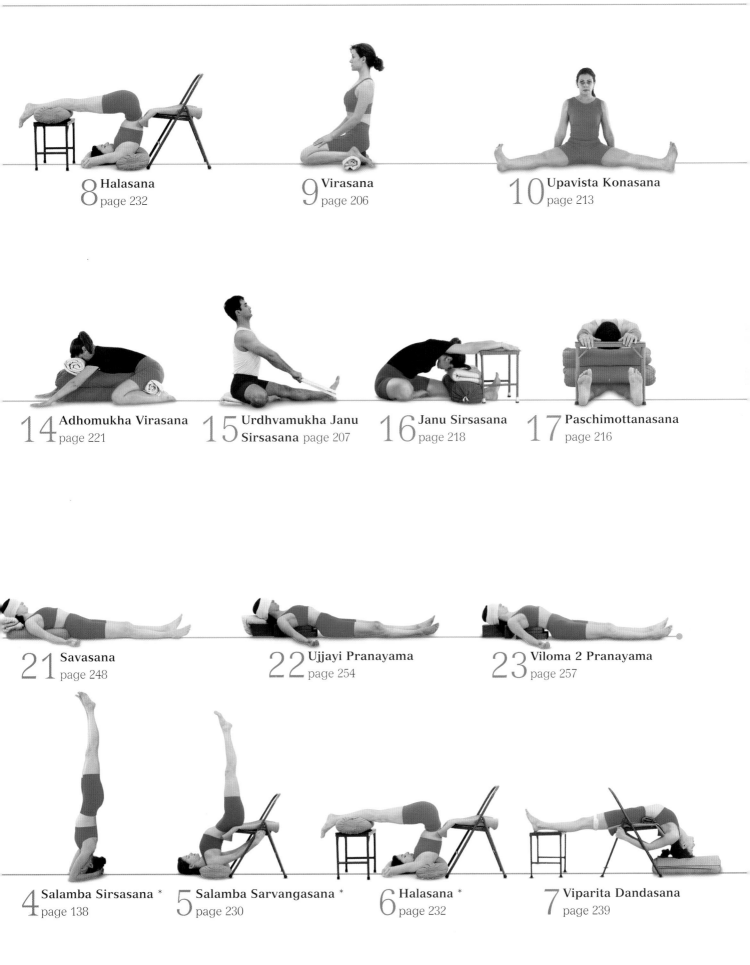

8 **Halasana**
page 232

9 **Virasana**
page 206

10 **Upavista Konasana**
page 213

14 **Adhomukha Virasana**
page 221

15 **Urdhvamukha Janu Sirsasana** page 207

16 **Janu Sirsasana**
page 218

17 **Paschimottanasana**
page 216

21 **Savasana**
page 248

22 **Ujjayi Pranayama**
page 254

23 **Viloma 2 Pranayama**
page 257

4 **Salamba Sirsasana** *
page 138

5 **Salamba Sarvangasana** *
page 230

6 **Halasana** *
page 232

7 **Viparita Dandasana**
page 239

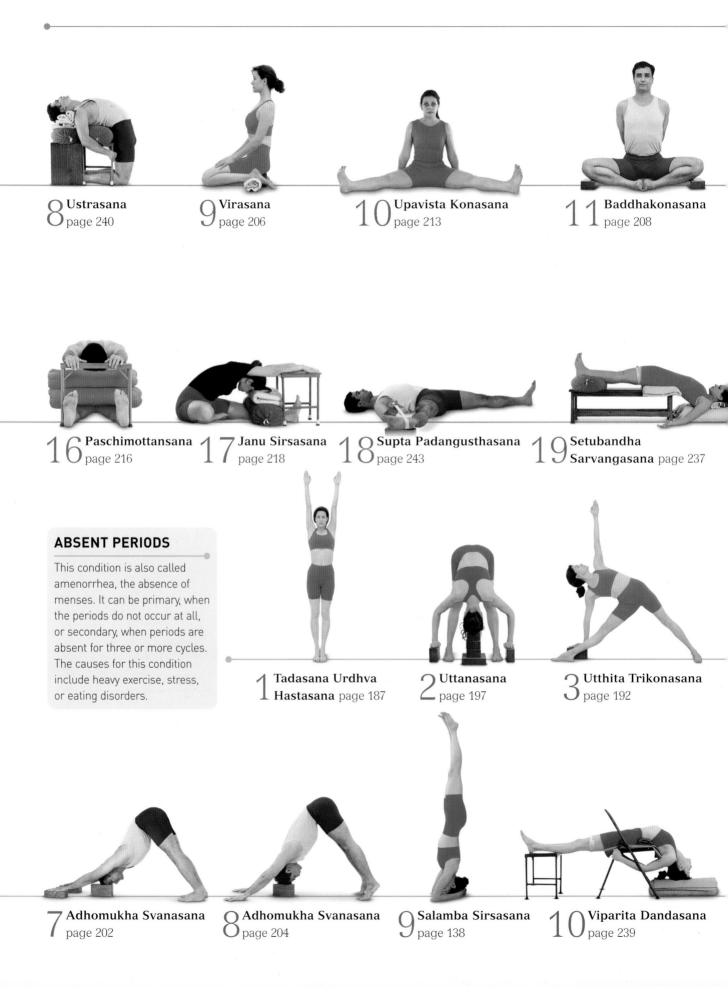

8 **Ustrasana**
page 240

9 **Virasana**
page 206

10 **Upavista Konasana**
page 213

11 **Baddhakonasana**
page 208

16 **Paschimottansana**
page 216

17 **Janu Sirsasana**
page 218

18 **Supta Padangusthasana**
page 243

19 **Setubandha**
Sarvangasana page 237

ABSENT PERIODS

This condition is also called amenorrhea, the absence of menses. It can be primary, when the periods do not occur at all, or secondary, when periods are absent for three or more cycles. The causes for this condition include heavy exercise, stress, or eating disorders.

1 **Tadasana Urdhva**
Hastasana page 187

2 **Uttanasana**
page 197

3 **Utthita Trikonasana**
page 192

7 **Adhomukha Svanasana**
page 202

8 **Adhomukha Svanasana**
page 204

9 **Salamba Sirsasana**
page 138

10 **Viparita Dandasana**
page 239

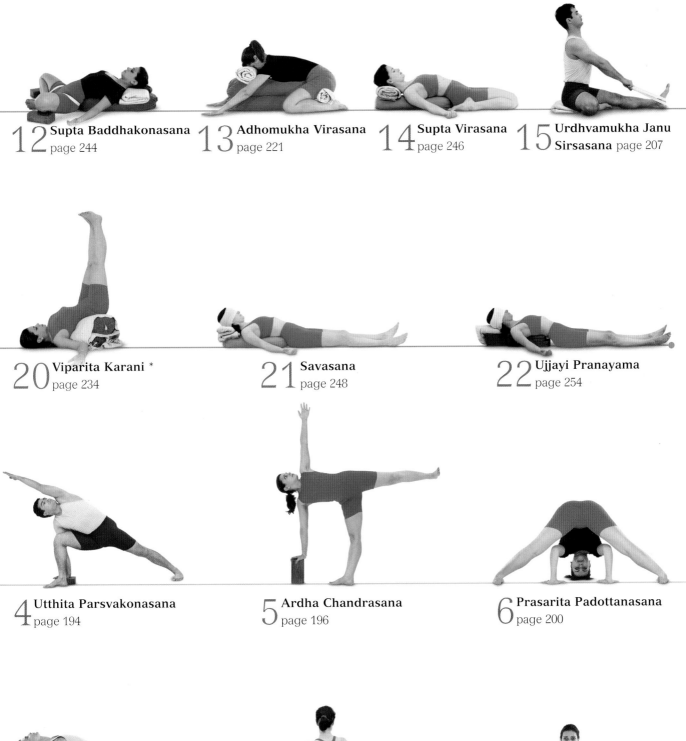

12 **Supta Baddhakonasana** page 244

13 **Adhomukha Virasana** page 221

14 **Supta Virasana** page 246

15 **Urdhvamukha Janu Sirsasana** page 207

20 **Viparita Karani** * page 234

21 **Savasana** page 248

22 **Ujjayi Pranayama** page 254

4 **Utthita Parsvakonasana** page 194

5 **Ardha Chandrasana** page 196

6 **Prasarita Padottanasana** page 200

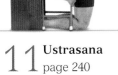

11 **Ustrasana** page 240

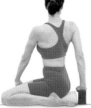

12 **Parsva Virasana** page 228

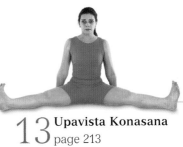

13 **Upavista Konasana** page 213

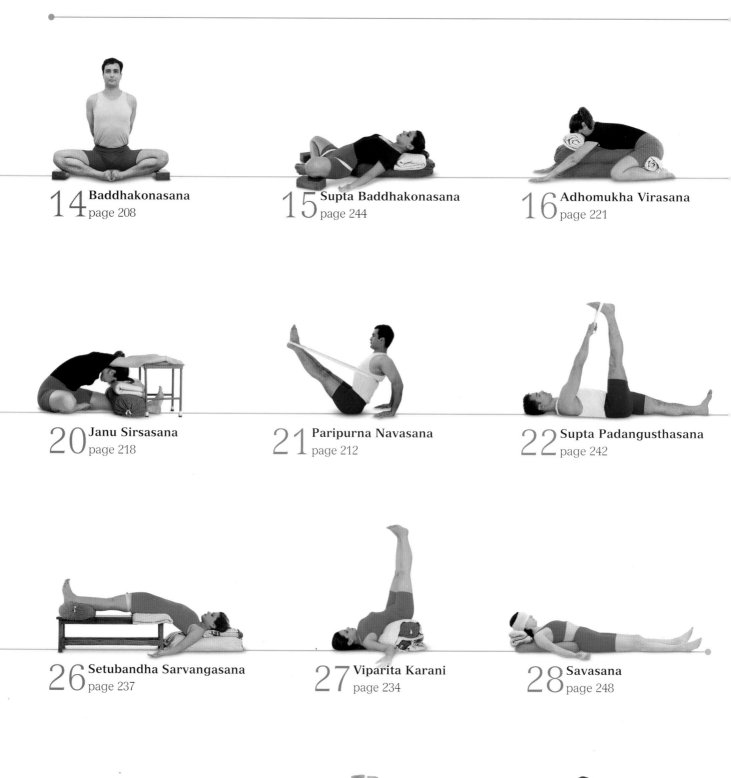

14 **Baddhakonasana**
page 208

15 **Supta Baddhakonasana**
page 244

16 **Adhomukha Virasana**
page 221

20 **Janu Sirsasana**
page 218

21 **Paripurna Navasana**
page 212

22 **Supta Padangusthasana**
page 242

26 **Setubandha Sarvangasana**
page 237

27 **Viparita Karani**
page 234

28 **Savasana**
page 248

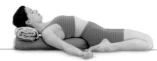

4 **Supta Virasana**
page 246

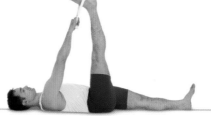

5 **Supta Padangusthasana**
page 242

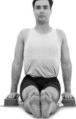

6 **Dandasana**
page 205

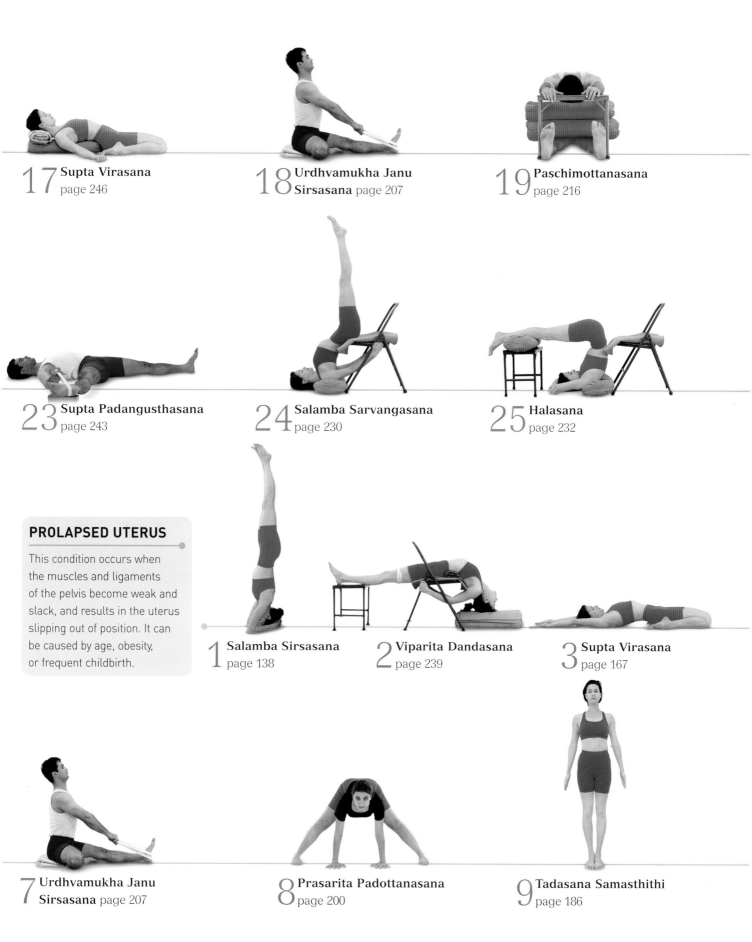

17 **Supta Virasana**
page 246

18 **Urdhvamukha Janu Sirsasana** page 207

19 **Paschimottanasana**
page 216

23 **Supta Padangusthasana**
page 243

24 **Salamba Sarvangasana**
page 230

25 **Halasana**
page 232

PROLAPSED UTERUS

This condition occurs when the muscles and ligaments of the pelvis become weak and slack, and results in the uterus slipping out of position. It can be caused by age, obesity, or frequent childbirth.

1 **Salamba Sirsasana**
page 138

2 **Viparita Dandasana**
page 239

3 **Supta Virasana**
page 167

7 **Urdhvamukha Janu Sirsasana** page 207

8 **Prasarita Padottanasana**
page 200

9 **Tadasana Samasthithi**
page 186

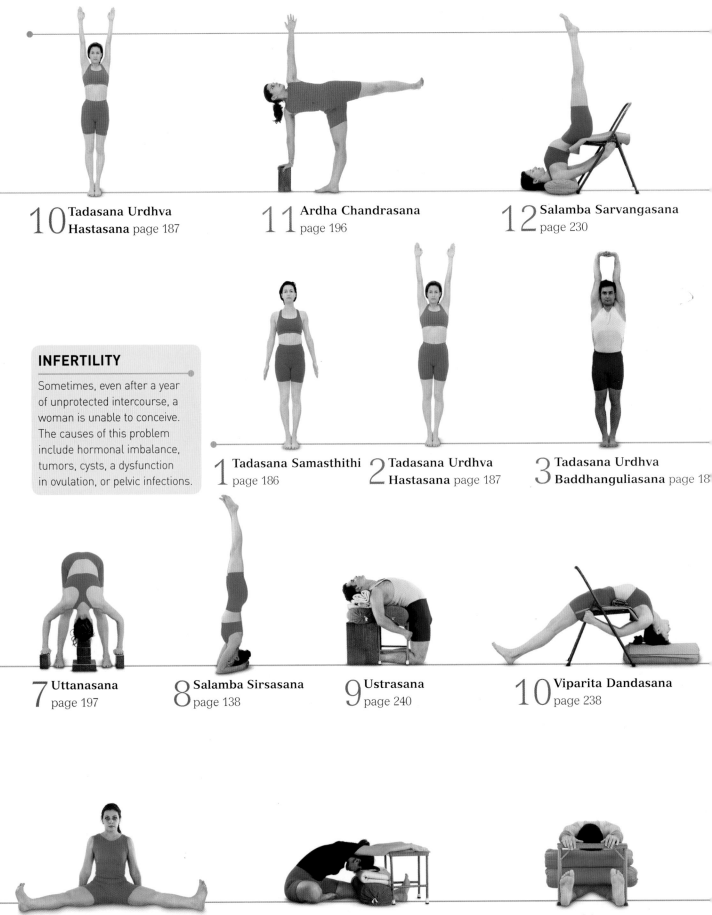

10 **Tadasana Urdhva Hastasana** page 187

11 **Ardha Chandrasana** page 196

12 **Salamba Sarvangasana** page 230

INFERTILITY

Sometimes, even after a year of unprotected intercourse, a woman is unable to conceive. The causes of this problem include hormonal imbalance, tumors, cysts, a dysfunction in ovulation, or pelvic infections.

1 **Tadasana Samasthithi** page 186

2 **Tadasana Urdhva Hastasana** page 187

3 **Tadasana Urdhva Baddhanguliasana** page 18

7 **Uttanasana** page 197

8 **Salamba Sirsasana** page 138

9 **Ustrasana** page 240

10 **Viparita Dandasana** page 238

14 **Upavista Konasana** page 213

15 **Janu Sirsasana** page 218

16 **Paschimottanasana** page 216

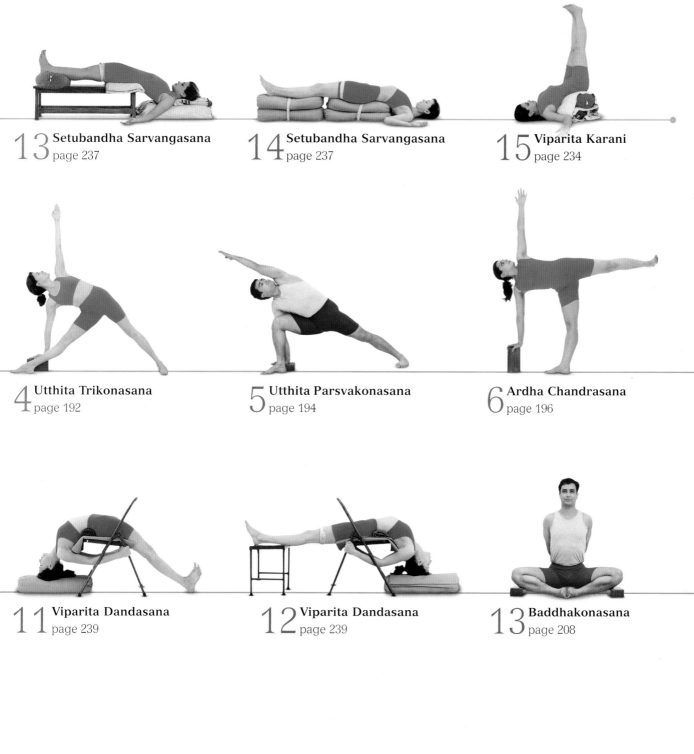

13 **Setubandha Sarvangasana** page 237

14 **Setubandha Sarvangasana** page 237

15 **Viparita Karani** page 234

4 **Utthita Trikonasana** page 192

5 **Utthita Parsvakonasana** page 194

6 **Ardha Chandrasana** page 196

11 **Viparita Dandasana** page 239

12 **Viparita Dandasana** page 239

13 **Baddhakonasana** page 208

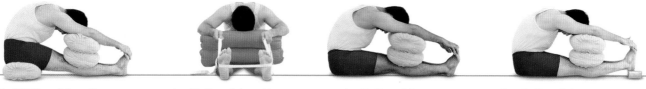

17 **Paschimottanasana** page 215

18 **Paschimottanasana** page 216

19 **Paschimottanasana** page 214

20 **Paschimottanasana** page 215

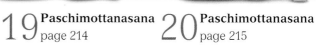

"Do not stop trying just because perfection eludes you."

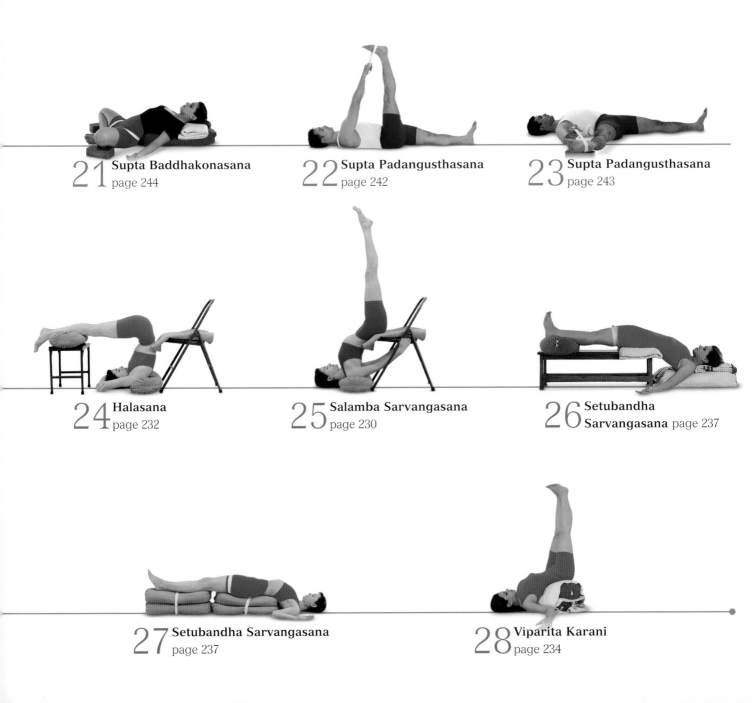

21 **Supta Baddhakonasana**
page 244

22 **Supta Padangusthasana**
page 242

23 **Supta Padangusthasana**
page 243

24 **Halasana**
page 232

25 **Salamba Sarvangasana**
page 230

26 **Setubandha
Sarvangasana** page 237

27 **Setubandha Sarvangasana**
page 237

28 **Viparita Karani**
page 234

MEN'S HEALTH

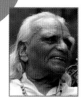

Nearly half of all adult men face some form of impotence at some time in their lives. The treatment of this, and many other disorders that relate to the male reproductive organs and glands, is helped by regular practice of the prescribed sequences of asanas. The enlargement of the prostate gland and various forms of hernia are common problems that affect men above the age of 50. These ailments respond to the practice of yoga.

IMPOTENCE

This is the inability, often temporary, to achieve or maintain an erection. The causes can be structural, hormonal, neurological, or psychological. It can also be caused by the side effects of medicines or substance abuse.

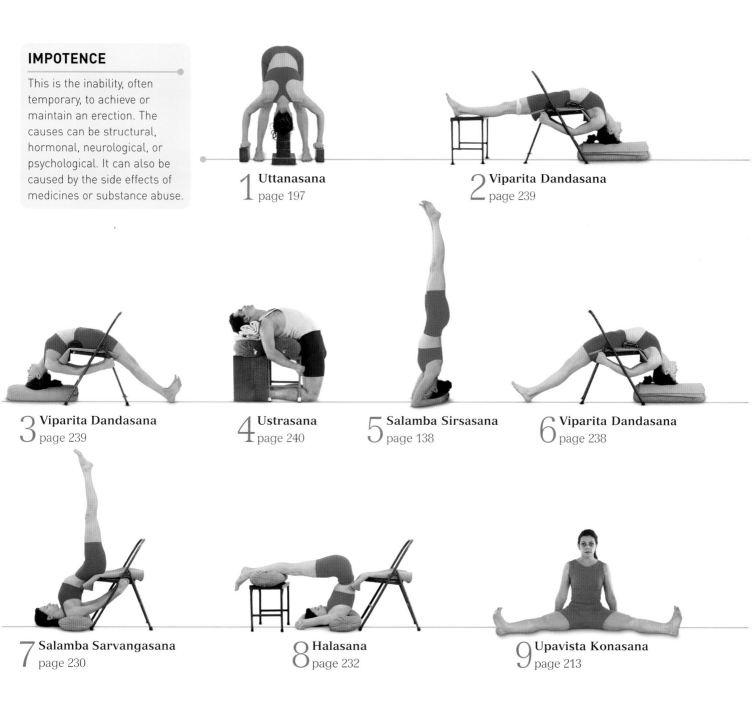

1 **Uttanasana**
page 197

2 **Viparita Dandasana**
page 239

3 **Viparita Dandasana**
page 239

4 **Ustrasana**
page 240

5 **Salamba Sirsasana**
page 138

6 **Viparita Dandasana**
page 238

7 **Salamba Sarvangasana**
page 230

8 **Halasana**
page 232

9 **Upavista Konasana**
page 213

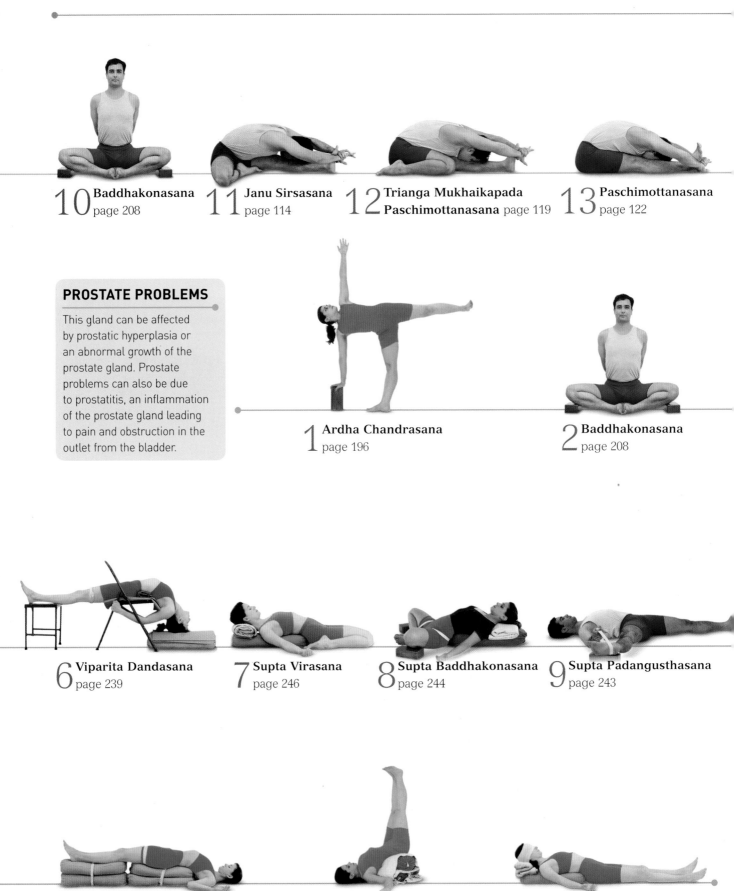

10 **Baddhakonasana**
page 208

11 **Janu Sirsasana**
page 114

12 **Trianga Mukhaikapada**
Paschimottanasana page 119

13 **Paschimottanasana**
page 122

PROSTATE PROBLEMS

This gland can be affected by prostatic hyperplasia or an abnormal growth of the prostate gland. Prostate problems can also be due to prostatitis, an inflammation of the prostate gland leading to pain and obstruction in the outlet from the bladder.

1 **Ardha Chandrasana**
page 196

2 **Baddhakonasana**
page 208

6 **Viparita Dandasana**
page 239

7 **Supta Virasana**
page 246

8 **Supta Baddhakonasana**
page 244

9 **Supta Padangusthasana**
page 243

13 **Setubandha Sarvangasana**
page 237

14 **Viparita Karani**
page 234

15 **Savasana**
page 248

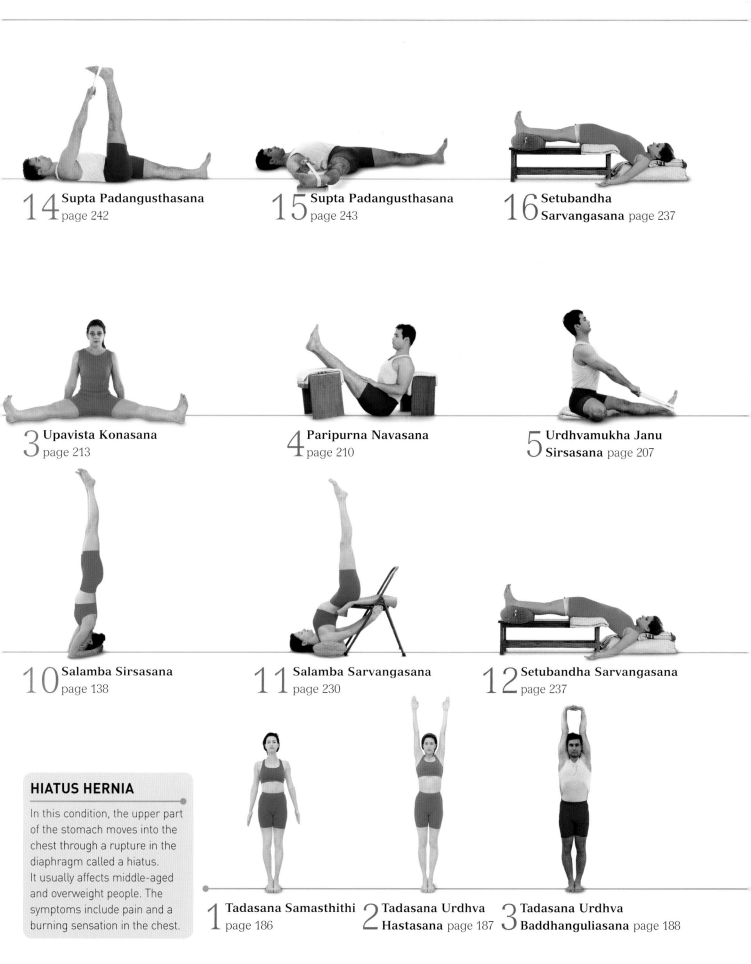

14 **Supta Padangusthasana** page 242

15 **Supta Padangusthasana** page 243

16 **Setubandha Sarvangasana** page 237

3 **Upavista Konasana** page 213

4 **Paripurna Navasana** page 210

5 **Urdhvamukha Janu Sirsasana** page 207

10 **Salamba Sirsasana** page 138

11 **Salamba Sarvangasana** page 230

12 **Setubandha Sarvangasana** page 237

HIATUS HERNIA

In this condition, the upper part of the stomach moves into the chest through a rupture in the diaphragm called a hiatus. It usually affects middle-aged and overweight people. The symptoms include pain and a burning sensation in the chest.

1 **Tadasana Samasthithi** page 186

2 **Tadasana Urdhva Hastasana** page 187

3 **Tadasana Urdhva Baddhanguliasana** page 188

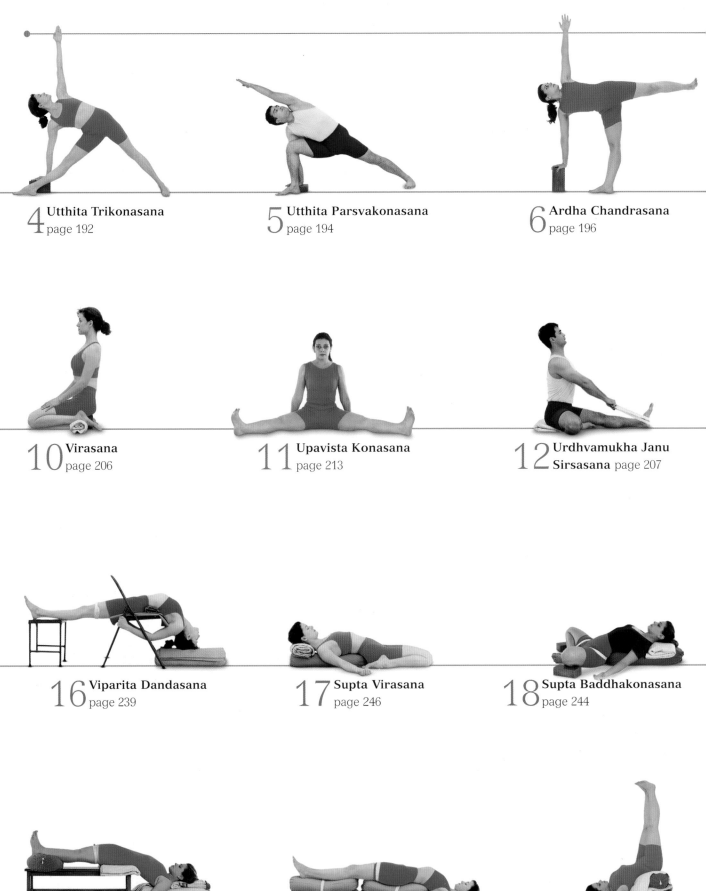

4 **Utthita Trikonasana** page 192

5 **Utthita Parsvakonasana** page 194

6 **Ardha Chandrasana** page 196

10 **Virasana** page 206

11 **Upavista Konasana** page 213

12 **Urdhvamukha Janu Sirsasana** page 207

16 **Viparita Dandasana** page 239

17 **Supta Virasana** page 246

18 **Supta Baddhakonasana** page 244

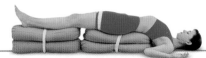

22 **Setubandha Sarvangasana** page 237

23 **Setubandha Sarvangasana** page 237

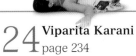

24 **Viparita Karani** page 234

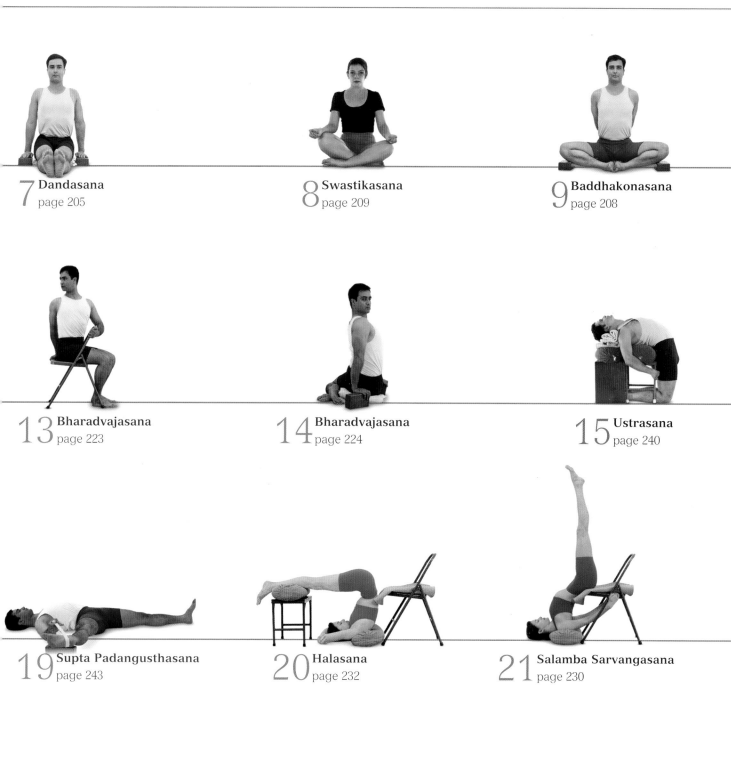

7 **Dandasana**
page 205

8 **Swastikasana**
page 209

9 **Baddhakonasana**
page 208

13 **Bharadvajasana**
page 223

14 **Bharadvajasana**
page 224

15 **Ustrasana**
page 240

19 **Supta Padangusthasana**
page 243

20 **Halasana**
page 232

21 **Salamba Sarvangasana**
page 230

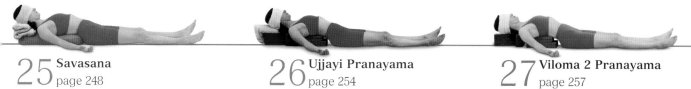

25 **Savasana**
page 248

26 **Ujjayi Pranayama**
page 254

27 **Viloma 2 Pranayama**
page 257

INGUINAL HERNIA

This occurs when the intestine protrudes through a weak point or tear into the lower layers of the abdominal wall. A direct inguinal hernia creates a bulge in the groin area, while an indirect inguinal hernia descends into the scrotum.

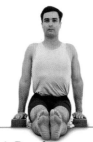

1 **Dandasana**
page 205

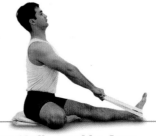

2 **Urdhvamukha Janu Sirsasana** page 207

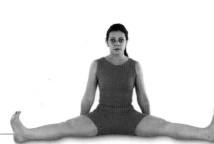

6 **Upavista Konasana**
page 213

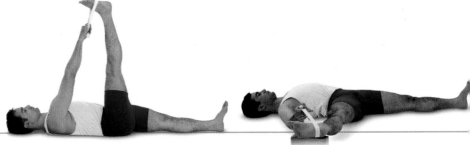

7 **Supta Padangusthasana**
page 242

8 **Supta Padangusthasana**
page 243

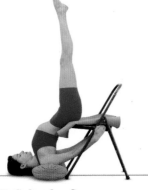

12 **Salamba Sarvangasana**
page 230

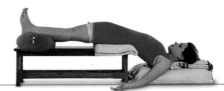

13 **Setubandha Sarvangasana** page 237

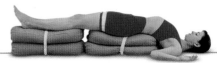

14 **Setubandha Sarvangasana** page 237

UMBILICAL HERNIA

This condition sometimes affects infants, and occurs in the region of the umbilicus. It usually corrects itself naturally. It also occurs in adults when the intestine protrudes through the abdominal wall at the navel.

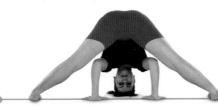

1 **Prasarita Padottanasana**
page 200

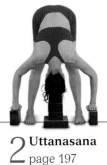

2 **Uttanasana**
page 197

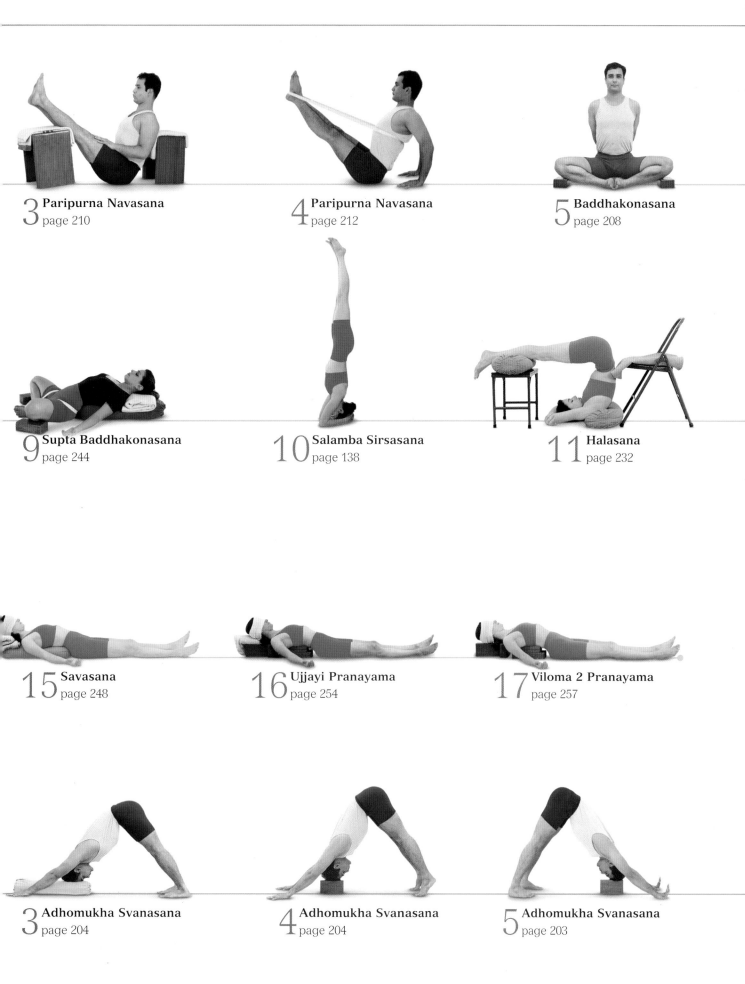

3 **Paripurna Navasana**
page 210

4 **Paripurna Navasana**
page 212

5 **Baddhakonasana**
page 208

9 **Supta Baddhakonasana**
page 244

10 **Salamba Sirsasana**
page 138

11 **Halasana**
page 232

15 **Savasana**
page 248

16 **Ujjayi Pranayama**
page 254

17 **Viloma 2 Pranayama**
page 257

3 **Adhomukha Svanasana**
page 204

4 **Adhomukha Svanasana**
page 204

5 **Adhomukha Svanasana**
page 203

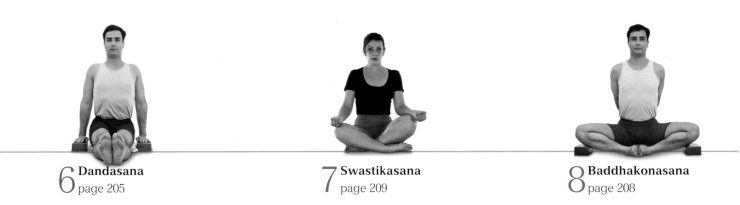

6 **Dandasana**
page 205

7 **Swastikasana**
page 209

8 **Baddhakonasana**
page 208

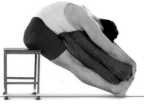

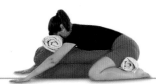

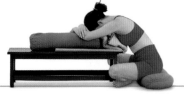

12 **Adhomukha Paschimottanasana**
page 217

13 **Adhomukha Virasana**
page 221

14 **Adhomukha Swastikasana**
page 222

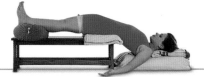

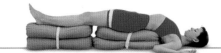

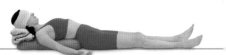

18 **Setubandha Sarvangasana**
page 237

19 **Setubandha Sarvangasana**
page 237

20 **Savasana**
page 248

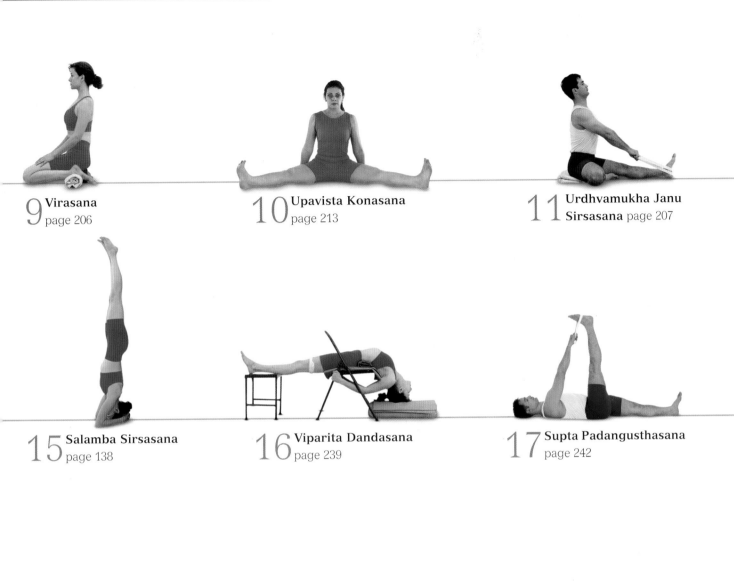

9 **Virasana** page 206

10 **Upavista Konasana** page 213

11 **Urdhvamukha Janu Sirsasana** page 207

15 **Salamba Sirsasana** page 138

16 **Viparita Dandasana** page 239

17 **Supta Padangusthasana** page 242

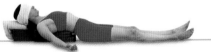

21 **Ujjayi Pranayama** page 254

22 **Viloma 2 Pranayama** page 257

"Asanas will help transform an individual by taking the person away from an awareness of just the body, toward the consciousness of the soul."

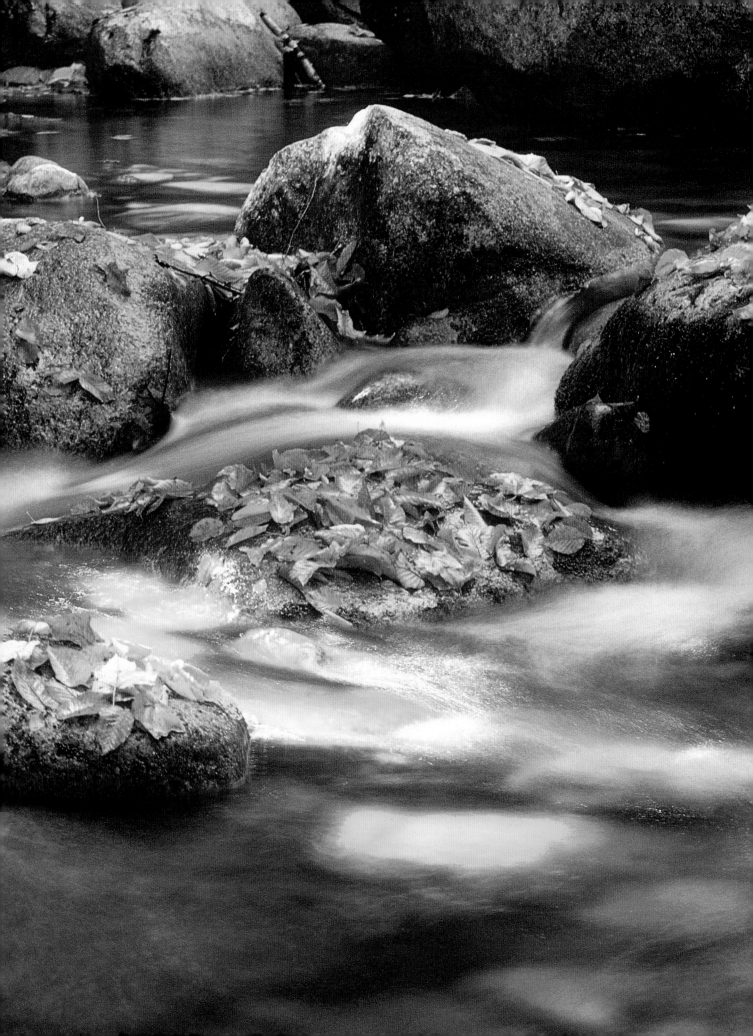

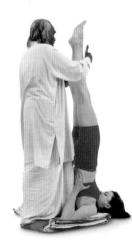

CHAPTER 8

IYENGAR YOGA COURSE

*"Our **body** is the bow and the **asanas** are the arrows to hit the target—the **soul**."*

Learning a new subject requires dedication and perseverance. In yoga, the physical body, the sense organs, the emotions, mind, and consciousness are trained slowly and gradually. A beginner starts with simple asanas and progresses to more complex ones by building up strength and concentration. Advanced students of yoga, too, should practice asanas in a logical sequence that allows them to experience the full effectiveness of each asana. Understanding sequencing is a gradual process. Just as a car cannot pick up speed in first gear, we require time and patience to understand the subtleties and technical requirements of asanas.

Guide to your Yoga Practice

This course takes you from simple to complex asanas. Follow the sequence listed for each week, as this not only makes your practice more effective, but also minimizes the possibility of injury or strain.

People start yoga with many preconceptions; some expect instant cures to ailments, others assume that the simplest of asanas will be difficult to achieve. These are usually people whose muscles are stiff, and whose posture is often faulty. Even the physically fit may not possess the stability of body or mind needed to practice correctly. A beginner must, therefore, practice asanas at a very basic level at first, then continue practicing regularly, until the intelligence penetrates all the sheaths of his or her body (*see page* 46).

Advice for beginners

Initially, practice as many asanas of the sequence as you feel comfortable with. Do not exhaust your strength or stamina. Begin with small expectations. Restructuring muscles, bones, tissues, posture, and internal organs takes time. In yoga, basic movements, such as turning out the right foot or interlocking the fingers, are called "motions." More subtle movements as, for example, lifting the kneecap, tightening the groin, and drawing in the kidneys, are regarded as "actions." Motions get you into a pose, actions refine it. Understand the motions first. Learn *how* to observe, rather than *what* you must observe. Grasping the essence of the asana is more important than getting the movements right. Some instructions may seem absurd—even impossible—to beginners. Gradually, however, you will become aware of the complexity and subtlety of the body's movements in each increasingly simple maneuver, not as an abstraction, but as a necessity.

Eventually, understanding the actions of an asana will establish the rhythm and pace of your practice.

The yoga course begins with simple asanas, which prepare the body to perform the more complicated asanas with ease. You will learn to access levels of yourself that you were unaware existed. The asana connects you to the inner world within you.

Scheduling your practice

Practice asanas when you feel fresh and energetic. Early in the morning, if your muscles are not stiff, or early evenings, when the muscles are supple and free, is advisable. Do not practice just after a heavy meal. The duration of your practice is flexible. Learn to know when to stop.

Make your yoga sessions a daily practice. If you are tired or a part of your body is aching, practicing asanas will relieve your body of tension and strain. Just keep the cautions at the beginning of each asana in mind.

General guidelines

If you do not get a particular asana right, practice one with similar movements. The physical body, sense organs, emotions, mind, and consciousness are trained gradually in yoga. If you stop practicing a particular asana, the body loses a part of its intelligence. Practice different types of asanas. If your legs ache, for instance, do not avoid your yoga session. Locate the discomfort, think about its cause, and understand how to remove it. Through your intelligence, introduce a soothing sensation into that area.

Holding the pose
Concentrate completely when you are in the final pose

Delve deep into your consciousness and extend a feeling of calm to the part of your body that needs it most.

Your environment

Coordinate your practice with the state of your body and mind. Hot summer days can make you feel exhausted or dehydrated. Practice with props to relax. For example, perform Salamba Sarvangasana with the help of a chair and a bolster. Reclining asanas, inversions, and resting asanas are also suitable since they slow down the metabolism, calm all parts of the body and mind, and conserve energy. In winter, standing asanas, back bends, and inversions help to combat colds, arthritis, and seasonal depression. Twists, forward bends, and inversions help to counter the effects of damp conditions.

Sequence

Practicing asanas in the prescribed order enhances their effectiveness as well as your experience of each asana. Understanding the significance of sequencing takes time. Grasp the subtleties and movements of each asana and its impact on your body, before attempting to formulate an order which suits your personal needs. Follow the 20-Week Yoga Course until you feel confident enough to develop your own sequence. Those suffering from specific ailments, however, should follow the asana sequences appropriate to their condition, given in Chapter 6 (*see pages* 260–383).

Timing

As much as possible, hold the final pose for the recommended time to maximize the benefits and build strength. However, timing also depends on attention. The intelligence of the brain rises and drops very fast, but the body's intelligence cannot be awakened at the same speed. You have to bring awareness to all parts of the body for the whole time you are in the pose.

Ultimately, use your discrimination to decide the sequence, timing, and nature of the asanas you want to practice, according to your age and physical condition. Keep your progress in developing an awareness and understanding of the asanas in mind. First, stretch and awaken your body and mind to the logic behind a series of asanas. Do not begin your session with a back bend, for instance. For those in perfect physical condition, cycles of asanas can be figured out fairly easily. If your condition is less than perfect, evolve a sequence which suits your body's requirements. There should be a physical, physiological, psychological, and spiritual rhythm in your practice of yoga.

Balance and harmony
Yogacharya Iyengar in a variation of Bharadvajasana

Formulating your own practice

All the asanas listed in the 20-Week Yoga Course are simple poses, made even easier with props. Practice Virabhadrasana 1 and 2 (*see pages* 96 and 76), against a wall for the first few weeks. Once you feel comfortable in the pose, practice without the support of the wall. Similarly, after about six months (this can vary from person to person) of practicing Utthita Trikonasana, place your hand on the floor, instead of on the block. Attempt Halasana, Salamba Sarvangasana, Janu Sirsasana, Trianga Mukhaikapada Paschimottanasana, Paschimottanasana, and Paripurna Navasana without props after six months. Attempt Salamba Sirsasana against the wall after eight months. It might take up to eight months to achieve Salamba Sirsasana without the support of the wall. Attempt Supta Virasana, Ustrasana, Urdhva Dhanurasana, Bharadvajasana, and Marichyasana (*page* 133) without suppport after eight months. As your muscles and joints become supple, props will become a hindrance, and you will progress smoothly to the classic poses without them.

20-WEEK YOGA COURSE

WEEK 1

ASANAS	PAGE
1. **Tadasana Samasthithi** against a wall	186
2. **Tadasana Urdhva Hastasana** against a wall	187
3. **Tadasana Urdhva Baddhanguliasana** against a wall	188
4. **Uttanasana** 1 foam block and 5 wooden blocks	197
5. **Adhomukha Svanasana** 3 blocks*	202
6. **Dandasana** 1 blanket and 2 blocks	205
7. **Virasana** 2 blankets and 2 bolsters	206
8. **Adhomukha Virasana** 2 blankets and 2 bolsters	221
9. **Paschimottanasana** 1 stool and 2 bolsters (legs apart)	216
10. **Bharadvajasana** 1 blanket and 2 blocks	224
11. **Setubandha Sarvangasana** 4 bolsters	237
12. **Savasana**	170

WEEK 2

ASANAS	PAGE
1. **Tadasana Samasthithi** against a wall	186
2. **Tadasana Urdhva Hastasana** against a wall	187
3. **Tadasana Urdhva Baddhanguliasana** against a wall	188
4. **Paschima Baddha Hastasana**	189
5. **Utthita Trikonasana** 1 block	192
6. **Uttanasana** 1 foam block and 5 wooden blocks	197
7. **Adhomukha Svanasana** 3 blocks	202
8. **Dandasana** 1 blanket and 2 blocks	205
9. **Virasana** 2 blankets and 2 bolsters	206
10. **Urdhvamukha Janu Sirsasana** 1 belt	207
11. **Baddhakonasana** 2 blocks and 1 bolster (parallel to the hips)	208
12. **Adhomukha Virasana** 2 blankets and 2 bolsters	221
13. **Paschimottanasana** 2 bolsters and 1 belt (legs apart)	216
14. **Bharadvajasana** 1 chair (sitting sideways)	223
15. **Supta Baddhakonasana** 1 blanket, 1 bolster, 2 blocks, and 1 belt	244
16. **Setubandha Sarvangasana** 4 bolsters	237
17. **Savasana**	170

WEEK 3

ASANAS	PAGE
1. **Tadasana Samasthithi** against a wall	186
2. **Tadasana Urdhva Hastasana** against a wall	187
3. **Tadasana Urdhva Baddhanguliasana** against a wall	188
4. **Paschima Baddha Hastasana**	189
5. **Utthita Trikonasana** 1 block	192
6. **Uttanasana** 1 foam block and 5 wooden blocks	197
7. **Adhomukha Svanasana** 1 block (heels against a wall)	204
8. **Dandasana** 1 blanket and 2 blocks	205
9. **Virasana** 2 blankets and 2 bolsters	206
10. **Urdhvamukha Janu Sirsasana** 1 belt	207
11. **Baddhakonasana** 2 blocks and 1 bolster (parallel to the hips)	208
12. **Adhomukha Virasana** 2 blankets and 2 bolsters	221
13. **Paschimottanasana** 2 bolsters and 1 belt (legs apart)	216
14. **Bharadvajasana** 1 chair (sitting sideways)	223
15. **Utthita Marichyasana** 1 stool, 1 rounded block, and a wall	226
16. **Supta Baddhakonasana** 1 blanket, 1 bolster, 2 blocks, and 1 belt	244
17. **Setubandha Sarvangasana** 4 bolsters	237
18. **Savasana**	170

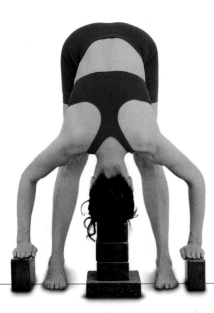

*blocks are wooden unless otherwise specified

WEEK 4

ASANAS	PAGE
1. **Tadasana Samasthithi** against a wall	186
2. **Tadasana Urdhva Hastasana** against a wall	187
3. **Tadasana Urdhva Baddhanguliasana** against a wall	188
4. **Paschima Baddha Hastasana**	189
5. **Tadasana Gomukhasana**	191
6. **Utthita Trikonasana** 1 block	192
7. **Utthita Parsvakonasana** 1 block	194
8. **Uttanasana** 1 foam block and 5 wooden blocks	197
9. **Adhomukha Svanasana** 1 block (heels against a wall)	204
10. **Dandasana** 1 blanket and 2 blocks	205
11. **Virasana** 1 rolled blanket and 1 block	206
12. **Urdhvamukha Janu Sirsasana** 1 belt	207
13. **Swastikasana**	209
14. **Baddhakonasana** 2 blocks and 1 bolster (parallel to the hips)	208

ASANAS	PAGE
15. **Upavista Konasana**	213
16. **Adhomukha Virasana** 2 blankets and 2 bolsters	221
17. **Paschimottanasana** 2 bolsters and 1 belt (legs apart)	216
18. **Janu Sirsasana** 1 stool, 1 blanket, and 1 bolster	218
19. **Paschimottanasana** 3 bolsters	215
20. **Bharadvajasana** 1 chair (sitting sideways)	223
21. **Bharadvajasana** 1 chair (legs through chair back)	223
22. **Utthita Marichyasana** 1 stool, 1 rounded block, and a wall	226
23. **Parsva Virasana** 1 rolled blanket and 2 blocks	228
24. **Supta Baddhakonasana** 1 blanket, 1 bolster, 2 blocks, and 1 belt	244
25. **Supta Padangusthasana** 1 belt	242
26. **Setubandha Sarvangasana** 4 bolsters	237
27. **Savasana**	170

WEEK 5

ASANAS	PAGE
1. **Tadasana Samasthithi** against a wall	186
2. **Tadasana Urdhva Hastasana** against a wall	187
3. **Tadasana Urdhva Baddhanguliasana** against a wall	188
4. **Paschima Baddha Hastasana**	189
5. **Tadasana Gomukhasana**	191
6. **Utthita Trikonasana** 1 block	192
7. **Utthita Parsvakonasana** 1 block	194
8. **Virabhadrasana 1**	96
9. **Virabhadrasana 2**	76
10. **Adhomukha Svanasana** 1 block (heels against a wall)	204
11. **Prasarita Padottanasana.** 1 block or 1 bolster	201
12. **Uttanasana (concave back)**	199
13. **Dandasana** 1 blanket and 2 blocks	205
14. **Virasana** 1 rolled blanket and 1 block	206
15. **Urdhvamukha Janu Sirsasana** 1 belt	207
16. **Swastikasana**	209
17. **Baddhakonasana** 2 blocks and 1 bolster (parallel to the hips)	208
18. **Upavista Konasana**	213
19. **Adhomukha Virasana** 2 blankets and 2 bolsters	221
20. **Adhomukha Swastikasana** 1 bench, 1 blanket, and 2 bolsters	222
21. **Paschimottanasana** 3 bolsters	215
22. **Janu Sirsasana** 1 stool, 1 blanket, and 1 bolster	218

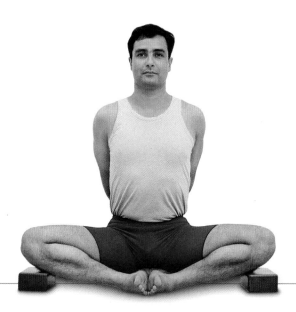

WEEK 6

ASANAS	PAGE
23. Paschimottanasana 1 stool and 2 bolsters	216
24. Bharadvajasana 1 chair (sitting sideways)	223
25. Bharadvajasana 1 chair (legs through chair back)	223
26. Bharadvajasana 1 blanket and 2 blocks	224
27. Utthita Marichyasana 1 stool, 1 rounded block, and a wall	226
28. Parsva Virasana 1 rolled blanket, and 2 blocks	229
29. Supta Baddhakonasana 1 blanket, 1 bolster, 2 blocks, and 1 belt	244
30. Supta Padangusthasana 1 belt	242
31. Supta Padangusthasana 1 block and 1 belt	243
32. Setubandha Sarvangasana 1 bench, 1 blanket, and 2 bolsters	237
33. Savasana	170

ASANAS	PAGE
1. Tadasana Samasthithi against a wall	186
2. Tadasana Urdhva **Hastasana** against a wall	187
3. Tadasana Urdhva **Baddhanguliasana** against a wall	188
4. Tadasana Paschima **Namaskarasana**	190
5. Tadasana Gomukhasana	191
6. Utthita Trikonasana 1 block	192
7. Utthita Parsvakonasana 1 block	194
8. Virabhadrasana 1	96
9. Virabhadrasana 2	76
10. Ardha Chandrasana 1 block	196
11. Adhomukha Svanasana 1 bolster	204
12. Prasarita Padottanasana 1 block or 1 bolster	201
13. Uttanasana 1 foam block and 5 wooden blocks	197
14. Adhomukha **Paschimottanasana** 1 stool and 2 bolsters	217
15. Dandasana 1 blanket and 2 blocks	205
16. Virasana 2 blankets and 2 bolsters	206
17. Urdhvamukha Janu **Sirsasana** 1 belt	207
18. Swastikasana	209
19. Baddhakonasana 2 blocks and 1 bolster	208
20. Upavista Konasana	213
21. Paripurna Navasana 2 stools and 3 mats	210
22. Adhomukha Virasana 2 blankets and 2 bolsters	221

ASANAS	PAGE
23. Adhomukha Swastikasana 1 bench, 1 blanket, and 2 bolsters	222
24. Paschimottanasana 1 stool and 2 bolsters (legs apart)	216
25. Janu Sirsasana 1 stool, 1 blanket, and 1 bolster	218
26. Paschimottanasana 1 block and 2 bolsters	215
27. Bharadvajasana 1 chair (sitting sideways)	223
28. Bharadvajasana 1 chair (legs through chair back)	223
29. Bharadvajasana 1 blanket and 2 blocks	224
30. Marichyasana 1 blanket and 1 block	225
31. Utthita Marichyasana 1 stool, 1 rounded block, and a wall	226
32. Parsva Virasana 1 blanket and 1 block	228
33. Supta Baddhakonasana 1 blanket, 1 bolster, 2 blocks, and 1 belt	244
34. Supta Virasana 1 blanket and 1 bolster	246
35. Supta Padangusthasana 1 belt	242
36. Supta Padangusthasana 1 belt and 1 block	243
37. Halasana 1 stool, 1 chair, 1 blanket, and 2 bolsters	232
38. Setubandha Sarvangasana 1 bench, 1 blanket, and 2 bolsters	237
39. Savasana	170

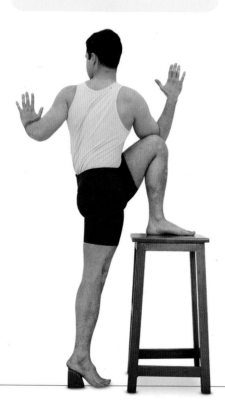

WEEK 7

ASANAS	PAGE
1. Tadasana Samasthithi against a wall	186
2. Tadasana Urdhva Hastasana against a wall	187
3. Tadasana Urdhva Baddhanguliasana against a wall	188
4. Tadasana Paschima Namaskarasana	190
5. Tadasana Gomukhasana	191
6. Utthita Trikonasana 1 block	192
7. Utthita Parsvakonasana 1 block	194
8. Virabhadrasana 1	96
9. Virabhadrasana 2	76
10. Ardha Chandrasana 1 block	196
11. Parsvottanasana	84
12. Adhomukha Svanasana 1 bolster	204
13. Prasarita Padottanasana 1 block or 1 bolster	201
14. Uttanasana 1 foam block and 5 wooden blocks	197
15. Adhomukha Paschimottanasana 1 stool and 2 bolsters	217
16. Dandasana 1 blanket and 2 blocks	205
17. Virasana 2 blankets and 2 bolsters	206
18. Urdhvamukha Janu Sirsasana 1 belt	207

ASANAS	PAGE
19. Swastikasana	209
20. Baddhakonasana 2 blocks and 1 bolster	208
21. Upavista Konasana	213
22. Paripurna Navasana 2 stools and 3 mats	210
23. Adhomukha Virasana 2 blankets and 1 bolster	220
24. Adhomukha Swastikasana 1 bench, 1 blanket, and 1 bolster	222
25. Paschimottanasana 1 stool and 2 bolsters (legs together)	216
26. Janu Sirsasana 1 stool, 1 blanket, and 1 bolster	218
27. Paschimottanasana 1 block and 2 bolsters	215
28. Bharadvajasana 1 chair (sitting sideways)	223
29. Bharadvajasana 1 chair (legs through chair back)	223
30. Bharadvajasana 1 blanket and 2 blocks	224
31. Marichyasana 1 blanket and 1 block	225
32. Utthita Marichyasana 1 stool, 1 rounded block, and a wall	226
33. Parsva Virasana 1 blanket and 1 block	228
34. Supta Baddhakonasana 1 blanket, 1 bolster, 2 blocks, and 1 belt	244

ASANAS	PAGE
35. Supta Virasana 1 blanket and 1 bolster	246
36. Supta Padangusthasana 1 belt	242
37. Supta Padangusthasana 1 belt and 1 block	243
38. Halasana 1 stool, 1 chair, 1 blanket, and 2 bolsters	232
39. Setubandha Sarvangasana 1 bench, 3 blankets, and 1 bolster	236
40. Savasana 1 blanket, 1 bolster, and 1 bandage	248

WEEK 8

ASANAS	PAGE
1. Tadasana Samasthithi against a wall	186
2. Tadasana Urdhva Hastasana against a wall	187
3. Tadasana Urdhva Baddhanguliasana against a wall	188
4. Tadasana Paschima Namaskarasana	190
5. Tadasana Gomukhasana	191
6. Utthita Trikonasana 1 block	192
7. Utthita Parsvakonasana 1 block	194
8. Virabhadrasana 1	96
9. Virabhadrasana 2	76
10. Ardha Chandrasana 1 block	196
11. Parsvottanasana	84
12. Adhomukha Svanasana 1 bolster	204
13. Prasarita Padottanasana 1 block or 1 bolster	201
14. Uttanasana 1 foam block and 5 wooden blocks	197

ASANAS	PAGE
15. Adhomukha Paschimottanasana 1 stool and 2 bolsters	217
16. Dandasana 1 blanket and 2 blocks	205
17. Virasana 2 blankets and 2 bolsters	206
18. Urdhvamukha Janu Sirsasana 1 belt	207
19. Swastikasana	209
20. Baddhakonasana 2 blocks and 1 bolster	208
21. Upavista Konasana	213
22. Paripurna Navasana 2 stools and 3 mats	210
23. Adhomukha Virasana 2 blankets and 1 bolster	220
24. Adhomukha Swastikasana 1 bench, 1 blanket, and 1 bolster	222
25. Paschimottanasana 1 stool, 1 blanket, and 2 bolsters (legs together)	216
26. Janu Sirsasana 1 stool and 1 bolster	218
27. Paschimottanasana 2 bolsters	214
28. Bharadvajasana 1 chair (sitting sideways)	223
29. Bharadvajasana 1 chair (legs through chair back)	223
30. Bharadvajasana 1 blanket and 2 blocks	224
31. Marichyasana 1 blanket and 1 block	225
32. Utthita Marichyasana 1 stool, 1 rounded block, and a wall	226
33. Parsva Virasana 1 blanket and 1 block	228
34. Supta Baddhakonasana 1 blanket, 1 bolster, 2 blocks, and 1 belt	244

ASANAS	PAGE
35. Supta Virasana 1 blanket and 1 bolster	246
36. Supta Padangusthasana 1 belt	242
37. Supta Padangusthasana 1 belt and 1 block	243
38. Salamba Sarvangasana 1 chair, 1 blanket, and 1 bolster	230
39. Halasana 1 chair, 1 stool, 1 blanket, and 2 bolsters	232
40. Setubandha Sarvangasana 1 bench, 3 blankets, and 1 bolster	236
41. Savasana 1 blanket, 1 bolster, and 1 bandage	248

WEEK 9

ASANAS	PAGE
1. Tadasana Samasthithi against a wall	186
2. Tadasana Urdhva Hastasana against a wall	187
3. Tadasana Urdhva Baddhanguliasana against a wall	188
4. Tadasana Paschima Namaskarasana	190
5. Tadasana Gomukhasana	191
6. Utthita Trikonasana 1 block	192
7. Utthita Parsvakonasana 1 block	194
8. Virabhadrasana 1	96
9. Virabhadrasana 2	76
10. Ardha Chandrasana 1 block	196
11. Parsvottanasana	84
12. Adhomukha Svanasana 1 bolster	204

ASANAS	PAGE
13. Prasarita Padottanasana 1 block or 1 bolster	201
14. Uttanasana 1 foam block and 5 wooden blocks	197
15. Adhomukha Paschimottanasana 1 stool and 2 bolsters	217
16. Dandasana 1 blanket and 2 blocks	205
17. Virasana 2 blankets and 2 bolsters	206
18. Urdhvamukha Janu Sirsasana 1 belt	207
19. Swastikasana	209
20. Baddhakonasana 2 blocks and 1 bolster	208
21. Upavista Konasana	213
22. Paripurna Navasana 2 stools and 3 mats	210
23. Adhomukha Virasana 2 blankets and 1 bolster	220
24. Adhomukha Swastikasana 1 bench, 1 blanket, and 1 bolster	222
25. Paschimottanasana 1 stool and 2 bolsters (legs together)	216
26. Janu Sirsasana 1 stool, 1 blanket, and 1 bolster	218
27. Paschimottanasana 2 bolsters	214
28. Bharadvajasana 1 chair (sitting sideways)	223
29. Bharadvajasana (legs through a chair back)	223
30. Bharadvajasana 1 blanket and 2 blocks	224
31. Marichyasana 1 blanket and 1 block	225
32. Utthita Marichyasana 1 stool, 1 rounded block, and a wall	226

WEEK 10

ASANAS	PAGE
33. Parsva Virasana 1 blanket and 1 block	228
34. Supta Baddhakonasana 1 blanket, 1 bolster, 2 blocks, and 1 belt	244
35. Supta Virasana 1 blanket and 1 bolster	246
36. Supta Padangusthasana 1 belt	242
37. Supta Padangusthasana 1 belt and 1 block	243
38. Salamba Sarvangasana 1 chair, 1 blanket, and 1 bolster	230
39. Halasana 1 chair, 1 stool, 1 blanket, and 2 bolsters	232
40. Setubandha Sarvangasana 1 bench, 3 blankets, and 1 bolster	236
41. Savasana 1 blanket, 1 bolster, and 1 bandage	248

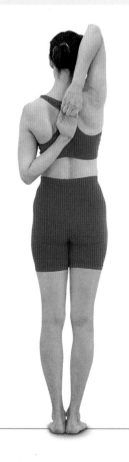

ASANAS	PAGE
1. Tadasana Samasthithi against a wall	186
2. Tadasana Urdhva Hastasana against a wall	187
3. Tadasana Urdhva Baddhanguliasana against a wall	188
4. Tadasana Paschima Namaskarasana	190
5. Tadasana Gomukhasana	191
6. Utthita Trikonasana 1 block	192
7. Utthita Parsvakonasana 1 block	194
8. Virabhadrasana 1	96
9. Virabhadrasana 2	76
10. Ardha Chandrasana 1 block	196
11. Parsvottanasana	84
12. Adhomukha Svanasana 1 bolster	204
13. Prasarita Padottanasana 1 block or 1 bolster	201
14. Uttanasana 1 foam block and 5 wooden blocks	197
15. Adhomukha Paschimottanasana 1 stool and 2 bolsters	217
16. Dandasana 1 blanket and 2 blocks	205
17. Virasana 2 blankets and 2 bolsters	206
18. Urdhvamukha Janu Sirsasana 1 belt	207
19. Swastikasana	209
20. Baddhakonasana 2 blocks and 1 bolster	208
21. Upavista Konasana	213
22. Paripurna Navasana 2 belts	212
23. Adhomukha Virasana 2 blankets and 1 bolster	220

ASANAS	PAGE
24. Adhomukha Swastikasana 1 bench, 1 blanket, and 1 bolster	222
25. Paschimottanasana 1 stool and 2 bolsters (legs together)	216
26. Janu Sirsasana 1 stool, 1 blanket, and 1 bolster	218
27. Paschimottanasana 2 bolsters	214
28. Bharadvajasana 1 chair (sitting sideways)	223
29. Bharadvajasana (legs through a chair back)	223
30. Bharadvajasana 1 blanket and 2 blocks	224
31. Marichyasana 1 blanket and 1 block	225
32. Utthita Marichyasana 1 stool, 1 rounded block, and a wall	226
33. Parsva Virasana 1 blanket and 1 block	228
34. Supta Baddhakonasana 1 blanket, 1 bolster, 2 blocks, and 1 belt	244
35. Supta Virasana 1 blanket and 1 bolster	246
36. Supta Padangusthasana 1 belt	242
37. Supta Padangusthasana 1 belt and 1 block	243
38. Salamba Sarvangasana 1 chair, 1 blanket, and 1 bolster	230
39. Halasana 1 chair, 1 stool, 1 blanket, and 2 bolsters	232
40. Setubandha Sarvangasana 1 bench, 3 blankets, and 1 bolster	236
41. Viparita Karani 1 blanket, 1 block, and 2 bolsters	234
42. Savasana 1 blanket, 1 bolster, and 1 bandage	248

WEEK 11

ASANAS	PAGE
1. **Tadasana Samasthithi** against a wall	186
2. **Tadasana Urdhva Hastasana** against a wall	187
3. **Tadasana Urdhva Baddhanguliasana** against a wall	188
4. **Tadasana Paschima Namaskarasana**	190
5. **Tadasana Gomukhasana**	191
6. **Utthita Trikonasana** 1 block	192
7. **Utthita Parsvakonasana** 1 block	194
8. **Virabhadrasana 1**	96
9. **Virabhadrasana 2**	76
10. **Ardha Chandrasana** 1 block	196
11. **Parsvottanasana**	84
12. **Adhomukha Svanasana** 1 bolster	204
13. **Prasarita Padottanasana** 1 block or 1 bolster	201
14. **Uttanasana** 1 foam block and 5 wooden blocks	197
15. **Adhomukha Paschimottanasana** 1 stool and 2 bolsters	217
16. **Dandasana** 1 blanket and 2 blocks	205
17. **Virasana** 2 blankets and 2 bolsters	206

ASANAS	PAGE
18. **Urdhvamukha Janu Sirsasana** 1 belt	207
19. **Swastikasana**	209
20. **Baddhakonasana** 2 blocks and 1 bolster	208
21. **Upavista Konasana**	213
22. **Paripurna Navasana** 1 long yoga belt	212
23. **Adhomukha Virasana** 2 blankets and 1 bolster	220
24. **Adhomukha Swastikasana** 1 bench, 1 blanket, and 1 bolster	222
25. **Paschimottanasana** 1 stool and 2 bolsters (legs together)	216
26. **Janu Sirsasana** 1 stool, 1 blanket and 1 bolster	218
27. **Paschimottanasana** 2 bolsters	214
28. **Bharadvajasana** 1 chair (sitting sideways)	223
29. **Bharadvajasana** (legs through a chair back)	223
30. **Bharadvajasana** 1 blanket and 2 blocks	224
31. **Marichyasana** 1 blanket and 1 block	225
32. **Utthita Marichyasana** 1 stool, 1 rounded block, and a wall	226
33. **Parsva Virasana** 1 blanket and 1 block	228

ASANAS	PAGE
34. **Supta Baddhakonasana** 1 blanket, 1 bolster, 2 blocks, and 1 belt	244
35. **Supta Virasana** 1 blanket and 1 bolster	246
36. **Supta Padangusthasana** 1 belt	242
37. **Supta Padangusthasana** 1 belt and 1 block	243
38. **Salamba Sarvangasana** 1 chair, 1 blanket, and 2 bolsters	230
39. **Halasana** 1 chair, 1 stool, 1 blanket, and 1 bolster	232
40. **Setubandha Sarvangasana** 1 bench, 3 blankets, and 1 bolster	236
41. **Viparita Karani** 1 blanket, 1 block, and 2 bolsters	234
42. **Savasana** 1 blanket, 1 bolster and 1 bandage	248

WEEK 12

ASANAS	PAGE
1. **Tadasana Samasthithi** against a wall	186
2. **Tadasana Urdhva Hastasana** against a wall	187
3. **Tadasana Urdhva Baddhanguliasana** against a wall	188
4. **Tadasana Paschima Namaskarasana**	190
5. **Tadasana Gomukhasana**	191
6. **Utthita Trikonasana** 1 block	192
7. **Utthita Parsvakonasana** 1 block	194
8. **Virabhadrasana 1**	96
9. **Virabhadrasana 2**	76

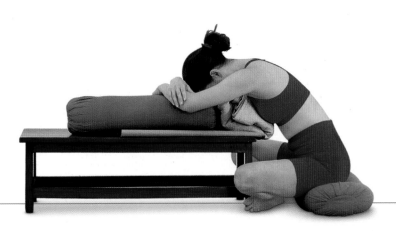

WEEK 13

ASANAS	PAGE
10. Ardha Chandrasana 1 block	196
11. Parsvottanasana	84
12. Adhomukha Svanasana 1 bolster	204
13. Prasarita Padottanasana 1 block or 1 bolster	201
14. Uttanasana 1 foam block and 5 wooden blocks	197
15. Adhomukha **Paschimottanasana** 1 stool and 2 bolsters	217
16. Dandasana 1 blanket and 2 blocks	205
17. Virasana 2 blankets and 2 bolsters	206
18. Urdhvamukha Janu **Sirsasana** 1 belt	207
19. Swastikasana	209
20. Baddhakonasana 2 blocks and 1 bolster	208
21. Upavista Konasana	213
22. Paripurna Navasana 1 long yoga belt	212
23. Adhomukha Virasana 2 blankets and 1 bolster	220
24. Adhomukha Swastikasana 1 bench, 1 blanket, and 1 bolster	222
25. Paschimottanasana 1 stool and 2 bolsters (legs together)	216
26. Janu Sirsasana 1 stool, 1 blanket, and 1 bolster	218

ASANAS	PAGE
27. Paschimottanasana 2 bolsters	214
28. Bharadvajasana 1 chair (sitting sideways)	223
29. Bharadvajasana (legs through a chair back)	223
30. Bharadvajasana 1 blankets and 2 blocks	224
31. Marichyasana 1 blanket and 1 block	225
32. Utthita Marichyasana 1 stool, 1 block, and a wall	226
33. Parsva Virasana 1 blanket and 1 block	228
34. Supta Baddhakonasana 1 blanket, 1 bolster, 2 blocks, and 1 belt	244
35. Supta Virasana 1 blanket and 1 bolster	246
36. Supta Padangusthasana 1 belt	242
37. Supta Padangusthasana 1 belt and 1 block	243
38. Salamba Sarvangasana 1 chair, 1 blanket, and 1 bolster	230
39. Halasana 1 chair, 1 stool, 1 blanket, and 2 bolsters	232
40. Setubandha Sarvangasana 1 bench, 3 blankets, and 1 bolster	236
41. Viparita Karani 1 blanket, 1 block, and 2 bolsters	234
42. Savasana 1 blanket, 1 bolster, and 1 bandage	248

ASANAS	PAGE
1. Tadasana Samasthithi against a wall	186
2. Tadasana Urdhva **Hastasana** against a wall	187
3. Tadasana Urdhva **Baddhanguliasana** against a wall	188
4. Tadasana Paschima **Namaskarasana**	190
5. Tadasana Gomukhasana	191
6. Utthita Trikonasana 1 block	192
7. Utthita Parsvakonasana 1 block	194
8. Virabhadrasana 1	96
9. Virabhadrasana 2	76
10. Ardha Chandrasana 1 block	196
11. Parsvottanasana	84
12. Adhomukha Svanasana 1 bolster	204
13. Prasarita Padottanasana 1 block or 1 bolster	201
14. Uttanasana 1 foam block and 5 wooden blocks	197
15. Adhomukha **Paschimottanasana** 1 stool and 2 bolsters	217
16. Dandasana 1 blanket and 2 blocks	205
17. Virasana 2 blankets and 2 bolsters	206
18. Urdhvamukha Janu **Sirsasana** 1 belt	207
19. Swastikasana	209
20. Baddhakonasana 2 blocks and 1 bolster	208
21. Upavista Konasana	213
22. Paripurna Navasana 1 long yoga belt	212
23. Adhomukha Virasana 2 blankets and 1 bolster	220

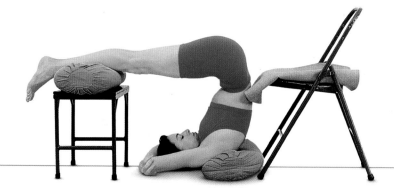

WEEK 14

ASANAS	PAGE
24. Adhomukha Swastikasana 1 bench, 1 blanket, and 1 bolster	222
25. Paschimottanasana 1 stool and 2 bolsters (legs together)	216
26. Janu Sirsasana 1 stool, 1 blanket, and 1 bolster	218
27. Paschimottanasana 2 bolsters	214
28. Bharadvajasana 1 chair (sitting sideways)	223
29. Bharadvajasana (legs through a chair back)	223
30. Bharadvajasana 1 blanket and 2 blocks	224
31. Marichyasana 1 blanket and 1 block	225
32. Utthita Marichyasana 1 stool, 1 rounded block, and a wall	226
33. Parsva Virasana 1 blanket and 1 block	228
34. Supta Baddhakonasana 1 blanket, 1 bolster, 2 blocks, and 1 belt	244
35. Supta Virasana 1 blanket and 1 bolster	246
36. Supta Padangusthasana 1 belt	242
37. Supta Padangusthasana 1 belt and 1 block	243
38. Salamba Sirsasana against a wall	138
39. Salamba Sarvangasana 1 chair, 1 blanket, and 1 bolster	230
40. Halasana 1 chair, 1 stool, 1 blanket, and 2 bolsters	232
41. Setubandha Sarvangasana 1 bench, 3 blankets, and 1 bolster	236
42. Viparita Karani 1 blanket, 1 block, and 2 bolsters	234
43. Savasana 1 blanket, 1 bolster, and 1 bandage	248

ASANAS	PAGE
1. Tadasana Samasthithi against a wall	186
2. Tadasana Urdhva Hastasana against a wall	187
3. Tadasana Urdhva **Baddhanguliasana** against a wall	188
4. Tadasana Paschima **Namaskarasana**	190
5. Tadasana Gomukhasana	191
6. Utthita Trikonasana 1 block	192
7. Utthita Parsvakonasana 1 block	194
8. Virabhadrasana 1	96
9. Virabhadrasana 2	76
10. Ardha Chandrasana 1 block	196
11. Parsvottanasana	84
12. Adhomukha Svanasana 1 bolster	204
13. Prasarita Padottanasana 1 block or 1 bolster	201
14. Uttanasana 1 foam block and 5 wooden blocks	197
15. Adhomukha **Paschimottanasana** 1 stool and 2 bolsters	217
16. Dandasana 1 blanket and 2 blocks	205
17. Virasana 2 blankets and 2 bolsters	206
18. Urdhvamukha Janu **Sirsasana** 1 belt	207
19. Swastikasana	209
20. Baddhakonasana 2 blocks and 1 bolster	208
21. Upavista Konasana	213
22. Paripurna Navasana 1 long yoga belt	212
23. Adhomukha Virasana 2 blankets and 1 bolster	220

ASANAS	PAGE
24. Adhomukha Swastikasana 1 bench, 1 blanket, and 1 bolster	222
25. Paschimottanasana 1 stool and 2 bolsters (legs together)	216
26. Janu Sirsasana 1 stool, 1 blanket, and 1 bolster	218
27. Paschimottanasana 2 bolsters	214
28. Bharadvajasana 1 chair (sitting sideways)	223
29. Bharadvajasana (legs through a chair back)	223
30. Bharadvajasana 1 blanket and 2 blocks	224
31. Marichyasana 1 blanket and 1 block	225
32. Utthita Marichyasana 1 stool, 1 rounded block, and a wall	226
33. Parsva Virasana 1 blanket and 1 block	228
34. Supta Baddhakonasana 1 blanket, 1 bolster, 2 blocks, and 1 belt	244
35. Supta Virasana 1 blanket and 1 bolster	246
36. Supta Padangusthasana 1 belt	242

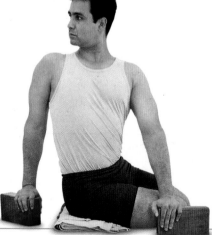

ASANAS	PAGE
37. **Supta Padangusthasana** 1 belt and 1 block	243
38. **Salamba Sirsasana** against a wall	138
39. **Salamba Sarvangasana** 1 chair, 1 blanket, and 1 bolster	230
40. **Halasana** 1 chair, 1 stool, 1 blanket, and 2 bolsters	232
41. **Setubandha Sarvangasana** 1 bench, 3 blankets, and 1 bolster	236
42. **Viparita Karani** 1 blanket, 1 block, and 2 bolsters	234
43. **Savasana** 1 blanket, 1 bolster, and 1 bandage	248

WEEK 15

ASANAS	PAGE
1. **Tadasana Samasthithi** against a wall	186
2. **Tadasana Urdhva** **Hastasana** against a wall	187
3. **Tadasana Urdhva** **Baddhanguliasana** against a wall	188
4. **Tadasana Paschima** **Namaskarasana**	190
5. **Tadasana Gomukhasana**	191
6. **Utthita Trikonasana** 1 block	192
7. **Utthita Parsvakonasana** 1 block	194
8. **Virabhadrasana 1**	96
9. **Virabhadrasana 2**	76
10. **Ardha Chandrasana** 1 block	196
11. **Parsvottanasana**	84
12. **Adhomukha Svanasana** 1 bolster	204

ASANAS	PAGE
13. **Prasarita Padottanasana** 1 block or 1 bolster	201
14. **Uttanasana** 1 foam block and 5 wooden blocks	197
15. **Adhomukha** **Paschimottanasana** 1 stool and 2 bolsters	217
16. **Dandasana** 1 blanket and 2 blocks	205
17. **Virasana** 2 blankets and 2 bolsters	206
18. **Urdhvamukha Janu** **Sirsasana** 1 belt	207
19. **Swastikasana**	209
20. **Baddhakonasana** 2 blocks and 1 bolster	208
21. **Upavista Konasana**	213
22. **Paripurna Navasana** 1 long yoga belt	212
23. **Adhomukha Virasana** 2 blankets and 1 bolster	220
24. **Adhomukha Swastikasana** 1 bench, 1 blanket, and 1 bolster	222
25. **Paschimottanasana** 1 stool and 2 bolsters (legs together)	216
26. **Janu Sirsasana** 1 stool, 1 blanket, and 1 bolster	218
27. **Paschimottanasana** 2 bolsters	214
28. **Bharadvajasana** 1 chair (sitting sideways)	223
29. **Bharadvajasana** (legs through a chair back)	223
30. **Bharadvajasana** 1 blanket and 2 blocks	224

ASANAS	PAGE
31. **Marichyasana** 1 blanket and 1 block	225
32. **Utthita Marichyasana** 1 stool, 1 rounded block, and a wall	226
33. **Parsva Virasana** 1 blanket and 1 block	228
34. **Viparita Dandasana** 1 chair, 1 stool, 2 blankets, 1 bolster, and 1 belt	239
35. **Supta Baddhakonasana** 1 blanket, 1 bolster, 2 blocks, and 1 belt	244
36. **Supta Virasana** 1 blanket and 1 bolster	246
37. **Supta Padangusthasana** 1 belt	242
38. **Supta Padangusthasana** 1 belt and 1 block	243
39. **Salamba Sirsasana** against a wall	138
40. **Salamba Sarvangasana** 1 chair, 1 blanket, and 1 bolster	230
41. **Halasana** 1 chair, 1 stool, 1 blanket, and 2 bolsters	232
42. **Setubandha Sarvangasana** 1 bench, 3 blankets, and 1 bolster	236
43. **Viparita Karani** 1 blanket, 1 block, and 2 bolsters	234
44. **Savasana** 1 blanket, 1 bolster, and 1 bandage	248
45. **Ujjayi Pranayama** 2 blankets, 2 foam blocks, 2 wooden blocks, and 1 bandage	252

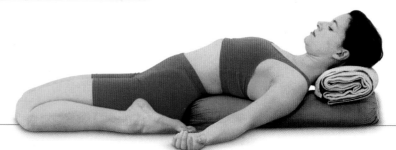

WEEK 16

ASANAS	PAGE
1. **Tadasana Samasthithi** against a wall	186
2. **Tadasana Urdhva Hastasana** against a wall	187
3. **Tadasana Urdhva Baddhanguliasana** against a wall	188
4. **Tadasana Paschima Namaskarasana**	190
5. **Tadasana Gomukhasana**	191
6. **Utthita Trikonasana** 1 block	192
7. **Utthita Parsvakonasana** 1 block	194
8. **Virabhadrasana 1**	96
9. **Virabhadrasana 2**	76
10. **Ardha Chandrasana** 1 block	196
11. **Parsvottanasana**	84
12. **Adhomukha Svanasana** 1 bolster	204
13. **Prasarita Padottanasana** 1 block or 1 bolster	201
14. **Uttanasana** 1 foam block and 5 wooden blocks	197
15. **Adhomukha Paschimottanasana** 1 stool and 2 bolsters	217
16. **Dandasana** 1 blanket and 2 blocks	205
17. **Virasana** 2 blankets and 2 bolsters	206
18. **Urdhvamukha Janu Sirsasana** 1 belt	207
19. **Swastikasana**	209
20. **Baddhakonasana** 2 blocks and 1 bolster	208
21. **Upavista Konasana**	213
22. **Paripurna Navasana** 1 long yoga belt	212
23. **Adhomukha Virasana** 2 blankets and 1 bolster	220

ASANAS	PAGE
24. **Adhomukha Swastikasana** 1 bench, 1 blanket, and 1 bolster	222
25. **Paschimottanasana** 1 stool and 2 bolsters (legs together)	216
26. **Janu Sirsasana** 1 stool, 1 blanket, and 1 bolster	218
27. **Paschimottanasana** 2 bolsters	214
28. **Bharadvajasana** 1 chair (sitting sideways)	223
29. **Bharadvajasana** (legs through a chair back)	223
30. **Bharadvajasana** 1 blanket and 2 blocks	224
31. **Marichyasana** 1 blanket and 1 block	225
32. **Utthita Marichyasana** 1 stool, 1 rounded block, and a wall	226
33. **Parsva Virasana** 1 blanket and 1 block	228
34. **Viparita Dandasana** 1 chair, 1 stool, 2 blankets, 1 bolster, and 1 belt	239
35. **Ustrasana** 2 stools, 1 blanket, and 2 bolsters	240
36. **Supta Baddhakonasana** 1 blanket, 1 bolster, 2 blocks, and 1 belt	244
37. **Supta Virasana** 1 blanket and 1 bolster	246
38. **Supta Padangusthasana** 1 belt	242
39. **Supta Padangusthasana** 1 belt and 1 block	243
40. **Salamba Sirsasana** against a wall	138
41. **Salamba Sarvangasana** 1 chair, 1 blanket, and 1 bolster	230
42. **Halasana** 1 chair, 1 stool, 1 blanket, and 2 bolsters	232

ASANAS	PAGE
43. **Setubandha Sarvangasana** 1 bench, 3 blankets, and 1 bolster	236
44. **Viparita Karani** 1 blanket, 1 block, and 2 bolsters	234
45. **Savasana** 1 blanket, 1 bolster, and 1 bandage	248
46. **Ujjayi Pranayama** 2 blankets, 2 foam blocks, 2 wooden blocks, and 1 bandage	254

WEEK 17

ASANAS	PAGE
1. **Tadasana Samasthithi** against a wall	186
2. **Tadasana Urdhva Hastasana** against a wall	187
3. **Tadasana Urdhva Baddhanguliasana** against a wall	188
4. **Tadasana Paschima Namaskarasana**	190
5. **Tadasana Gomukhasana**	191
6. **Utthita Trikonasana** 1 block	192
7. **Utthita Parsvakonasana** 1 block	194
8. **Virabhadrasana 1**	96
9. **Virabhadrasana 2**	76
10. **Ardha Chandrasana** 1 block	196
11. **Parsvottanasana**	84

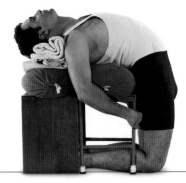

ASANAS	PAGE
12. **Adhomukha Svanasana** 1 bolster	204
13. **Prasarita Padottanasana** 1 block or 1 bolster	201
14. **Uttanasana** 1 foam block and 5 wooden blocks	197
15. **Adhomukha** **Paschimottanasana** 1 stool and 2 bolsters	217
16. **Dandasana** 1 blanket and 2 blocks	205
17. **Virasana** 2 blankets and 2 bolsters	206
18. **Urdhvamukha Janu** **Sirsasana** 1 belt	207
19. **Swastikasana**	209
20. **Baddhakonasana** 2 blocks and 1 bolster	208
21. **Upavista Konasana**	213
22. **Paripurna Navasana** 1 long yoga belt	212
23. **Adhomukha Virasana** 2 blankets and 1 bolster	220
24. **Adhomukha Swastikasana** 1 bench, 1 blanket, and 1 bolster	222
25. **Paschimottanasana** 1 stool and 2 bolsters (legs together)	216
26. **Janu Sirsasana** 1 stool, 1 blanket, and 1 bolster	218
27. **Paschimottanasana** 2 bolsters	214
28. **Bharadvajasana** 1 chair (sitting sideways)	223
29. **Bharadvajasana** (legs through a chair back)	223
30. **Bharadvajasana** 1 blanket and 2 blocks	224
31. **Marichyasana** 1 blanket and 1 block	225
32. **Utthita Marichyasana** 1 stool, 1 rounded block, and a wall	226

ASANAS	PAGE
33. **Parsva Virasana** 1 blanket and 1 block	228
34. **Viparita Dandasana** 1 chair, 2 blankets, and 1 bolster (feet against a wall)	239
35. **Ustrasana** 2 stools, 1 blanket, and 2 bolsters	240
36. **Supta Baddhakonasana** 1 blanket, 1 bolster, 2 blocks, and 1 belt	244
37. **Supta Virasana** 1 blanket and 1 bolster	246
38. **Supta Padangusthasana** 1 belt	242
39. **Supta Padangusthasana** 1 belt and 1 block	243
40. **Salamba Sirsasana** against a wall	138
41. **Salamba Sarvangasana** 1 chair, 1 blanket, and 1 bolster	230
42. **Halasana** 1 chair, 1 stool, 1 blanket, and 2 bolsters	232
43. **Setubandha Sarvangasana** 1 bench, 3 blankets, and 1 bolster	236
44. **Viparita Karani** 1 blanket, 1 block, and 2 bolsters	234
45. **Savasana** 1 blanket, 1 bolster, and 1 bandage	248
46. **Ujjayi Pranayama** 2 blankets, 2 foam blocks, 2 wooden blocks, and 1 bandage	254

WEEK 18

ASANAS	PAGE
1. **Tadasana Samasthithi** against a wall	186
2. **Tadasana Urdhva** **Hastasana** against a wall	187
3. **Tadasana Urdhva** **Baddhanguliasana** against a wall	188

ASANAS	PAGE
4. **Tadasana Paschima** **Namaskarasana**	190
5. **Tadasana Gomukhasana**	191
6. **Utthita Trikonasana** 1 block	192
7. **Utthita Parsvakonasana** 1 block	194
8. **Virabhadrasana 1**	96
9. **Virabhadrasana 2**	76
10. **Ardha Chandrasana** 1 block	196
11. **Parsvottanasana**	84
12. **Adhomukha Svanasana** 1 bolster	204
13. **Prasarita Padottanasana** 1 block or 1 bolster	201
14. **Uttanasana** 1 foam block and 5 wooden blocks	197
15. **Adhomukha** **Paschimottanasana** 1 stool and 2 bolsters	217
16. **Dandasana** 1 blanket and 2 blocks	205
17. **Virasana** 2 blankets and 2 bolsters	206
18. **Urdhvamukha Janu** **Sirsasana** 1 belt	207
19. **Swastikasana**	209
20. **Baddhakonasana** 2 blocks and 1 bolster	208
21. **Upavista Konasana**	213
22. **Paripurna Navasana** 1 long yoga belt	212
23. **Adhomukha Virasana** 2 blankets and 1 bolster	220
24. **Adhomukha Swastikasana** 1 bench, 1 blanket, and 1 bolster	222
25. **Paschimottanasana** 1 stool and 2 bolsters (legs together)	216
26. **Janu Sirsasana** 1 stool, 1 blanket, and 1 bolster	218

WEEK 19

ASANAS	PAGE
27. **Paschimottanasana** 2 bolsters	214
28. **Bharadvajasana** 1 chair (sitting sideways)	223
29. **Bharadvajasana** (legs through a chair back)	223
30. **Bharadvajasana** 1 blanket and 2 blocks	224
31. **Marichyasana** 1 blanket and 1 block	225
32. **Utthita Marichyasana** 1 stool, 1 rounded block, and a wall	226
33. **Parsva Virasana** 1 blanket and 1 block	228
34. **Viparita Dandasana** 1 chair, 2 blankets, and 1 bolster (feet against a wall)	239
35. **Ustrasana** 2 stools, 1 blanket, and 2 bolsters	240
36. **Supta Baddhakonasana** 1 blanket, 1 bolster, 2 blocks, and 1 belt	244
37. **Supta Virasana** 1 blanket and 1 bolster	246
38. **Supta Padangusthasana** 1 belt	242
39. **Supta Padangusthasana** 1 belt and 1 block	243
40. **Salamba Sirsasana** against a wall	138
41. **Salamba Sarvangasana** 1 chair, 1 blanket, and 1 bolster	230
42. **Halasana** 1 chair, 1 stool, 1 blanket, and 2 bolsters	232
43. **Setubandha Sarvangasana** 1 bench, 3 blankets, and 1 bolster	236
44. **Viparita Karani** 1 blanket, 1 block, and 2 bolsters	234
45. **Savasana** 1 blanket, 1 bolster, and 1 bandage	248
46. **Ujjayi Pranayama** 2 blankets, 2 foam blocks, 2 wooden blocks, and 1 bandage	254

ASANAS	PAGE
1. **Tadasana Samasthithi** against a wall	186
2. **Tadasana Urdhva Hastasana** against a wall	187
3. **Tadasana Urdhva Baddhanguliasana** against a wall	188
4. **Tadasana Paschima Namaskarasana**	190
5. **Tadasana Gomukhasana**	191
6. **Utthita Trikonasana** 1 block	192
7. **Utthita Parsvakonasana** 1 block	194
8. **Virabhadrasana 1**	96
9. **Virabhadrasana 2**	76
10. **Ardha Chandrasana** 1 block	196
11. **Parsvottanasana**	84
12. **Adhomukha Svanasana** 1 bolster	204
13. **Prasarita Padottanasana** 1 block or 1 bolster	201
14. **Uttanasana** 1 foam block and 5 wooden blocks	197
15. **Adhomukha Paschimottanasana** 1 stool and 2 bolsters	217
16. **Dandasana** 1 blanket and 2 blocks	205
17. **Virasana** 2 blankets and 2 bolsters	206
18. **Urdhvamukha Janu Sirsasana** 1 belt	207
19. **Swastikasana**	209
20. **Baddhakonasana** 2 blocks and 1 bolster	208
21. **Upavista Konasana**	213
22. **Paripurna Navasana** 1 long yoga belt	212

ASANAS	PAGE
23. **Adhomukha Virasana** 2 blankets and 1 bolster	220
24. **Adhomukha Swastikasana** 1 bench, 1 blanket, and 1 bolster	222
25. **Paschimottanasana** 1 stool and 2 bolsters (legs together)	216
26. **Janu Sirsasana** 1 stool, 1 blanket, and 1 bolster	218
27. **Paschimottanasana** 2 bolsters	214
28. **Bharadvajasana** 1 chair (sitting sideways)	223
29. **Bharadvajasana** (legs through a chair back)	223
30. **Bharadvajasana** 1 blanket and 2 blocks	224
31. **Marichyasana** 1 blanket and 1 block	225
32. **Utthita Marichyasana** 1 stool, 1 rounded block, and a wall	226
33. **Parsva Virasana** 1 blanket and 1 block	228
34. **Viparita Dandasana** 1 chair, 2 blankets, and 1 bolster (feet against a wall)	239
35. **Ustrasana** 2 stools, 1 blanket, and 2 bolsters	240
36. **Supta Baddhakonasana** 1 blanket, 1 bolster, 2 blocks, and 1 belt	244
37. **Supta Virasana** 1 blanket and 1 bolster	246
38. **Supta Padangusthasana** 1 belt	242
39. **Supta Padangusthasana** 1 belt and 1 block	243
40. **Salamba Sirsasana** against a wall	138
41. **Salamba Sarvangasana** 1 chair, 1 blanket, and 1 bolster	230
42. **Halasana** 1 chair, 1 stool, 1 blanket, and 2 bolsters	232

ASANAS	PAGE
43. Setubandha Sarvangasana 1 bench, 3 blankets, and 1 bolster	236
44. Viparita Karani 1 blanket, 1 block, and 2 bolsters	234
45. Savasana 1 blanket, 1 bolster, and 1 bandage	248
46. Ujjayi Pranayama 2 blankets, 2 foam blocks, 2 wooden blocks, and 1 bandage	254

WEEK 20

ASANAS	PAGE
1. Tadasana Samasthithi against a wall	186
2. Tadasana Urdhva Hastasana against a wall	187
3. Tadasana Urdhva Baddhanguliasana against a wall	188
4. Tadasana Paschima Namaskarasana	190
5. Tadasana Gomukhasana	191
6. Utthita Trikonasana 1 block	192
7. Utthita Parsvakonasana 1 block	194

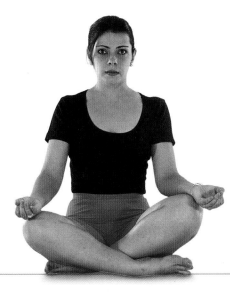

ASANAS	PAGE
8. Virabhadrasana 1	96
9. Virabhadrasana 2	76
10. Ardha Chandrasana 1 block	196
11. Parsvottanasana	84
12. Adhomukha Svanasana 1 bolster	204
13. Prasarita Padottanasana 1 block or 1 bolster	201
14. Uttanasana 1 foam block and 5 wooden blocks	197
15. Adhomukha Paschimottanasana 1 stool and 2 bolsters	217
16. Dandasana 1 blanket and 2 blocks	205
17. Virasana 2 blankets and 2 bolsters	206
18. Urdhvamukha Janu Sirsasana 1 belt	207
19. Swastikasana	209
20. Baddhakonasana 2 blocks and 1 bolster	208
21. Upavista Konasana	213
22. Paripurna Navasana 1 long yoga belt	212
23. Adhomukha Virasana 2 blankets and 1 bolster	220
24. Adhomukha Swastikasana 1 bench, 1 blanket, and 1 bolster	222
25. Paschimottanasana 1 stool and 2 bolsters (legs together)	216
26. Janu Sirsasana 1 stool, 1 blanket, and 1 bolster	218
27. Paschimottanasana 2 bolsters	214
28. Bharadvajasana 1 chair (sitting sideways)	223
29. Bharadvajasana (legs through a chair)	223

ASANAS	PAGE
30. Bharadvajasana 1 blankets and 2 blocks	224
31. Marichyasana 1 blankets and 1 block	225
32. Utthita Marichyasana 1 stool, 1 rounded block, and a wall	226
33. Parsva Virasana 1 blanket and 1 block	228
34. Viparita Dandasana 1 chair, 2 blankets, and 1 bolster (feet against a wall)	239
35. Ustrasana 2 stools, 1 blanket, and 2 bolsters	240
36. Supta Baddhakonasana 1 blanket, 1 bolster, 2 blocks, and 1 belt	244
37. Supta Virasana 1 blanket and 1 bolster	246
38. Supta Padangusthasana 1 belt	242
39. Supta Padangusthasana 1 belt and 1 block	243
40. Salamba Sirsasana against a wall	138
41. Salamba Sarvangasana 1 chair, 1 blanket, and 1 bolster	230
42. Halasana 1 chair, 1 stool, 1 blanket, and 2 bolsters	232
43. Setubandha Sarvangasana 1 bench, 3 blankets, and 1 bolster	236
44. Viparita Karani 1 blanket, 1 block, and 2 bolsters	234
45. Savasana 1 blanket, 1 bolster, and 1 bandage	248
46. Ujjayi Pranayama 2 blankets, 2 foam blocks, 2 wooden blocks, and 1 bandage	254
47. Viloma 2 Pranayama 1 blanket, 2 foam blocks, 2 wooden blocks, and 1 bandage	257

SKELETAL SYSTEM

Collar bone

Costal cartilage

Elbow joint

Pelvic rim

Hip joint

Sternum

Rib

Floating rib

Vertebra

Knee joint

Ankle joint

THE SPINE

Cervical vertebrae

Thoracic vertebrae

Lumbar vertebrae

Sacrum

Tailbone or coccyx

INTERNAL ORGANS

Trachea

Lung

Liver

Large intestine

Pharynx

Esophagus

Stomach

Pancreas

Small intestine

Rectum

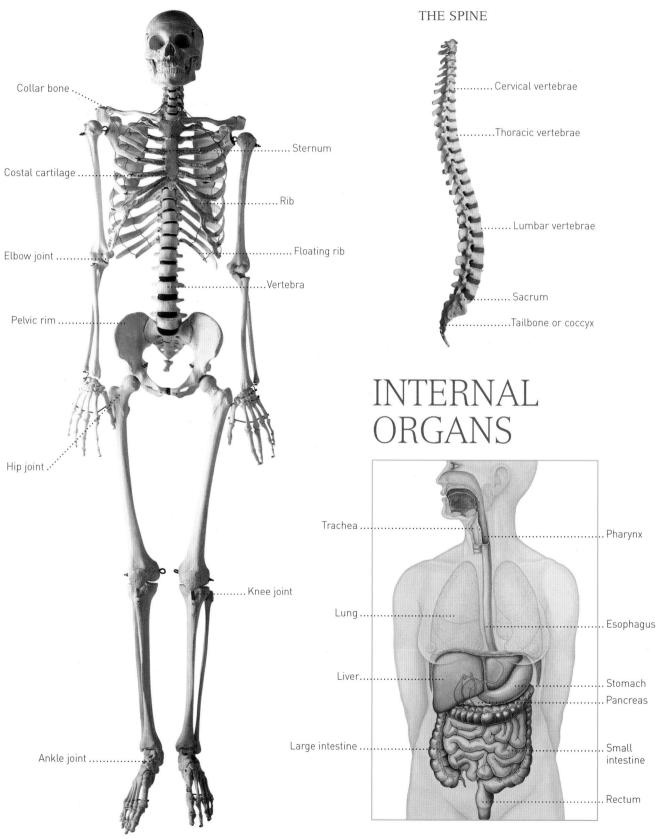

MUSCULAR SYSTEM

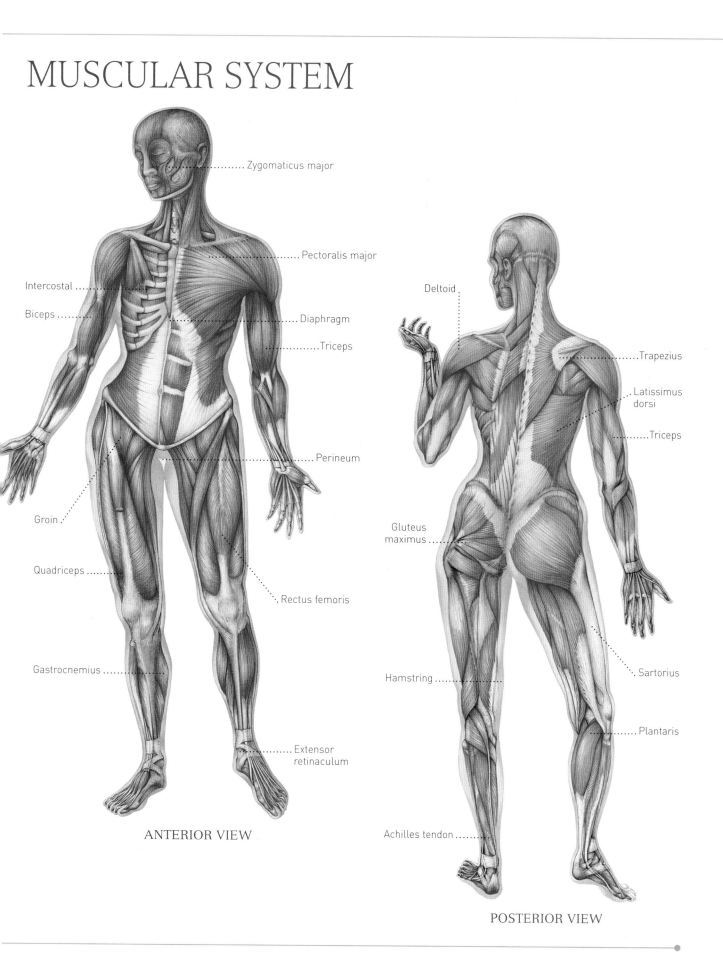

Zygomaticus major

Pectoralis major

Intercostal

Biceps

Diaphragm

Triceps

Perineum

Groin

Quadriceps

Rectus femoris

Gastrocnemius

Extensor
retinaculum

ANTERIOR VIEW

Deltoid

Trapezius

Latissimus
dorsi

Triceps

Gluteus
maximus

Hamstring

Sartorius

Plantaris

Achilles tendon

POSTERIOR VIEW

GLOSSARY

Abhyantara inhalation

Ahankara false pride

Ahimsa creed of nonviolence

Ajna chakra energy or command chakra

Alabdha bhumikatva indisposition

Alasya laziness

Anahata chakra spiritual heart chakra

Anandamaya kosha the sheath of bliss, the most important of the 5 sheaths of the body, reached by the practice of yoga

Angamejayatva unsteadiness in the body

Annamaya kosha anatomical sheath, one of 5 sheaths of the body

Antara-kumbhaka suspension of breath with full lungs

Antaranga-sadhana emotional and mental discipline gained through following the 8 limbs or steps of yoga

Antaratma-sadhana quest for the soul gained through following the 8 limbs or steps of yoga

Anusasanam discipline

Aparigraha freedom from desire

Arambhavastha beginners' stage of yoga, practiced at the level of the physical body alone

Asmita egoism

Astanga yoga eight limbs: the steps to self-realization through the practice of yoga

Asteya freedom from avarice

Atman the self or soul

Avirati desire for sensual satisfaction

Ayama expansion or distribution of energy

Bahya exhalation

Bahya-kumbhaka suspension of breath with empty lungs

Bahiranga-sadhana one of 3 yogic disciplines, comprising the practice of ethics

Bhakti marg path of love and devotion

Bharadvaja a sage, the father of the warrior Dronacharya

Bhranti darshana false knowledge

Brahmacharya chastity

Buddhi intelligence

Chitta the restraint of consciousness

Chittavritti an imbalance in the mental state

Chakras critical junctions in the body, notionally located along the spine, which, when activated by asanas and pranayama, transform cosmic energy into spiritual energy

Dharana concentration, the sixth limb or step of Astanga yoga

Dhyana the seventh stage of the 8 limbs or steps of Astanga yoga

Dronacharya son of the sage Bharadvaja and a major character in the epic, *Mahabharata*

Dorsal region the upper part of the body, relating especially to the back

Duhkha misery or pain

Ekagra a focused state of mind

Floating ribs the last 2 pairs of ribs which are not attached to the sternum

Ghatavastha intermediate stage of yoga, when the mind and body learn to move together

Gheranda Samhita text on yoga, written by the sage Gheranda in the 15th century

Guru teacher; one who hands down a system of knowledge to a disciple

Guru-sishya parampara the tradition of teaching, dating back centuries, of teacher and student

Hatha yoga sighting the soul through the restraint of energy

Hathayoga Pradipika treatise on yoga compiled in the 15th century by the sage Svatmarama

Isvara pranidhana devotion to God

Jivatma the individual self

Jnana marg path of knowledge whereby the seeker learns to discriminate between the real and the unreal

Kaivalya freedom of emancipation

Karma marg path of selfless service without thought of reward

Karana sharira causal body, one of the 3 layers of the body

Karya sharira gross body, one of the 3 layers of the body

Kathopanishad ancient text circa 300-400 BC

Klesha sorrow caused by egoism, desire, ignorance, attachment, and hatred

Ksipta a distracted mind

Kundalini divine, cosmic energy which is latent in every human being

Kumbhaka retention of energy

Leukorrhea excessive white vaginal discharge

Manas the mind

Manava (manusya) an intelligent and conscious human being

Mahabharata the most ancient of the Indian epics, dating to the first millennium BC

Manipuraka chakra site of the sense of fear and apprehension

Manomaya kosha psychological sheath, one of the 5 sheaths of the body

Marichi a sage, son of Brahma, the creator of the universe

Menorrhagia abnormally heavy or long periods

Metrorrhagia bleeding in between periods

Mudha a dull, inert mind

Muladhara chakra controls sexual energy

Nadi notional channels which distribute energy from the chakras through the body

Nirbija seedless

Niruddha a controlled and restrained mind

Nishpattyavastha ultimate stage of yoga practice, the state of perfection

Niyama self-restraint

Parmatama the universal self

Parichayavastha third stage of yoga practice, when the intelligence and the body become one

Parigraha possessiveness

Patanjala Yoga Darshana corpus of aphorisms on yoga, compiled between 300 BC–AD 300 and usually attributed to the sage Patanjali

Patanjali, a sage, the founder of yoga; believed to have lived sometime between 300 BC–AD 300

Perineum the area between the thighs, behind the genital organs and in front of the anus

Pramada indifference

Prakriti shakti energy of nature

Prana vital energy or life-force

Pranamaya kosha life-force sheath, one of the 5 sheaths of the body

Pranayama control of energy through breathing

Pratyahara mental detachment from the external world

Psoriasis an ailment leading to dry and scaly patches on the skin

Purusha shakti energy of the soul

Raja yoga sighting the soul through the restraint of consciousness

Rajasic spicy, pungent foods that overstimulate the body and mind

Sahasrara chakra the most important chakra—when uncoiled, it brings the seeker to freedom

Samadhi self-realization

Samshaya doubt

Samyama integration of the body, breath, mind, intellect, and self

Santosha contentment

Sarvanga sadhana holistic practice which integrates the body, mind and the self

Sattvic natural, organic vegetarian food

Satya truth

Saucha cleanliness

Scoliosis a curved spine

Shakti vital energy and the sense of self, which determine a person's emotions, will power, and discrimination

Shvasa-prashvasa uneven respiration or unsteadiness

Styana reluctance to work

Suksma sharira the subtle body, one of the 3 layers of the body

Svadhyaya to study one's body, mind, intellect, and ego

Svatmarama sage, author of *Hathayoga Pradipika*

Swadhishtana chakra site of worldly desires

Tamasic food containing meat or alcohol

Tapas austerity gained through the committed practice of yoga

Vijnanamaya kosha intellectual sheath, one of the 5 sheaths of the body

Viksipta a scattered, fearful mind

Virabhadra a legendary warrior

Vishuddhi chakra seat of intellectual awareness

Vyadhi physical ailments

Yama ethical codes for daily life

Yoga the path which integrates the body, senses, mind, and the intelligence, with the self

Yogacharya a teacher and a master of yogic traditions

Yoga-agni the fire of yoga which, when lit, ignites the kundalini

Yogabhrastha falling from the grace of yoga

Yoga marg the journey to self-realization, when the mind and its actions are brought under control

Yoga Sutras a collection of aphorisms on the practice of yoga, attributed to the sage Patanjali

Yogi a student, a seeker of truth

NAMES OF ASANAS

Name	Translation
Adhomukha Paschimottanasana	Downward-facing intense back stretch
Adhomukha Svanasana	Downward-facing dog stretch
Adhomukha Swastikasana	Downward-facing cross-legged pose
Adhomukha Virasana	Downward-facing hero pose
Ardha Chandrasana	Half moon pose
Baddhakonasana	Fixed angle pose
Bharadvajasana	Torso stretch
Bharadvajasana on a chair	Lateral twist of the spine
Dandasana	Staff pose
Halasana	Plough pose
Janu Sirsasana	Head on knee pose
Marichyasana	Torso and leg stretch
Paripurna Navasana	Complete boat pose
Parsva Virasana	Side twist in the hero pose
Parsvottanasana	Intense torso stretch
Paschimottanasana	Intense back stretch
Prasarita Padottanasana	Intense leg stretch
Salamba Sarvangasana	Shoulderstand
Salamba Sirsasana	Headstand
Savasana	Corpse pose
Setubandha Sarvangasana	Bridge pose
Supta Baddhakonasana	Reclining fixed angle pose
Supta Padangusthasana	Reclining leg, foot, and toe stretch
Supta Virasana	Reclining hero pose
Swastikasana	Cross-legged pose
Tadasana	Mountain pose
Tadasana Samasthithi	Steady and firm mountain pose
Tadasana Gomukhasana	Mountain pose with hands held in the shape of a cow's face
Tadasana Paschima Baddha Hastasana	Mountain pose with the arms folded behind the back
Tadasana Paschima Namaskarasana	Mountain pose with hands folded behind the back
Tadasana Urdhva Baddhanguliasana	Mountain pose with fingers interlocked
Tadasana Urdhva Hastasana	Mountain pose with arms stretched up
Trianga Mukhaikapada Paschimottanasana	Three parts of the body stretch
Ujjayi Pranayama	Conquest of energy
Upavista Konasana	Seated wide-angle pose
Urdhva Dhanurasana	Bow pose
Urdhvamukha Janu Sirsasana	Upward-facing bent knee pose
Ustrasana	Camel pose
Uttanasana	Intense forward stretch
Utthita Marichyasana	Intense torso and leg stretch
Utthita Parsvakonasana	Intense side stretch
Utthita Trikonasana	Extended triangle pose
Viloma 2 Pranayama	Interrupted breathing cycle
Viparita Dandasana	Inverted staff pose
Viparita Karani	Inverted pose
Virabhadrasana 1	Warrior pose 1
Virabhadrasana 2	Warrior pose 2
Virasana	Hero pose

INDEX

A

Abdomen, 186–87
  blood circulation, 211
  stretching, 167
  toning and activating 188
Abdominal cramps, 157
Abdominal hernia, 84
Abdominal muscles, 97, 211, 223, 229
Abdominal organs, 85, 103, 115, 119, 133, 151, 161, 193, 195, 198, 201, 207–08, 211, 225, 237
Abdominal blood circulation, 225
Abdominal pain during menstruation, 93
Abdominal walls, sagging, 103
Abhyantara, 55
Absent periods, 390–93
Acidity, 73, 92, 97, 167, 193, 195, 198, 201, 217, 221, 247, 287–89
Acne, 344–47
Adhomukha Paschimottanasana, 217
Adhomukha Svanasana, 62, 88–91, 202–84
Adhomukha Swastikasana, 222
Adhomukha Virasana, 220–21
Adrenal glands, 123, 215, 219, 239, 241
Aging, 69
Ahankara, 47, 50
Ahimsa, 52
Ajna chakra, 49, 57
Alabdha bhumikatva, 47
Alasya, 47
Alcohol abuse, 240
Alcoholism, 217, 368–71
Anahata chakra, 57
Anandamaya kosha, 48
Angamejayatva, 36, 47
Angina pain, 189, 215, 228, 272–74
Ankles, 241
  arthritis, 166
  joint flexibility, 204
  osteoarthritis, 338–41
  pain, 224, 229
  stiffness, 157
  strengthening, 73, 89
Annamaya kosha, 48
Anorexia, 217, 372–75
Antara-kumbhaka, 55
Antaranga-sadhana, 47
Antaratma-sadhana, 47
Anxiety, 170, 204, 233, 364–66
Aparigraha, 52–53
Appetite loss, 217, 228
Arambhavastha, stage of yoga, 37–38, 62
Arches of feet, 119, 204, 206, 229
Ardha Chandrasana, 196
Asanas,
  Adhomukha Paschimottanasana, 217
  Adhomukha Svanasana, 88–91, 202–204
  Adhomukha Swastikasana, 222
  Adhomukha Virasana, 221–21
  Ardha Chandrasana, 196
  back bends, 65, 154–63
  Baddhakonasana, 108–11, 208

benefits of poses in, 40
Bharadvajasana, 128–31, 224
Bharadvajasana on a chair, 223
brain of pose, 65
classic poses, 62–65
concept, 63
Dandasana, 102–03, 205
forward bends, 64, 112–25
Halasana, 150–53, 232–33
importance of, 40
inversions, 64–65, 136–53
Janu Sirsasana, 114–17, 218–19
Marichyasana, 132–35, 225
Paripurna Navasana, 210–12
Parsva Virasana, 228–29
Parsvottanasana, 84–87
Paschimottanasana, 122–25, 214–16
poses, *see* classic poses
practice against wall, 183
pranayama, 36, 250–53
Prasarita Padottanasana, 200–01
props for, 184–85
reclining, 65, 164–73
Salamba Sarvangasana, 144–49, 230–31
Salamba Sirsasana, 138–43
Savasana, 170–72, 248–49
Setubandha Sarvangasana, 236–37
sitting, 64, 100–11
standing, 64, 66–99
stress, asanas for, 175, 180–81, 186–249
Supta Baddhakonasana, 244–45
Supta Padangusthasana, 242–43
Swastikasana, 209
  Tadasana, 68–69,
  variations of, 186–91
  Trianga Mukhaikapada Paschimottanasana, 118–21
twists, 64, 126–35
Ujjayi Pranayama, 254–56
Upavista Konasana, 213
Urdhva Dhanurasana, 160–63
Urdhvamukha Janu Sirsasana, 207
Ustrasana, 156–59, 240–41
Uttanasana, 92–95, 197–99
Utthita Marichyasana, 226–27
Utthita Parsvakonasana, 80–83, 194–95
Utthita Trikonasana, 70–75, 192–93
Viloma 2 Pranayama, 257
Viparita Dandasana, 238–39
Viparita Karani, 234–35
Virabhadrasana, 96–99
Virabhadrasana, 76–79
Virasana, 104–09, 206
with props, 12, 24, 25,173–83
Astanga yoga, 47, 52, 53
Asteya, 52–53
Arms, arthritis, 188–89
  flexibility,190
  ligaments, 193
Arterial blockage, 237, 239
Arteries, blood circulation, 236
Arteries of heart, thickening, 160
Arthritic pain, 81
Arthritic pain in back, 241
Arthritis of 187, 235
  ankles, 166

arms, 188–89
back, 233, 241
elbows, 105
fingers, 105, 188–89, 204
hips, 213
lower back, 223
shoulder, 188–89, 204
shoulder joints, 89
spine, 233
wrist, 204
Asthma, 102, 144, 150, 167, 205, 208, 210, 213–14, 217–218, 231, 233, 235, 242, 256, 282–84
Asthmatic attack, 118, 122
Asthmatics, 103
Avirati, 47
Ayama, 53, 54, 250

B

Back flexibility, 129
Back pain 129, 167, 221
  during menstruation, 93
Back muscles, 97, 157
Back stiffness, 157
Back stretching, 167
Back toning and activating, 187–88
Backache, 73, 77, 97, 105, 133, 138, 170, 188, 190–91, 193, 195, 201, 210, 232, 237, 243, 254, 257
Baddhakonasana, 43, 108–09, 208
Bahiranga-sadhana, 47
Bahya, 55
Bahya-kumbhaka, 55
Bellur Initiative, 27–31
Bellur Krishnamachar and Seshamma Smaraka Nidhi Trust, 30
Bhakti marg, 46, 251
Bharadvaja, 128
Bharadvajasana, 64, 128–31, 224
Bharadvajasana on a chair, 223
Bhranti darshana, 47
Bile formation, 204
Bile secretion, 119
Bladder control, 186, 219, 245
Bladder toning and strengthening, 97, 123
Blocked arteries, 223, 226, 242, 246–47, 273
Blocked fallopian tubes, 109
Blood circulation, 157, 161
  in knee, 222
  in pelvic area, 215
  in ovarian region, 245
  to abdominal organs, 225
  to arteries, 237
  to ovaries, 241
Blood, hemoglobin content, 121
Blood pressure, 115, 160, 198, 201, 204, 215, 228, 235, 237, 245, 254–55
Body alignment, 69
  alignment, 69
  and brain, 263
  and mind, 22–33, 37, 39
  harmony with mind, 39
  metabolic rate, 211
  relaxation, 171
Bolster, 184
Bowel movement, 145

Brahmacharya, 52–53
Brain
  blood flow to, 198
  body and, 263
  calm, 89
  cells, 128
  cooling, 85
  soothing, 198, 201, 237–39
Brain and nervous system ailments
  asanas for, 351–58
  epilepsy, 356–58
  eye strain, 351–53
  headache, 351–52
  memory impairment, 352–55
  migraine, 354–56
  sciatica, 356–57
  stress-related headache, 352–53
Breathing, 171, 191
  capacity, 77
  difficulties, 150
  ease, 275
Breathlessness, 103, 145, 204–05, 208, 210, 220–22, 226, 233, 235, 277–79
Bronchitis, 145, 205, 208, 210, 214, 217–18, 220, 223, 226, 228, 231, 233, 235, 242, 280–83
Buddhi, 50
Bulimia, 186–90, 194, 205, 217, 370–73
Buttock muscles toning, 69

C

Calcaneal spurs, 105, 204, 206, 229
  softening, 89
Calf muscles, stretching, 243
Calves, pain, 206, 224, 229
Camel pose asana, 156–59, 240–41
Cardiac arrest, 237
Cardiac condition, 84, 104, 191, 160, 188, 210, 224–26, 243
Cardiac disorders, 167, 256
Cervical spondylosis, 80, 138, 150, 189–92, 194, 210, 214, 225, 231–32, 235, 326–27
Chair, as prop, 184
Chakras, 56–57
Chest
  congestion, 224–25, 228
  expanding, 237
  muscles, 103
Chitta, 48, 50
Chittavritti, 36, 176
Choking, 103
Chronic constipation, 231
Chronic fatigue syndrome, 171, 194, 196, 210, 224–26, 228
Chronic headache, 215, 219
Classic poses,
  bow pose, 160–63
  camel pose, 156–59
  corpse pose, 170–73
  downward-facing dog stretch, 88–91
  extended triangle pose, 70–75
  fixed angle pose, 108–11
  head-on-knee pose, 114–17
  headstand, 138–43
  hero pose, 104–07
  intense chest stretch, 84–87

intense forward stretch, 92–95
intense side stretch, 80–84
intense torso stretch, 122–25
mountain pose, 68–69
plough pose 150–53
reclining hero stretch, 166–69
shoulderstand, 144–49
staff pose, 102–08
three parts of the body stretch, 120–21
torso and leg stretch, 132–35
torso stretch, 128–31
warrior pose 96–99
warrior pose 76–79
Cold, 132, 141, 145, 210, 224–25, 228, 233, 257, 276–77
Cold extremities, 264–66
Colitis, 145, 231
Confidence boosting, 188–91, 201, 256
Congestion,
chest, 210, 231, 233
in ovaries, 145
Constipation, 119, 156, 204, 225–26, 238, 240, 254, 257, 289–91
Coronary blood flow, 247
Cosmic energy awakening, 56
Coughs, 141, 257
Cramps in legs, 206
Crepe bandage, 184

D

Dandasana, 102–03, 205
Depression, 186–92, 194, 198, 201, 204, 221, 224–26, 228, 237, 256, 367–69
Dharana, 47, 52, 53
Dhyana, 22, 47, 52, 53, 252
Diaphragm, 215
Diarrhea, 76, 118, 122, 128, 132, 150, 156, 160, 186–88, 190–92, 194, 196–97, 202, 206–07, 210, 214, 217–18, 220, 222–26, 228, 235, 238, 240, 242, 257, 290
Digestion, 81, 85, 97, 119, 151, 167, 193, 195, 205, 223, 225, 229, 237
Digestive system ailments, 123, 141, 285–99
acidity, 287–89
asanas for, 285–99
constipation, 289–91
diarrhea, 290
duodenal ulcers, 292–95
gastric ulcers, 294–97
indigestion, 285–87
irritable bowel syndrome, 292–93
ulcerative colitis, 296–99
Disciple, 59
Displaced bladder, 239
Displaced uterus, 97, 108, 189, 191
Dizziness, 92, 221
Dizzy spells, 70
Dorsal spine area, 129
Dreamless sleep, 249
Dronacharya, 128
Dropped arches, 119
Drug addiction, 375–77
Dryness and itching in vagina, 219
Duhkha, 38
Duodenal ulcers, 292–95
Dysentery, 76, 84, 128, 132

E

Ear ailments, 235, 237
Eczema, 346–49
Ekagra, state of mind, 51
Elbows, arthritis 85, 105
flexibility of, 190
osteoarthritis of, 330–31
pain or cramps of, 151
stiffness of, 115
Eliminatory problem, 141
Emotional stability, 239
Endocrine glands, blood supply to, 215
Energy level, 133, 151
Epilepsy, 356–58
Excess menstrual flow, 161
Extreme fatigue, 204
Eye ailments, 235, 237
Eye strain, 130, 186–87, 189, 191–92, 196, 207, 215, 228, 223–24, 226, 228, 238, 240, 242, 257, 351–53

F

Facial muscles, 215
Fallopian tube blockage, 109
Fat around
hips, 77, 81
waist, 81, 133
Fatigue, 151, 192, 196, 198, 201, 204, 210, 215, 221–26, 228, 233, 257, 312–15, 360–63
Faulty posture, 193
Feet
ache, 222
circulation in, 105
degenerative effect of aging on, 69
pain, 247
revitalization, 186
Fibroids, 228
Fingers
arthritic, 105, 188–89, 204
joints, stiffness of, 115
osteoarthritis of, 332–33
pain or cramps of, 151
Flat feet, 119, 186–87, 206
Flat feet, correction, 229, 247
Flatulence, 73, 103, 119, 193, 195, 211, 221, 224–25, 227, 229, 245, 247
Foam blocks, as props 185
Folded blankets, as props, 185
Food and nourishment, 178

G

Gall bladder disorder, 224
Gastric ulcers, 294–97
Gastritis, 73, 193, 195
Ghatavastha stage of yoga, 38, 62–63
Gheranda, 53
Gheranda Samhita, 53
Gout, 105, 206
in knees, 224, 229
pain, 247
Groin
stiffness, 105
supple, 209, 245
Guru, 58–59
Guru-sishya parampara, 58

H

Halasana, 150–53, 232–33
Half-Halasana stool, 184
Halitosis, 141
Hamstrings muscle, 119, 186, 195, 198, 204, 206, 241
Hamstrings, stretching, 243
supple, 224, 229
Hands, pain or cramps of, 151
Hatha yoga, 48
Hathayoga Pradipika, 48–49, 54–55, 64
Headache, 88, 128, 138, 150, 156, 160, 186–92, 194, 196, 198, 201–04, 206–07, 215, 219–25, 228, 231, 235, 236–38, 242, 255, 257, 351–52
Health, and yoga, 39
Heart and circulation ailments,
angina, 272–74
asanas for, 264–65
blocked arteries, 271–73
cold extremities, 264–66
heart attack, 274–76
high blood pressure, 268–70
low blood pressure, 270–71
varicose veins, 266–68
Heart attack, 156, 274–75
Heart, energizing, 201
Heart massage, strengthening, 123, 239, 247
Heart muscles, toning, 81, 237
Heart rate, 204
Heart rest and massage, 123, 215
Heart stress, 115
Heartbeat, 89, 93
Heartburn, 76, 103
Heart stimulation, 208
Heels, pain of, 89, 206, 224, 229
Hemoglobin content of blood, 141
Hemorrhoids, 145, 151, 186, 201, 231, 245
Hernia, 109, 145, 151, 208, 213, 225, 243, 247, 399–401
Herniated discs, 105
Hiatus hernia, 399–401
High blood pressure, 70, 80, 84, 88, 96, 138, 144, 150, 187–88, 190, 192, 202, 221, 223–26, 228, 240, 242, 249, 268–70
High stool as prop, 184–85
Hips,
arthritis, 213,
fat around, 77, 81
flexibility of joints, 129, 198, 204
Hips, joint
flexibility, 129, 198, 204
pain, 222, 224, 227, 229
stiffness, 105, 206
strengthening, 243
supple, 195, 201, 209
Hips, osteoarthritis, 232, 243, 334–36
stiffness, 115
supple, 245
Hormonal system ailment
asanas for, 302–07
diabetes, 304–07
obesity, 302–06
Hot flashes during menopause, 89
Hypertension, 145, 151, 156, 194, 196, 231, 233, 237
Hyperventilation, 366–67

I

Immune system, asanas for, 308–09
Impotence, 123, 397–99
Incontinence, 300–01
Indigestion, 204, 211, 224, 227, 235, 239, 245, 247, 285–87
Infections resistance, 241, 247
Infertility, 394–96
Inflammation, in blood vessels of legs, 206
in knees, 209
of veins in legs, 209
Inguinal hernia, 402–03
Inner eye, 22
Insomnia, 141, 145, 171, 186–91, 194, 196, 198, 207, 210, 224–26, 228, 231, 233, 237–38, 240, 362–64
Internal organs, 424
Intestines, 133
Irregular menstruation, 109
Irritable bowel syndrome, 292–93
Irritability, 359–61
Ischemia, 150, 160
Isvara pranidhana, 53
Iyengar, B.K.S.
humble beginnings, 16, 18, 19
family life, 19, 20
legacy, 24–31
message from, 32–33

J

Janu Sirsasana, 114–17, 218–19
Jivatma, 46
Jnana marg, 46
Jogging, 204
Junk food, 178

K

Kalidasa, 76
Kaivalya, 49
Karana sharira, 48
Karma marg, 46
Karya sharira, 48
Kathopanishad, 47
Klesha, 41
Kidneys, 109, 133, 205, 207, 211, 217
disorder, 224–25, 235
toning, 93, 123, 241, 245
Knees
cartilage of, 204, 206, 209
gout and rheumatism of, 224, 229
inflammation in, 206, 209, 247
joints of, 119, 186–87
joints, flexibility of, 204
joints, strengthening of, 188–91, 198, 201
ligaments, injuries of, 104
osteoarthritis of, 166, 186–91, 194, 196–97, 207, 220, 223–26, 240, 243, 336–39
pain in, 206, 209
rheumatism of, 223
stiffness of, 105, 193
strengthening of, 195, 243
Krishnamarcharya, Tirumalai, 11–13

Ksipta, state of mind, 51
Kumarasambhava, 76
Kundalini, 56–57

L

Legs,
    blood vessels, inflammation of, 206
    degenerative effects of aging, 69
    ligaments of, 193, 204
    muscles of, 103, 115, 205, 227
    shortening of, 227
    toning of, 103
    pain in, 247
    stiffness of, 115
    strengthening of, 195
    tendons of, 204
    toning of, 89, 241
    veins, inflammation of, 209
Leukorrhea, 186–91, 194, 208, 245, 387–89
Ligaments and tendons of legs, 204
Ligaments of legs, strengthening, 103
Ligaments of spine, 215
Ligaments of body, 255
Liver, 123, 133, 217
    disorder of, 224–25
    toning of, 85, 93, 241
Long hours standing, effects of, 247
Low blood pressure, 138, 186–74, 197, 200, 207, 210, 223–26, 228, 240, 270–71
Low immune system, asanas for, 308–11
Low open stool as prop, 184
Lower back
    arthritis, 223
    pain, 224, 227
    stiffness, 224, 227, 243
Lower backache, 77, 167, 201, 204, 207, 211, 217, 225, 227, 229, 241, 245, 247, 318–21
Lower spine, strengthening, 225
Lumbago, 97, 133, 233
Lumbar spine,
    excessive curvature, 197,
    painful, stiff, sprained and fused, 129
Lungs,
    capacity of, 81, 157, 239, 241
    energizing of, 141, 201
    tissue elasticity of, 241, 247

M

Mahabharata, 128
Manas, 50
Manava (manusa), 50
Manipuraka chakra, 57
Manomaya kosha, 48
Marichi, 132
Marichyasana, 132–34, 225
Memory impairment, 352–55
Memory sharpening, 215, 228
Men's health ailments,
    asanas for, 397–405
    hiatus hernia, 399–401
    impotence, 397–99
    inguinal hernia, 402–03
    prostate gland, 398–99
    umbilical hernia, 402–03
Menopause, 245, 257, 383–86
    hot flashes during, 31, 89
    symptoms of, 239, 241,
Menorrhagia, 76, 257, 388–91

Menstrual cramps, 135, 161, 228
Menstrual discomfort, 243
Menstrual disorders, 193, 195, 207, 210, 213, 234
Menstrual flow, 89, 145, 157, 161, 201, 207, 213, 219
Menstrual pain, 85, 97, 167, 208, 221, 239, 241, 245, 280–81
Menstruation, 30, 93, 128, 138, 144, 150, 166, 192, 194, 205, 221, 223–26, 228, 230, 232, 234, 378–80
    abdominal and back pain during, 93
    discomfort, 73
    heavy, 97
Mental exhaustion, 89, 93
Mental faculties, 50
Mental fatigue, 150, 249, 360–63
Menuhin, Yehudi, 12
Metrorrhagia, 76, 257, 386–87
Middle backache, 167, 207, 320–23
Migraine, 128, 138, 150, 156, 160, 171, 186–92, 194, 196, 198, 201, 206–07, 210, 215, 219–20, 222–26, 228, 231, 233, 235, 237–38, 240, 242, 354–57
Mind,
    body and, 22–23, 37
    body harmony, 39
    nature, 50
    peace of, 171
    serenity of, 257
    states of, 50–51
    stress on, 115
Mind and emotions, ailments,
    alcoholism, 368–71
    anorexia, 372–75
    anxiety, 364–65
    asanas for, 359–77
    bulimia, 370–73
    depression, 365–73
    drug addiction, 375–77
    fatigue, 150, 257, 360–63
    hyperventilation, 366–67
    insomnia, 362–64
    irritability, 359–61
    mental fatigue, 360–63
Mood swings, 257
Mudha, 50
Muladhara chakra, 57
Muscles, bones, and joints ailments,
    asanas for, 312–43
    lower backache, 318–21
    middle backache, 320–32
    muscle cramps, 314–21
    osteoarthritis of
        ankles, 338–41
        elbows, 330–31
        fingers, 332–33
        hips, 334–35
        knee, 336–39
        shoulders, 328–29
        wrist, 332–33
    physical fatigue, 312–15
    rheumatoid arthritis, 340–43
    upper backache, 322–25
Muscular system, 424–25

N

Nadi, 57
Nausea, 222, 235
Neck
    arthritis, 85
    pain, 129, 221
    sprains, 195
    stiffness, 105, 193, 207, 223–24, 227

strain, 237
Negative stress, 179
Nerves,
    soothing, 85, 145,
    stimulation, 89
Nervous disorder, 231
Nervous exhaustion, 237
Nervous system, 171, 198, 204, 256
Nervous tension, 171
Nirbija (seedless) samadhi, 49
Niruddha, 51, 176
Nishpattyavastha, 38, 63
Niyama, 47, 52–53

O

Osteoarthritis of,
    ankles, 338–41
    elbows, 330–31
    fingers, 332–33
    hips, 232, 243, 334–36
    knees, 167, 169, 186–91, 194–97, 207, 220, 223–26, 240, 242, 336–39
    shoulders, 328–29
    wrist, 332–33
Ovarian cysts, 145
Ovarian region, blood circulation in, 245
Ovaries, 109, 123, 213
    blood circulation in, 241
    congestion and heaviness, 145
    disorders, 167

P

Padmasana, 54
Pain during menstruation, 243
Palpitation, 76, 145, 204, 222, 231, 233, 235
Pancreas, 123, 133
Parathyroid glands, 145, 231, 233
Paramatama, 46
Parichayavastha, 38, 63
Parigraha, 52
Paripoorna Matsyendrasana, 260
Paripurna Navasana, 210–12
Parkinson's disease, 68
Parsva Virasana, 228–29
Parsvottanasana, 84–85
Paschima Baddha Hastasana, 189
Paschimottanasana, 65, 122–25, 116–18
Patanjali, 37, 40, 41, 46–47, 48–49, 50, 52–53, 55, 176, 260
Patanjala Yoga Darshana, 37
Peace of mind, 171
Pelvic area
    alignment, 243
    blood circulation, 215
    massage and toning, 73
    stretching, 241
Pelvic organs, 161, 193, 195, 207–08, 215, 247
Pelvic, 186–88
Perception, organs of, 179
Perriera, Father Joe, 22
Peptic ulcers, 208, 232
Physical exhaustion, 93
Physical fatigue, 150, 249, 312–15
Pineal glands, 141, 161, 239, 241
Pituitary glands, 141, 161, 239, 241
Polio, 188–89, 191
Positive stress, 179
Posture correction, 157, 186
Prakriti shakti, 57

Prana, 48, 49, 53, 54, 57, 252, 253
Pranamaya kosha, 48
Pranayama, 15, 22,23, 32, 36, 47, 50–55, 250–57
    asanas, and, 36, 251
    between material and spiritual world, 55, 252
    breath in, 54–55, 252–53
    final goal, 54–55
    with props, 254–57
Prasarita Padottanasana, 200–01
Pratyahara, 47, 52–53
Pregnancy, advanced stage of, 88
Premenstrual stress, 194, 205, 208, 232
Premenstrual syndrome, 382–83
Prolapsed bladder, 213
Prolapsed disc, 77
Prolapsed uterus, 108, 145, 161, 188, 190, 207, 213, 239, 241, 245, 247, 392–95
Props
    asanas with 181, 184
    help from, 23, 25, 182–83
    therapy and, 183
    types of, 184–85
Prostate gland, 109, 207, 228, 398–99
Psoriasis, 194, 349–50
Puberty, 245
Pulse rate, 215
Purusha, 250
Purusha shakti, 57

R

Raja yoga, 48
Rajasic food, 179
Ramaamani Iyengar Memorial Yoga Institute, 25
Recuperation after illness, 249
Recurrent headache, 202
Refreshing, 279
Reproductive system, organs of, 123, 207, 213
Respiratory system ailments,
    asanas for, 170, 276–84
    asthma, 228–84
    breathlessness, 277–79
    bronchitis, 280–83
    colds, 276–77
    sinusitis, 279–81
    symptoms, 249
Rheumatic fever, 194
Rheumatic pain, 206, 247
Rheumatism, 167, 223–24, 229
    in knees, 223–24, 229
Rheumatoid arthritis, 192, 197, 202, 205, 208, 240, 340–43
Rolled blankets as props, 185
Rounded wooden block as prop, 185

S

Sahasrara chakra, 57
Salamba Sarvangasana, 40, 65, 144–49, 230–31
Salamba Sirsasana, 65, 138–43
Samadhi, 46, 47, 48–49, 52, 53
Samyama, 53
Santosha, 53
Sarvanga sadhana, 42, 48
Sattvic food, 20, 178
Satya, 52
Saucha, 52, 53

Savasana, 65, 170–72, 248–49
Sciatica, 97, 208, 227, 245, 356–57
    pain, 81, 109, 186–91, 205, 213, 243
Sedentary lifestyle, 193
Self-confidence, 187, 239
Self-realization, 46, 52–53
Senses, control of, 177
Serious illness, recovery from, 171
Setubandha Sarvangasana, 236–37
Severe backache, 210, 257
Severe constipation, 156
Shakti, 56
Shvasa-prashvasa, 36, 47
Shoulders,
    alignment, 73
    arthritis, 85, 188–89, 204
    blades, misalignment of, 195
    blades, stiffness of, 89
    cramps, 151
    dislocation, 88
    misalignment, 195
    pain, 129, 151, 231
    osteoarthritis, 328–29
    round, 115
    stiffness, 105, 115, 157, 193,
    223–24, 227
    supple, 128
Sinus blockage, 145
Sinusitis, 231, 279–81
Skeletal system, 425
Skin ailments
    acne, 344–47
    asanas for, 344–50
    eczema, 346–49
    psoriasis, 349–50
    temperature, 215
Sleep disorders, 249
Slipped disc, 77, 188–91
Sluggish liver, 123
Soham, 250
Spinal column, alignment, 227
Spinal column, supple, 195
Spinal disc disorder, 68, 92, 166
Spinal disorders, 188
Spinal muscles, 211
    supple, 223
    toning, 103
Spine, 151, 161, 208
    arthritis, 233
    curvature, 115
    degenerative effect of aging on, 69
    flexibility, 73, 239
    ligaments, 215
    muscle, 157
    stiffness, 202
    straightening, 69
    strengthening, 237
    stretching, 221
    supple, 129
    tendency to sag, 102
    toning, 221, 241
Spiritual pranayama, 55, 250–53
Spiritual void, and yoga, 38
Spleen, 133
    disorder, 224
    toning, 85, 93, 241
Stamina, 141
Stiff spine, 202
Stiffness in neck, 223
Stomach ulcers, 167
Stomachache, 93, 198, 201
Stress,
    active and passive practice, 181
    asanas,
        Adhomukha
            Paschimottanasana, 217
        Adhomukha Svanasana,

220–22
        Adhomukha Swastikasana,
        240
        Adhomukha Virasana, 220–21
        alleviating of, 179
        Ardha Chandrasana, 196
        Bharadvajasana, 224
        Bharadvajasana on a chair,
        223
        Dandasana, 205
        Marichyasana, 225
        Paripurna Navasana, 210–12
        Parsva Virasana, 228–29
        Paschimottanasana, 214–16
        Prasarita Padottanasana,
        200–01
        Sequencing and timing of, 181
        Setubandha Sarvangasana,
        236–37
        Supta Baddhakonasana,
        244–45
        Supta Padangusthasana,
        242–43
        Swastikasana, 209
        Tadasana Gomukhasana, 191
        Paschima Baddha
        Hastasana, 189
        Tadasana Paschima
       Namaskarasana, 190
        Tadasana Samasthithi, 186
        Tadasana Urdhva
        Baddhanguliasana, 188
        Tadasana Urdhva Hastasana,
        187
        Ujjayi Pranayama, 254–56
        Upavista Konasana, 213
        Urdhvamukha Janu
        Sirsasana, 207
        Uttanasana, 197
        Utthita Parsvakonasana,
        194–95
        Utthita Trikonasana, 192–93
        Viloma 2 Pranayama, 257
        Viparita Dandasana, 238–39
        Viparita Karani, 234–35
        with props 181–83
    causes of, 176
    food and nourishment, impact
    on, 179
    learning to deal with, 180
    modern world and, 178
    on heart and mind, 115
    origin of, 41
    positive and negative, 179
    reactions to, 179
    related appetite loss, 217, 228
    related compression, 215
    related headache, 128, 188–92,
        194, 196, 198, 201, 207, 220,
        222, 230, 233, 235, 237–38,
        240, 242, 249, 352–53
    relief from, 41, 179
    types of, 179
    understanding, 176–77
    yoga and, 41
Suksma sharira, 48
Sunstroke, 204
Supta Baddhakonasana, 244–45
Supta Padangusthasana, 242–43
Supta Virasana, 166–68, 246–47
Svadhyaya, 53
Svatmarama, 48–49, 64
Swadhishtana chakra, 57
Swastikasana, 209
Sympathetic nervous system, 198,
    201, 215, 222, 257

T

Tadasana, 68–69
Tadasana Gomukhasana, 191
Tadasana Paschima Namaskarasana,
    190
Tadasana Urdhva
    Baddhanguliyasana, 188
Tadasana Urdhva Hastasana, 187
Tailbone (broken, fused or deviated),
    77, 105
Tailbone pain, 227
Tamasic food, 178
Tapas, 53
Testicles, heaviness and pain, 109
Thickening of arteries of heart, 161
Throat ailments, 145, 235
Throat congestion, 103
Throat tightness, feeling of, 215
Thyroid gland, 145, 161, 211, 215,
    219, 231, 233, 239, 241
Tired feet, 209
Tired legs, 222, 237
Tiredness in feet, 205
Tonsillitis, 141, 257
Torso, 187–88
Trianga Mukhaikapada
    Paschimottanasana, 118–21

U

Ujjayi Pranayama, 254–56
Ulcerative colitis, 296–99
Ulcers, 205, 217, 231
Umbilical hernia, 402–05
Upavista Konasana, 213
Upper backache, 167, 322–25
Upper body flexibility, 190
Urdhva Dhanurasana, 46, 65,
    160–63
Urdhvamukha Janu Sirsasana,
    207
Urinary system ailments, asanas for,
    109, 145, 300–01
Ustrasana, 156–58, 240–41
Uterine fibroids 145
Uterus, 123, 161
    displaced, 99
    muscles, 224
    prolapsed, 145, 207, 239, 241,
        245, 247, 392–95
Uttanasana, 92–95, 197–99
Utthita Marichyasana, 226–27
Utthita Parsvakonasana, 63, 65,
    80–83, 194–95
Utthita Trikonasana, 70–75, 192–93

V

Vagina, 219
Vaginal irritation, 109
Varicose veins, 192, 194, 196,
    202, 208, 231, 235, 237, 241,
    245, 266–68
Vertebral joints, 215
Vertigo, 70
Vijnanamaya kosha, 48
Viksipta, 51
Viloma 2 Pranayama, 257
Viparita Dandasana, 65, 238–39
Viparita Karani, 234–35
Virabhadra, 96
Virabhadrasana 96–99
Virabhadrasana 76–79

Virasana, 104–09, 206
Vishuddhi chakra, 57
Vomiting, 222
Vyadhi, 36, 37, 47

W

Waist, fat around, 81, 133
Waist, stretching, 167
Waste, elimination of, 81
Women's health, ailments,
    absent periods, 390–93
    asanas for, 378–96
    infertility, 394–96
    leukorrhea, 387–89
    menopause, 383–86
    menorrhagia, 388–91
    menstrual pain, 380–81
    menstruation, 378–80
    metrorrhagia, 386–87
    premenstrual syndrome, 382–83
    prolapsed uterus, 392–95
Wooden bench as prop, 184
Wooden blocks as props, 185
Wrists
    arthritis of, 85, 188–89, 204
    flexibility of, 190
    joint pain, 189, 191
    osteoarthritis of, 332–33
    pain or cramps in, 151
    stiffness of, 115

Y

Yama, 52–53
Yoga,
    advice for beginners, 408
    aim, 36–38, 47
    asanas, *see* Asanas
    belt, 185
    can be practiced at any age,
        43
    chakras, 56–57
    course, 407–23
    eight limbs, 52–53
    environment for, 409
    fills spiritual void, 38
    fitness and, 42–43
    for ailments, 259–405
    for everyone, 32, 35–43
    freedom of, 38
    guidelines, 408–09
    history, 48–49
    impact, 49
    learning of, 62–63
    meaning of, 46–47
    mind, 24, 32, 50–51
    philosophy of, 45–49
    pranayama, 54–55, 250–57
    scheduling of practice, 408
    sequence of, 409
    stages of, 37–38
    stimulative exercise, 42–43
    stress and, 41
    therapy, 260–61
    timing, 409
    way to health, 39
    20 week, course on 310–23
Yoga-agni, 59
Yoga Marsg, 46
Yoga Sutras, 30, 37, 40–41, 46–47,
    49, 53, 55, 176
Yogi, and Guru, 58–59

ACKNOWLEDGMENTS

Publishers' Acknowledgments
Dorling Kindersley would like to thank the Ramamani Memorial Yoga Institute, Pune, for their permission to use photographs of B.K.S. Iyengar from their archives. The publishers also extend their thanks to Sudha Malik, the yoga consultant for the project; Amit Kharsani for the Sanskrit calligraphy; and R.C. Sharma for indexing. The publishers would also like to thank Clare Sheddon and Salima Hirani for their help and advice during the early stages of the project; and Abhijeet Mukherjee for production support.

Revised edition 2008 Dorling Kindersley would like to thank photographer John Freeman and his assistant, Jamie Laing; Ruth Hope for her art direction; Nita Patel for her help and support before and during photography, and for writing the text in Chapter One, pp8–29 (DK copyright); Arunesh Talapatra and Rohan Sinha for their help during photography; and models Kobra Gulnaaz Dashti, Jake Clennell, Raya Umadatta, Firooza M. Ali, Rajvi H. Mehta, Arti H. Mehta, Birjoo Mehta, Uday V. Bhosale, and Mrs. N. Rajlaxmi. The publishers also extend thanks

to Chandru Melwani for his help throughout the compilation of both editions of this book. Thanks to the Ramamani Memorial Yoga Institute, Pune, for their permission to use additional photographs from their archives. Thanks to the Life Centre, 15 Edge Street, London W8 7PN, www.thelifecentre.com, and to agoy, www.agoy.com, for supplying the mats used on pp100–101, 112–113, 126–127, 136–137, 154–155, and 164–165. Special thanks go to Dr. Prakash Kalmadi at the Kare Ayurvedic Retreat, Mulshi Lake, Pune, India, www. karehealth.com, for his help and hospitality on location.

Updated edition 2014 Dorling Kindersley would like to thank Aparna Sharma for her guidance and support during the project; Glenda Fernandes for her support during the course of the project and for the research trip to Bellur, and Divya Chandok for proofreading. The publishers also extend their thanks to Aditya Kapoor for the new photography in Chapter 1, and Raya U.D. for the photograph on p16 and the children's yoga class at the Ramamani Iyengar Memorial Yoga Institute, Pune, on p26 and p31.

Picture Credits Dorling Kindersley would like to thank the following for their kind permission to reproduce their photographs: National Museum, New Delhi p36, p49 t, p55 t, & b, p56 b, p57; American Institute of Indian Studies, New Delhi p36 tl, p37, p48, p50 t, p59; Max Alexander 48; Joe Cornish p54; Ashok Dilwali p34; John Freeman p43, p248; Ashim Ghosh p60; Steve Gorton p37 tr; Alistair Hughes p50; Subir Kumedan p406; Chandru Melwani, Pune, India p29 t; Stephen Parker p6; Janet Peckam p46; Kim Sayer p177; Hashmat Singh p174; Pankaj Usrani p51 b; Amar Talwar p258; Colin Walton p178 tc. Punchstock: Digital Vision p261, t. DK Copyright pages (shot by Harminder Singh) 68-69, 96-97, 96-97, 195 b, 196, 200, 201 t, 202-203, 204 tr, 209-213, 217-221, 234-236, 237 t, 240-241, 244-245; (shot by John Freeman) 8, 14-28, 29c, 31, 33, 66-67, 100-101, 112-113, 126-127, 136-137, 154-155, 164-165, 250-251.

Every effort has been made to trace the copyright holders of photographs. The publisher apologizes for any omissions and will amend further editions. For further information see www.dk.images.com

KEY: t=top; r=right; l=left; c=center; b=bottom

USEFUL ADDRESSES

B.K.S. Iyengar website: www.bksiyengar.com

United Kingdom and Europe

Iyengar Yoga Institute (Maida Vale)
223a Randolph Avenue, London W9 1NL
www.iyi.org.uk

Iyengar Yoga Association of the UK (IYA (UK))
www.iyengaryoga.org.uk

Iyengar Yoga Silkeborg
Lyngbygade 8 Silkeborg 8600, Denmark
www.iyengaryoga-silkeborg.dk

Association Francaise de Yoga Iyengar
83 Boulevard Magenta, 75010, Paris, France
www.yoga-iyengar.asso.fr

Centre de Yoga Iyengar de Paris
Association Francaise de Yoga Iyengar
35, Avenue Victor Hugo, 75016 Paris, France
www.sfbiria.com

Light on Yoga Italy
(Iyengar Yoga Association Italy)
Via Leonardo Fibonacci, 27 - 50131, Firenze
www.iyengaryoga.it

B.K.S. Iyengar Yoga Vereinigung Deutschland e.V.
Pappelallee 24, 10437 Berlin, Germany
www.iyengar-yoga-deutschland.de

B.K.S Iyengar Yoga Vereniging Nederland
www.iyengaryoga.nl

The Iyengar Yoga Studio,
ul. Przyjaciol Zolnierza 88/10 71-670
Szczecin, Poland

Asociacion Espanola de Yoga Iyengar
C/Gran Vía, 40–9° pta 4 – 28013 Madrid,
Spain www.aeyi.org

Centro de Yoga Iyengar de Madrid
Carrera de San Jeronimo, 16–5 izda
Madrid 28014, Spain
www.eyimadrid.com

Institute of Iyengar Yoga and Physiotherapy
Fysikgrand 23, SE-907 03 Umea, Sweden

Iyengar-Yoga-Vereinigung Schweiz
CH-3000 Bern, Switzerland
www.iyengar.ch

Canada

B.K.S. Iyengar Yoga Association
(Vancouver)
P.O. Box 60639 Granville Park Post Office,
Vancouver, British Columbia V6H 4B9
www.iyengaryogavancouver.com

Iyengar Yoga Association of Canada
www.iyengaryogacanada.com

USA

B.K.S. Iyengar Yoga National Association of the United States
PO Box 538, Seattle, WA, 98111 USA
www.iynaus.org

The Iyengar Yoga Institute of New York
150 West 22nd Street, 11th floor, New York,
NY 10011
www.iyengarnyc.org

Australia and New Zealand

BKS Iyengar Association of Australia Ltd
PO Box 1280, Neutral Bay NSW 2089
www.iyengaryoga.asn.au

B.K.S. Iyengar Yoga Association of New Zealand
P.O. Box 4023, Nelson South 7045,
New Zealand
www.iyengar-yoga.org.nz